CU01020622

Oxford American Handbook of
Clinical Dentistry

Published and forthcoming Oxford American Handbooks

Oxford American Handbook of Clinical Medicine
Oxford American Handbook of Anesthesia
Oxford American Handbook of Clinical Dentistry
Oxford American Handbook of Clinical Surgery
Oxford American Handbook of Critical Care
Oxford American Handbook of Emergency Medicine
Oxford American Handbook of ENT and Head and Neck Surgery
Oxford American Handbook of Nephrology and Hypertension
Oxford American Handbook of Obstetrics & Gynecology
Oxford American Handbook of Pediatrics
Oxford American Handbook of Psychiatry
Oxford American Handbook of Respiratory Medicine

8   Oral and maxillofacial surgery   345

6 Restorative dentistry 223

Detailed contents

Acknowledgments

Editing and updating the *Oxford Handbook of Clinical Dentistry* was simplified by the recent revisions made for the fourth edition by David A. Mitchell and Laura Mitchell. I am indebted to them for all their work on this excellent text over the years. Creating an American version of the handbook required the expertise of several of my colleagues. I would like to thank the following individuals for their contributions to the editing of the following chapters:

Rachel Badovinac: Preventive and Community Dentistry
Dolrudee Jumlongras: Pediatric Dentistry
Chin-Yu Lin: Orthodontics
Sang Park: Restorative Dentistry, and Dental Materials
Ali A. Nasseh: Restorative Dentistry
David M. Kim and Paul A. Levi: Periodontology, Oral Medicine, and Practice Management

I would like to thank Bernard Friedland for writing new material for the chapter on Jurisprudence. I am sure that his insight and understanding of American law will provide the reader with an excellent primer.

OXFORD
UNIVERSITY PRESS

Great Clarendon Street, Oxford OX2 6DP

Oxford University Press is a department of the University of Oxford.
It furthers the University's objective of excellence in research, scholarship,
and education by publishing worldwide in

Oxford New York

Auckland Cape Town Dar es Salaam Hong Kong Karachi
Kuala Lumpur Madrid Melbourne Mexico City Nairobi
New Delhi Shanghai Taipei Toronto

With offices in

Argentina Austria Brazil Chile Czech Republic France Greece
Guatemala Hungary Italy Japan Poland Portugal Singapore
South Korea Switzerland Thailand Turkey Ukraine Vietnam

Oxford is a registered trade mark of Oxford University Press
in the UK and in certain other countries

Published in the United States
by Oxford University Press Inc., New York

© Oxford University Press, 2008

The moral rights of the authors have been asserted
Database right Oxford University Press (maker)

First published 2008

British Library Cataloguing in Publication Data

Data available

Library of Congress Cataloging in Publication Data

Da Silva, John D.

Oxford American Handbook of Clinical Dentistry/John D. Da Silva, David A. Mitchell, and Laura Mitchell.
    p.; cm. – (Oxford American handbooks)

Adapted from: Oxford Handbook of Clinical Dentistry / David Mitchell and Laura Mitchell. 4th ed. 2005.
Includes bibliographical references and index.
ISBN-13: 978-0-19-518964-3 (alk. paper)

1. Dentistry–Handbooks, manuals, etc. I. Mitchell, David A. II. Mitchell, Laura, 1958- III. Mitchell, David A.
Oxford Handbook of Clinical Dentistry. IV. Title. V. Title: Handbook of clinical dentistry. VI. Series.
[DNLM: 1. Mouth Diseases–therapy–Handbooks. 2. Tooth Diseases–therapy–Handbooks.
3. Dentistry–methods–Handbooks.
WU 49 D111o 2008]
  RK56.M58 2008   2007014456
  617.6–dc22

Typeset by Newgen Imaging Systems (P) Ltd., Chennai, India
printed in China
on acid-free paper by
Phoenix Offset

ISBN 978–0–19–518964–3 (Flexicover.: alk paper)

10 9 8 7 6 5 4 3 2 1

Oxford American Handbook of
Clinical Dentistry

Edited by

John D. Da Silva, D.M.D, M.P.H., Sc.M
Director of Advanced Graduate Education,
Harvard School of Dental Medicine

with

**David A Mitchell and
Laura Mitchell**

With contributions from
Paul Brunton

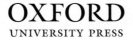
OXFORD
UNIVERSITY PRESS

Contents

10 Medicine relevant to dentistry   **473**
Medical theory

List of color plates

List of color plates

Symbols and abbreviations

►	this is important
Δ	diagnosis
$	supernumerary
−ve	negative
+ve	positive
↑	increased
↓	decreased
<	lesser than
>	greater than
~	approximately
#	fracture
μ	micro (e.g., μg, μm)
?	question/ask about (when ? appears alone)
∴	therefore
1°	primary
2°	secondary
3°	tertiary
$\overline{inc}$	lower incisor
$\underline{inc}$	upper incisor
AAO	American Association of Orthodontists
AAP	American Academy of Periodontology
Ab	antibody
ACS	American College of Surgeons
ACLS	Advanced Cardiac Life Support
ACTH	adrenocorticotrophic hormone
ADA	American Dental Association; Americans with Disabilities Act
ADH	antidiuretic hormone
ADM	acellular dermal matrix
AED	automated external defibrillator
Ag	antigen
AHA	American Heart Association
AIDS	acquired immune deficiency syndrome
ALS	amyotrophic lateral sclerosis
AMA	American Medical Association

AOB	anterior open bite
AP	anteroposterior
APTT	activated partial throbblastinin
ARF	acute renal failure
ASAP	as soon as possible
ATLS	advanced trauma life support
AZT	3'-azido-3'-deoxythimidine
BCC	basal cell carcinoma
BDA	British Dental Association
BDJ	*British Dental Journal*
bid	twice a day
BIDD	bismuth iodoform paraffin paste
BLS	basic life support
b/w	bitewing radiograph
BMA	British Medical Association
BMT	bone marrow transplant
BP	blood pressure
BSS	black silk suture
Ca^{2+}	calcium
CAD	computer-aided design
CAM	computer-aided manufacturing
CAL	clinical attachment loss
CAP	chronic adult periodontitis
CBC	complete blood count
CC	chief complaint
CDC	Centers for Disease Control and Prevention
CE	continuing education
CEJ	cementoenamel junction
CHD	Congenital Heart Disease
C/I	contraindication
Class I	Class I relationship
Class II/1	Class II division 1 relationship
Class II/2	Class II division 2 relationship
Class III	Class III relationship
CLD	certainly lethal dose
CLP	cleft lip and palate
cm	centimeter(s)
CMV	cytomegalovirus
CNS	central nervous system

CO	centric occlusion
C/O	complaining of
COPD	chronic obstructive pulmonary disease
CPR	cardiopulmonary resuscitation
CR	centric relation
C&S	culture and sensitivity
CSF	cerebrospinal fluid
CT	Computed tomography
CVA	cerebrovascular accident
CXR	chest X-ray
DA	dental assistant
DEA	Drug Enforcement Agency
DBS	dentin bonding system
deft	decayed, exfoliated, and filled deciduous teeth
DEJ	dentinoenamel junction
DHHS	Department of Health and Human Services
dl	deciliter(s)
DLE	discoid lupus erythematosus
DMFS	decayed, missing, and filled surfaced in permanent teeth
dmft	decayed, missing, filled deciduous teeth
DMFT	decayed, missing, filled permanent teeth
DVT	deep venous thrombosis
EBA	ethoxy benzoid acid
EBM/D	evidence-based medicine/dentistry
EBV	Epstein–Barr virus
ECG	electrocardiogram
ECM	electronic caries monitor
EDA	electronic dental anesthesia
EDTA	ethylene diamine tetraacetic acid
e.g.	for example
EMD	enamel matrix derivative
ENT	ear, nose, and throat
EOE	extraoral exam
ER	emergency room
ESR	erythrocyte sedimentation rate
EUA	examination under anesthesia
F	female
F/-	full upper denture (and -/F for lower)
FA	fixed appliance

FABP	flat anterior bite plane
FB	foreign body
FBC	full blood count
FDA	Food and Drug Administration
Fe	iron
F/F	full upper and lower dentures
FESS	functional endoscopic sinus surgery
fl	femtoliter(s)
FNAC	fine-needle aspiration cytology
FOP	functional occlusion plane
FOTI	fiber optic transillumination
f/s	fissure sealant
FWS	freeway space–interocclusal rest space
g	gram(s)
GA	general anesthesia
GAgP	generalized aggressive periodontis
GCF	gingival cervicular fluid
GI	glass ionomer
GKI	glucose, potassium, insulin
GP	gutta-percha
GT	greater taper
GTR	guided-tissue regeneration
h	hour(s)
H2	histamine 2 receptor antagonist
Hb	hemoglobin
HBeAg	hepatitis B e antigen (high-risk marker)
HBsAg	hepatitis B surface antigen
HCW	health-care worker
Hg	mercury
HIPAA	Health Insurance Portability and Accountability Act
HIV	human immunodeficiency virus
HLA	human leucocyte antigen
HMO	health maintenance organization
HPI	history of the present illness
HPV	human papilloma virus
HRT	hormone replacement therapy
HSV	herpes simplex virus
IAB	Inferior alveolar block
ICU	intensive care unit

ICP	intracranial pressure
i.e.	that is
IE	infective endocarditis
IFA	inferior alveolar nerve
Ig	Immunoglobulin (e.g., IgA, IgG, etc.)
IM	intramuscular
IMF	intermaxillary fixation
inc	incisor
INH	isonicotinyl hydrazine (isoniazid)
INR	International Normalized Ratio
IOE	intraoral examination
IOTN	Index of Orthodontic Treatment Need
ITP	idiopathic thrombocytopenic purpura
IU	international units
IV	intravenous
K^+	potassium
KCT	kaolin–cephalin clotting time
kg	kilogram
kV	kilovolt
l	liter(s)
LA	local anesthesia
LAgP	localized aggressive periodontitis
LED	light-emitting diode
LFH	lower face height
LFT	liver function test
LLS	lower labial segment
LMA	laryngeal mask airway
m	meter(s)
M	male
mand	mandible/mandibular
MAOI	monoamine oxidase inhibitor
max	maxilla/maxillary
MCV	mean corpuscular volume
MEN	multiple endocrine neoplasia
mg	milligram
MHz	megahertz
MI	myocardial infarction
MIH	molar incisor hypomineralization
MIP	maximal intercuspal position

micromol	micromoles
min	minute(s)
ml	milliliter(s)
mm	millimeter(s)
mmHg	millimeters of mercury
mmol	millimole(s)
MMPA	maxillary mandibular planes angle
NPDB	National Practitioner Data Bank
MRI	magnetic resonance imaging
MST	slow release morphine
MSU	mid-stream urine
MTA	mineral trioxide aggregate
NAD	nothing abnormal detected
NAI	non-accidental injury
NGT	nasogastric tube
NIH	National Institutes of Health
NPO	nothing by mouth
nm	nanometer(s)
nocte	at night
NSAID	nonsteroidal anti-inflammatory drug
NUG	necrotizing ulcerative gingivitis
NUP	necrotizing ulcerative periodontal disease
O_2	oxygen
o/b	overbite
od	once daily
OD	overdenture
O/E	on examination
OH	oral hygiene
OHCM	*Oxford Handbook of Clinical Medicine*
OHI	oral hygiene instruction
o/j	overjet
OP	outpatient
ORIF	open reduction and internal fixation
OSHA	Occupational Safety and Health Administration
OTC	over the counter
OVD	occlusal vertical dimension
P	pulse
P/-	partial upper denture (and -/P for lower)
PA	posteroanterior

PAC	plasma arc curing (light)
PAN	panoramic radiograph
PCA	patient-controlled analgesia
PCP	primary care physician
PCD	professional complementary to dentistry
PDH	past dental history
PDL	periodontal ligament
PEA	pulseless electrical activity
PEG	percutaneous endoscopic gastrostomy
PFM	porcelain fused to metal (crown)
PHI	protected health information
PJC	porcelain jacket crown
PLD	potentially lethal dose
PM	premolar
PMH	past medical history
PMMA	polymethylmethacrylate
PO	per orum (by mouth)
PPE	personal protective equipment
ppm	parts per million
PR	per rectum
prn	as required
PRR	preventive resin restoration
PTFE	(poly)tetrafluoroethene
PTT	partial thromboplastin time
PU	pass urine
qd	every day
qid	four times daily
QTH	quartz tungsten halogen
R	respiratory rate
RA	relative analgesia
RAS	recurrent aphthous stomatitis
RBC	red blood cell count
RCCT	randomized controlled clinical trial
RCP	retruded contact position
RCT	root canal treatment/therapy
RIG	radiologically inserted gastrostomy
RMGIC	resin-modified glass ionomer composite
RRF	retrograde root filling
Rx	treatment

SC	subcutaneous
SCC	squamous cell carcinoma
sec	second
SF	sugar-free
SLE	systemic lupus erythematosus
SS	stainless steel
STD	sexually transmitted disease; safely tolerated dose
TB	tuberculosis
TC	tungsten carbide
tid	three times a day
TENS	transcutaneous electrical nerve stimulation
TIA	transient ischemic attack
TIBC	total iron binding capacity
TMA	titanium molybdenum alloy
TMJ	temporomandibular joint
TMD	temporomandibular disorder
TMPDS	temporomandibular pain dysfuntion syndrome
TNF	tissue necrosis factor
TSH	thyroid-stimulating hormone
TTP	tender to percussion
ULS	upper labial segment
URA	upper removable appliance
URI	upper respiratory infection
URTI	upper respiratory tract infection
USS	ultrasound scanning
UTI	urinary tract infection
U&Es	urea and electrolytes
VDRL	Venereal Disease Research Laboratory (test)
VDO	vertical dimension of occlusion
VF	ventricular fibrillation
WHO	World Health Organization
Xbite	crossbite
X-rays	either X-rays or radiographs
yr	year(s)
ZOE	zinc oxide-eugenol

History and examination

Relevant pages in other chapters: It could, of course, be said that all pages are relevant to this section, because history and examination are the first steps in the care of any patient. However, as that is hardly helpful, the reader is referred specifically to the following: dental charting, p. 688; medical conditions, Chapter 10; the child with toothache, p. 62; preoperative management of the dental patient, p. 518; the cranial nerves, p. 492; ortho-dontic assessment, p. 128; pulpal pain, p. 228.

Principal sources: Experience.

Listen, look, and learn

Much of what you need to know about any individual patient can be obtained by watching them enter the operatory and sit in the chair, observing their body language during the interview, and asking a few well-chosen questions. One of the great secrets to providing good health care is developing the ability to actually listen to what your patients tell you and to use that information. Doctors and dentists are often concerned that if they allow patients to speak rather than answer questions, history taking will be inefficient and time consuming. In fact, most patients will give the information necessary to make an initial diagnosis along with other useful information, if given the opportunity. Most will lapse into silence after 2–3 minutes of monologue. History taking should be conducted with the patient sitting comfortably; this rarely equates with supine! In order to produce a complete history, however, it is customary and often necessary to resort to directed questioning; here are a few hints:

- Always introduce yourself to the patient and any accompanying person and explain, if it is not immediately obvious, what your role is in helping them.
- Introduce your dental assistant as well.
- Remember that patients are (usually) neither medically nor dentally trained, so use plain speech without speaking down to them.
- Questions are a key part of history taking, and the manner in which they are asked can lead to either a quick diagnosis and a trusting patient or to confusion. Leading questions should be avoided for the most part, as they convey a preconceived idea to the patient. This is also a problem when the question suggests the answer, e.g., "Is the pain worse when you drink hot drinks?" To avoid this situation, use open-ended questions that require a descriptive reply rather than a straight yes or no answer. However, with an uncommunicative patient, it may be necessary to ask leading questions to elicit relevant information.
- Occasionally it may be necessary to interrupt patients during a detailed monologue on an irrelevant topic, such as their grandmother's sick parrot. Try to do this tactfully, e.g., "How have things been in the last couple of days?" or "This is rather difficult—please slow down and let me understand how this affects the problem you've come to see me about today."

Specifics of a medical or dental history are described on p. 6 and p. 4. The objective is to elicit sufficient information to make an initial diagnosis while establishing rapport. This will help to facilitate further discussion and/or treatment.

Chief complaint (CC)

The aim of this part of the history is to begin to develop an initial differential diagnosis before examining the patient. The following is a suggested outline, which will require modification depending on the circumstances:

Chief complaint In the patient's own words. Use a general introductory question, e.g., "How can I help you today?" or "What is the problem?"

Avoid "What brought you here today?" unless you want to give the patient the chance to make a joke.

If symptoms are present:
Onset and pattern When did the problem start? Is it getting better, worse, or staying the same?

Frequency How often is it, how long does it last? Does it occur at any particular time of day or night?

Exacerbating and relieving factors What makes it better, what makes it worse? What started it?

If pain is the main symptom:
Origin and radiation Where is the pain and does it spread?

Character and intensity How would you describe the pain: sharp, shooting, dull, aching? This can be difficult, although patients with specific "organic" pain will often understand exactly what you mean, whereas patients with symptoms with a high behavioral overlay will be vague and prevaricate.

Associations Is there anything, in your own mind, that you associate with the problem?

Most dental problems can be quickly narrowed down using a simple series of questions such as these to create a provisional diagnosis and judge the urgency of the problem.

The dental history

It is important to assess the patient's dental awareness and the likelihood of raising it. A dental history may also provide invaluable clues toward the nature of the chief complaint and should not be ignored. This can be achieved by asking some simple, general questions:

How often do you go to the dentist?
  (gives information on motivation, likely attendance patterns, and whether patients change their dentist frequently)
When did you last see a dentist and what did he or she do?
  (may give clues toward the diagnosis of the presenting complaint, e.g., a recent root canal treatment [RCT])
How often do you brush your teeth and for how long?
  (motivation and likely gingival condition)
Have you ever had any pain or clicking from your jaw joints?
  (temporomandibular joint [TMJ] pathology)
Do you grind your teeth or bite your nails?
  (temporomandibular pain dysfunction syndrome [TMPDS], personality)
How do you feel about dental treatment?
  (dental anxiety)
What do you think about the appearance of your teeth?
  (motivation, need for orthodontic treatment)
What type of work do you do?
  (socioeconomic status, education)
Where do you live?
  (fluoride intake, travel time to the office)
What types of dental treatment have you had previously?
  (previous extractions, problems with local [LA] or general [GA] anesthesia, orthodontics, periodontal treatment)
What are your favorite drinks and foods?
  (caries rate, erosion)

Screening and medical history

Having patients complete a medical history is of value, as it encourages more accurate responses to sensitive questions. It is important to use this as a starting point and to clarify answers with the patient. The health history is a dynamic document that must be maintained and updated. It should be updated at the following times:

- For a new patient
- Annually
- For a patient of another office for which the dentist is covering emergencies

Since dental patients present for routine examinations every 6 months, dentists have a unique opportunity to screen patients for several health and social issues. Treatable problems should be screened as part of a dental visit. Particularly important is the detection of common asymptomatic medical problems such as hypertension.

Substance abuse is one of biggest public health problems worldwide. It is the responsibility of health care providers to provide substance abuse screening, brief intervention, and referrals. Patients should be screened for tobacco, alcohol, and drug use. Patients expect to be asked about their health and habits when they see a health care provider, so when they are not asked, they may feel that their treatment is suboptimal.

Screening tools

Several screening tools are available[1]:

- CAGE test[2]. One of the most commonly used alcohol screening tests. Four questions, 1 yes = positive. CAGE is a mnemonic for the screening questions.
  - Have you ever felt you should **C**ut down on your drinking?
  - Have people **A**nnoyed you by criticizing your drinking?
  - Have you ever felt bad or **G**uilty about your drinking?
  - Have you ever had a drink first thing in the morning (an **E**ye opener or **E**arly morning drink) to steady your nerves or get rid of a hangover or residual drug effect?
- CRAFFT questionnaire[3] for use with adolescents to screen for alcohol and drugs.[4]
- Six questions, 2 yes = positive, indicates a problem for follow-up.
  - Have you ever ridden in a **C**ar driven by someone (including yourself) who was high or had been using alcohol or drugs?
  - Do you ever use alcohol or drugs to **R**elax, feel better about yourself?
  - Do you ever use alcohol or drugs while you are by yourself (**A**lone)?
  - Do you ever **F**orget things you did while using alcohol or drugs?
  - Do your **F**amily or **F**riends ever tell you that you should cut down on your drinking or drug use?
  - Have you ever gotten into **T**rouble while you were using alcohol or drugs?

1 http://www.projectmainstream.net
2 J. A. Ewing 1984 *JAMA* **252** 1905.
3 http://www.ceasar-boston.org/clinicians/crafft.php
4 J. R. Knight *et al.* 1999 *Arch Pediatric Adolesc Med* **153**(6) 591–6.

States have agencies or departments responsible for the alcohol/drug-related programs, and resources. States vary widely in the titles of these agencies and in their organizational affiliation within state government structures. Addiction agencies are combined with mental health services in some states.

Example of a medical questionnaire

QUESTION   YES/NO

Are you healthy?

When was your last physical?

   Did you require any treatment or follow-up?

Have you ever been admitted to hospital?

   If yes, please give brief details:

Have you ever had an operation?

   If so, were there any problems?

Have you ever had any heart trouble or high blood pressure?

Have you ever had any chest trouble?

Have you ever had any problems with bleeding?

Have you ever had asthma, eczema, hay fever?

Are you allergic to penicillin?

Are you allergic to any other drug or substance?

Have you ever had

—rheumatic fever?

—diabetes?

—epilepsy?

—a diagnosis of tuberculosis?

   —a persistent cough greater than 3 weeks' duration?

   —a cough that produces blood?

—jaundice?

—hepatitis?

—other infectious disease?

Are you pregnant?

Are you taking any drugs, medications, or pills or herbal remedies?

   If yes, please give details:

Do you drink?

   If yes, how often and how much?

Who is your doctor?

▶ Check the medical history at each appointment.

▶ If in any doubt, contact the patient's primary care provider (PCP) or the specialist treating the patient before proceeding.

▶ The use of oral bisphosphonates has been found to be a risk factor for osteonecrosis of the jaw.[1] The use of these drugs and warfarin must be considered when reviewing a patient's medical history.

1 S. Ruggiero 2006 *J Oncol Pract* **2** 7.

Note: A complete medical history includes details of the patient's family history (for familial disease) and social history (for factors associated with disease, e.g., smoking, drinking, and for home support on discharge). It is part of a systematic review of systems:

Cardiovascular Chest pain, palpitations, breathlessness.

Respiratory Breathlessness, wheeze, cough—productive or not.

Gastrointestinal Appetite and eating, pain, distension, and bowel habit.

Genitourinary Pain, frequency (day and night), incontinence, straining, or dribbling.

Central nervous system seizures, fainting, and headaches.

Medical examination

For the vast majority of dental patients attending as outpatients a dentist's office, dental clinic, or hospital, simply recording a medical history should suffice to screen for any potential problems. The exceptions are patients who are to undergo GA and anyone with a positive medical history undergoing extensive treatment under sedation. For these patients the aim is to detect any gross abnormality so that it can be dealt with by consultation with relevant specialists.

A few basic things to check are as follows:

Cardiovascular system Check the pulse. Measure blood pressure.

Respiratory system Look at the respiratory rate (12–18/min). Is expansion equal on both sides?

Central nervous system Is the patient alert and correctly oriented in time, place, and person?

Musculoskeletal system Note limitations in movement and arthritis, especially those affecting the cervical spine, which may need to be hyperextended to intubate for anesthesia.

General jaundice Look at sclera in good light, the same for anemia. Cyanosis, peripheral: blue extremities; central: blue tongue. To test for dehydration, lift skin between thumb and forefinger.

If there is anything out of the ordinary ask the patient to consult with their PCP or a specialist for follow-up.

Examination of the head and neck

This is an aspect of examination that is both undertaught and overlooked in medical and dental training. In the former, the tendency is to approach the area in a rather cursory manner, partly because it is not well understood. In the latter, the clinician often forgets, despite otherwise extensive knowledge of the head and neck, to look beyond the mouth. For this reason the examination below is given in some detail; this thorough an inspection is only necessary, however, in selected cases, e.g., suspected oral cancer, facial pain of unknown origin, trauma, etc.

Head and facial appearance Look for specific deformities (p. 172), facial disharmony (p. 170), syndromes (p. 679), traumatic defects (p. 400–4), and facial palsy (p. 455). Assessment of the cranial nerves is covered on p. 492.

Skin Lesions of the face should be examined for color, scaling, bleeding, and crusting, palpated for texture and consistency and whether they are fixed to or arising from surrounding tissues.

Eyes Note obvious abnormalities such as exophthalmus and lid retraction (e.g., hyperthyroidism) and ptosis (drooping eyelid). Examine conjunctiva for chemosis (swelling), pallor, e.g., anemia or jaundice. Look at the iris and pupil. Ophthalmoscopy is the examination of the disc and retina via the pupil. It is a specialized skill requiring an adequate ophthalmoscope and is acquired by watching and practicing with a skilled supervisor. However, direct and consensual (contralateral eye) light responses of the pupils are straightforward and should always be assessed when head injury is suspected (p. 398).

Ears Gross abnormalities of the external ear are usually obvious. Further examination requires an otoscope, preferably a good one. Straighten the external auditory meatus by pulling upward, backward, and outward using the largest applicable speculum. Look for the pearly gray tympanic membrane; a plug of wax often intervenes.

Mouth p. 11.

Oropharynx and tonsils These can easily be seen by depressing the tongue with a tongue blade. **The hypopharynx and larynx** are seen by indirect laryngoscopy using a head light and mirror, and the **postnasal space** is similarly viewed.

Neck Inspect from in front and palpate from behind. Look for skin changes, scars, swellings, and arterial and venous pulsations. Palpate the neck systematically, starting at a fixed standard point, e.g., beneath the chin, working back to the angle of the mandible and then down the cervical chain, remembering the scalene and supraclavicular nodes. Swellings of the thyroid move with swallowing. Auscultation may reveal bruits over the carotids (usually due to atherosclerotic plaques).

TMJ Palpate both joints simultaneously. Have the patient open and close and move laterally while feeling for clicking, locking, and crepitus. Palpate the muscles of mastication for spasm and tenderness. Auscultation can also be used.

Examination of the mouth

Most dental textbooks include a detailed and comprehensive description of how to examine the mouth. Such descriptions are based on the premise that the examining dentist has until now never seen the patient, who has some exotic disease. Given the constraints of clinical practice, this approach needs to be altered to be as applicable to the routine dental patient who is healthy as it is to the patient presenting with pain of unknown origin.

The key to this is to develop a systematic approach that becomes almost automatic, so that when you are under pressure there is less likelihood of missing any pathology. Abnormal findings require further investigation.

Extraoral examination (EOE) (p. 10). For routine clinical practice this can usually be limited to a visual appraisal, e.g., swellings, asymmetry, patient's color, etc. More detailed examination can be carried out if indicated by the patient's symptoms.

Intraoral examination (IOE)
- Oral hygiene
- Soft tissues. The entire oral mucosa should be carefully inspected. Any ulcer of >3 weeks' duration requires further investigation (p. 468).
- Periodontal condition. This can be assessed rapidly, using a periodontal probe. Pockets >5 mm indicate the need for a more thorough assessment (p. 188).
- Chart the teeth present (p. 688).
- Examine each tooth in turn for caries (p. 26) and examine the integrity of any restorations present.
- Occlusion. This should involve not only getting the patient to close together and examining the relationship between the arches (p. 126), but also looking at the path of closure for any obvious prematurities (p. 154). Check for evidence of tooth wear (p. 276).

For those patients complaining of pain, a more thorough examination of the area related to their symptoms should then be carried out (p. 14).

Findings—general

▶ Do not perform or request a test you cannot interpret.

▶ Similarly, always look at, interpret, and act on any tests you have performed.

Temperature, pulse, blood pressure, and respiratory rate These are the nurses' stock in trade. You need to be able to interpret the results.

Temperature (35.5–37.5°C/95.9–99.5°F) ↑ physiologically postoperatively for 24 h, otherwise may indicate infection or a transfusion reaction. ↓ in hypothermia or shock.

Pulse Adult (60–80 beats/min); child is higher (up to 140 beats/min in infants). Should be regular.

Blood pressure (BP) (120–140/60–90 mmHg) ↑ with age. Falling BP may indicate a syncope, hypovolemia, or other form of shock. High BP may place the patient at risk from a GA and for transient ischemic attack (TIA)/stroke. An ↑ BP + ↓ pulse suggests ↑ intracranial pressure (p. 398).

Respiratory rate (12–18 breaths/min) ↑ in chest infections, pulmonary edema, and shock.

Urinalysis is routinely performed on all patients admitted to hospital. A positive result for

Glucose or ketones may indicate diabetes.

Protein suggests renal disease, especially infection.

Blood suggests infection or tumor.

Bilirubin indicates hepatocellular and/or obstructive jaundice.

Urobilinogen indicates jaundice of any type.

Blood tests (sampling techniques, p. 522) Reference ranges vary.

Complete blood count (EDTA, pink tube) measures the following:

Hemoglobin (males [M] 13–18 g/dl, females [F] 11.5–16.5 g/dl) ↓ in anemia, ↑ in polycythemia and myeloproliferative disorders.

Hematocrit (packed cell volume) (M 40–54%, F 37–47%). ↓ in anemia, ↑ in polycythemia and dehydration.

Mean cell volume (76–96 fl) ↑ in size (macrocytosis) in vitamin B12 and folate deficiency, ↓ (microcytosis) iron deficiency.

White cell count ($4-11 \times 10^9$/l) ↑ in infection, leukemia, and trauma, ↓ in certain infections, early leukemia and after cytotoxics.

Platelets ($150-400 \times 10^9$/l) See also p. 476.

Biochemistry Urea and electrolytes are the most important:

Sodium (135–145 mmol/l) Large fall causes fits.

Potassium (3.5–5 mmol/l) Must be kept within this narrow range to avoid serious cardiac disturbance. Watch carefully in diabetics, those in intravenous (IV) therapy, and the shocked or dehydrated patient. Succinylcholine (muscle relaxant) ↑ potassium.

Urea (2.5–7 mmol/l) Rising urea suggests dehydration, renal failure, or blood in the gut.

Creatinine (70–150 micromol/l) Rises in renal failure. Various other biochemical tests are available to aid specific diagnoses, e.g., bone, liver function, thyroid function, cardiac enzymes, folic acid, vitamin B12, etc.

Glucose (fasting 4–6 mmol/l) ↑ suspect diabetes, ↓ hypoglycemic drugs, exercise. Competently interpreted proprietary tests, e.g., BM stick = well to blood glucose (p. 514).

Virology Viral serology is costly and rarely necessary.

Immunology Similar to above but more frequently indicated in complex oral medicine patients

Bacteriology

Sputum and pus swabs are often helpful in dealing with hospital infections. Ensure they are taken with sterile swabs and transported immediately or put in an incubator.

Blood cultures are also useful if the patient has septicemia. These are taken when there is a sudden fever and incubated, with results available 24–48 h later. Take two samples from separate sites and put in paired bottles for aerobic and anaerobic culture (i.e., four bottles, unless your lab indicates otherwise).

Biopsy See p. 374.

Cytology With the exception of smears for candida and fine-needle aspiration, cytology is little used and not widely applicable in the dental specialties.

Findings—specific

Vitality testing It must be kept in mind that it is the integrity of the nerve supply that is being investigated here. However, the blood supply is more relevant to the continued vitality of a pulp. Test the suspect tooth and its neighbors.

Application of cold This is most practically carried out using ethyl chloride on a cotton pad. This is also an excellent test of the onset of local anesthetic.

Application of heat Vaseline should be applied first to the tooth under test to prevent the heated gutta percha (GP) sticking. No response suggests that the tooth is non-vital, but an ↑ response indicates that the pulp is hyperemic.

Electric pulp tester The tooth to be tested should be dry, and prophy paste or a proprietary lubricant is used as a conductive medium. Most machines ascribe numbers to the patient's reaction, but these should be interpreted with caution as the response can also vary with battery strength or the position of the electrode on the tooth. For the above methods misleading results may occur:

False positive	False negative
Multirooted tooth with vital +non-vital pulp	Nerve supply damaged, blood supply intact
Canal full of pus	Secondary dentine
Apprehensive patient	Large insulating restoration

Percussion is carried out by gently tapping adjacent and suspect teeth with the end of a mirror handle. A positive response indicates that a tooth is extruded from exudate in apical or lateral periodontal tissues.

Mobility of teeth is ↑ by ↓ in the bony support (e.g., due to periodontal disease or an apical abscess) and also by # of root or supporting bone.

Palpation of the buccal sulcus next to a painful tooth can help to determine if there is an associated apical abscess.

Biting onto gauze or rubber can be used to try and elicit pain from a cracked tooth.

Radiographs (pp. 16, 669).

Area under investigation	Radiographic view
General scan of teeth and jaws (retained roots, unerupted teeth)	Panoramic radiograph (PAN)
Localization of unerupted teeth	Periapicals
Crown of tooth and interproximal bone (caries, restorations)	Bitewing
Root and periapical area	Periapical
Submandibular gland	Lower occlusal view
Sinuses	Occipitomental, PAN
TMJ	PAN, computed tomography (CT)
Skull and facial bones	Occipitomental
	Posteroanterior (PA) and lateral skull
	Submentovertex

Local anesthesia can help localize organic pain.

Radiology and radiography

Radiography is the taking of radiographs, **Radiology** is their interpretation.

Radiographic images are produced by the differential attenuation of X-rays by tissues. Radiographic quality depends on the density of the tissues, the intensity of the beam, sensitivity of the emulsion, processing techniques, and viewing conditions.

Intraoral views

Use a stationary anode (tungsten), direct-current ↓ dose of self-rectifying machine. Use direct action film (↑ detail) at D or E speed. E speed is double the speed of D, hence ↓ dose to patient. Collimation ↓ unnecessary irradiation of tissues.

Periapical view shows all of tooth, root, and surrounding periapical tissues. Performed with the following techniques:

1 Paralleling technique Film is held in a film holder parallel to the tooth and the beam is directed (using a beam-aligning device) at right angles to the tooth and film. This is the most accurate and reproducible technique.

2 Bisecting angle technique Older technique that can be carried out without film holders. Film is placed close to the tooth and the beam is directed at right angles to the plane, bisecting the angle between the tooth and film. Normally held in place by film-holding device. This techniques is not as geometrically accurate.

Bitewings show crowns and crestal bone levels, and are used to diagnose caries, overhangs, calculus, and bone loss <4 mm. Patient bites on wing holding film against the upper and lower teeth and beam is directed between contact points perpendicular to the film in the horizontal plane.

Occlusal view demonstrates larger areas. May be oblique, true, or special. Used for localization of impacted teeth, salivary calculi. Film is held parallel to the occlusal plane. Oblique occlusal is similar to a large bisecting-angle periapical. True occlusal of the mandible gives a good cross-sectional view.

Key points
- Use paralleling technique
- Use film holders
- Collimation
- E speed film

Extraoral views

For skull and general facial views use a rotating anode and grid that ↓ scattered radiation reaching the film but ↑ dose to patient. Screen film is used for all extraorals (intensifying screens are now rare earth, e.g., gadolinium and lanthanum). X-rays act on screen, which fluoresces, and the light interacts with emulsion. There is loss of detail but ↓ the dose to patient. Dark-room techniques and film storage are affected due to the properties of the film.

Lateral oblique Largely superseded by panoramic but can use dental X-ray set.

PA mandible Patient has nose to forehead touching film. Beam is perpendicular to film. Used for diagnosing and assessing # mandible.

Reverse Townes position, as above, but beam 30° up to horizontal. Used for condyles.

Occipitomental Nose or chin touching the film beam parallel to horizontal unless OM prefixed by, e.g., 10°, 30°, which indicates angle of beam to horizontal.

Submentovertex Patient flexes neck vertex touching film, beam projected menton to vertex. ↓ use due to ↑ radiation and risk to cervical spine.

Cephalometry (pp. 130, 132) Cephalostat used for reproducible position. Use Frankfort plane or natural head position. Wedge (aluminum or copper and rare earth) to show soft tissues. Lead collimation to reduce unnecessary dose to patient and scatter leading to ↓ contrast.

Panoramic Generically referred to as PAN (dental panoramic tomograph). The technique is based on tomography (i.e., objects in focal trough are in focus, the rest is blurred). The state-of-the-art machine is a moving center of rotation (previously two or three centers) that accommodates the horseshoe shape of the jaws. Correct patient positioning is vital. Blurring and ghost shadows can be a problem (ghost shadows appear opposite to and above the real image due to 5–8° tilt of beam). Relatively low-dose technique and sectional images can be obtained. Useful as a screening tool for gross pathology. Cannot be used to diagnose caries.

Lead aprons (0.25 mm lead equivalent)
With well-maintained, well-collimated equipment where the beam does not point to the gonads, the risk of damage is minimal. Apply all normal principles to pregnant women (use lead apron if primary beam is directed at fetus), but otherwise do not treat any differently.

There is no risk in dentistry of deterministic/certainty effects (e.g., radiation burns). Stochastic/change effects are more important (e.g., tumor induction). The thyroid is the principal organ at risk. Follow principles of As Low As Reasonably Practicable.

Parralax technique involves two radiographs with a change in position of X-ray tube between them. The object furthest from the X-ray beam will appear to move in the same direction as the tube shift.

Advanced imaging techniques

Computerized Axial Tomography (CAT scan or CT)

Images are formed by scanning a thin cross section of the body with a narrow X-ray beam, measuring the transmitted radiation with detectors and obtaining multiple projections, which a computer then processes to reconstruct a cross-sectional image ("slice"). Three-dimensional reconstructions can be generated from the CT data acquired, using software designed specifically for this purpose. Modern scanners consist of either a fan beam with multiple detectors aligned in a circle, both rotating around the patient, or a stationary ring of detectors with the X-ray beam rotating within it. The image is divided into pixels that represent the average attenuation of blocks of tissue (voxels). The CT number (measured in Hounsfield units) compares the attenuation of the tissue with that of water. Typical values range from air at −1000 to bone at +400 to +1000 units. As the eye can only perceive a limited gray scale, the settings can be adjusted according to the main tissue of interest (i.e., bone or soft tissues). These "window levels" are set at the average CT number of the tissue being imaged and the "window width" is the range selected. The images obtained are very useful for assessing extensive trauma or pathology and planning surgery. The dose is, however, higher than that of conventional films. Smaller machines have been developed that take up very little space for use in the dental office. CT scans are widely used to plan implant placement.

Magnetic resonance imaging (MRI)

The patient is placed in a machine that is basically a large magnet. Protons then act like small bar magnets and point up or down, with a slightly greater number pointing up. When a radiofrequency pulse is directed across the main magnetic field, the protons "flip" and align themselves along it. When the pulse ceases the protons "relax" and as they realign with the main field they emit a signal. The hydrogen atom is used because of its high natural abundance in the body. The time taken for the protons to relax is measured by values known as T1 and T2. A variety of pulse sequences can be used to give different information. T1 is longer than T2 and times may vary depending on the fluidity of the tissues (e.g., in inflamed). MRI is not good for imaging cortical bone, as the protons are held firmly within the bony structure and give a signal void, i.e., black, although bone margins are visible. It is useful, however, for the TMJ and facial soft tissues.

Problems: Patient movement, expense, the claustrophobic nature of the machine, noise, magnetizing, and movement of instruments or metal implants and foreign bodies. Cards with magnetic strips (e.g., credit cards) near the machine may also be affected.

Digital imaging

This technique has been used extensively in general radiology, where it has great advantages over conventional methods in that there is a marked dose reduction and less concentrated contrast media may be used. The normal X-ray source is used but the receptor is a charged coupled device linked to a computer or a photostimulable phosphor plate that is scanned by a laser. The image is practically instantaneous and eliminates the problems of processing. However, the sensor is difficult to position and the film smaller than normal, which means the dose reduction is not always obtained. The CCD receiver is expensive.

Ultrasound

Ultra-high-frequency sound waves (1–20 MHz) are transmitted through the body using a piezoelectric material (i.e., the material distorts if an electric field is placed across it and vice versa). Good probe-to-skin contact is required (gel), as waves can be absorbed, reflected, or refracted. High-frequency (short wavelength) waves are absorbed more quickly whereas low-frequency waves penetrate further. Ultrasound has been used to image the major salivary glands and the soft tissues.

Doppler ultrasound is used to assess bloodflow, as the difference between the transmitted and returning frequency reflects the speed of travel of red cells. Doppler ultrasound has also been used to assess the vascularity of lesions and the patency of vessels prior to reconstruction.

Sialography

This is the imaging of the major salivary glands after infusion of contrast media under controlled rate and pressure using either conventional radiographic films or CT scanning. The use of contrast media will reveal the internal architecture of the salivary glands and show up radiolucent obstructions, e.g., calculi within the ducts of the imaged glands. This technique is particularly useful for inflammatory or obstructive conditions of the salivary glands. Patients allergic to iodine are at risk of anaphylactic reaction if an iodine-based contrast medium is used. Interventional sialography is now possible, e.g., for stone retrieval.

Arthrography

Just as the spaces within salivary glands can be outlined using contrast media, so can the upper and lower joint spaces of the TMJ. Although technically difficult, both joint compartments (usually the lower) can be injected with contrast media under fluoroscopic control and the movement of the meniscus can be visualized on video. Stills of the real-time images can be made, although interpretation is often unsatisfactory.

Differential diagnosis and treatment plan

Arriving at this stage is the whole point of taking a history and performing an examination, because by narrowing down your patient's symptoms into possible diagnoses you can, in most instances, formulate a series of tests and/or treatment that will benefit them.

Suggested approach

- History and examination (as above)
- Preliminary diagnostic tests
- Differential diagnosis
- Specific diagnostic test and examinations that confirm or refute the differential diagnoses
- Ideally, arrive at the definitive diagnosis(es).
- List in a logical progression the steps that can be undertaken to take the patient to oral health.
- Then carry them out.

Simple really!

This is the ideal, but life, as you are no doubt well aware, is far from ideal, and it is not always possible to follow this approach from beginning to end. The principles, however, remain valid and this general approach, even if much abbreviated, will help you deal with every new patient safely and sensibly.

An example

Mr. Ivor: Pain, age 25, an otherwise healthy young man has a "toothache." CC Pain, left side of mouth.

History of present illness (HPI) Lost large amalgam 20 3 weeks ago. Had twinges since then that seemed to go away, then 2 days ago tooth began to throb. Now whole jaw aches and he can't eat on that side. The pain radiates to his ear and is worse if he drinks tea. He has a foul taste in his mouth. Gets little relief from analgesics.

Past medical history (PMH) Well. Medical history, nothing abnormal detected (NAD), i.e., no "alarm bells" on questionnaire.

PDH Means well, but only presents when symptomatic, "had some bad experiences," "don't like needles."

Extra- and Intraoral examination

EOE Medical examination inappropriate in view of PMH. Some swelling on left side of face due to left submandibular lymphadenopathy. Looks distressed and anxious.

IOE Moderate oral hygiene (OH), generalized chronic gingivitis, no mucosal lesions, caries 2, 3, 12, 14, 18, 20, 29, 30, and 31. Partially erupted 17 with exudate present, 20 with large cavity, but periodontal probing depths <3 mm. No fluctuant soft tissue swelling. Otherwise complete dentition with Class I occlusion.

General diagnostics Temperature 100°F.

Differential diagnoses
- Acute apical abscess 20
- Acute pericoronitis 17
- Chronic gingivitis? Periodontitis
- Caries as charted

Specific diagnostic tests/examinations
- Vitality test 20 (non-vital)
- Periapical X-ray 20 (patent canal, apical area)

Rx plan
- Drain 20 via root canal. Administer LA to relieve pain and treat infection.
- Irrigate operculum of 17.
- Antibiotics (patient is febrile with two sources of infection, usually due to mixed anaerobic/aerobic organisms; use amoxicillin and metronidazole) and analgesics (NSAID for 24–48 h).
- Explain the problems and arrange a review appointment for oral hygiene instruction (OHI), periodontal charting, and full mouth series. PAN to screen third molars.

Future plan
- OHI, scaling
- RCT 20
- Plastic restorations as indicated
- Post/core crown 20
- Remove third molars as indicated (clinically and from PAN).

Treatment at the first visit is kept at a minimum to relieve patient's pain and thereby gain his trust and future attendance.

Preventive and community dentistry

Relevant pages in other chapters: Plaque control, p. 194; prevention of secondary caries, p. 195; prevention of trauma to anterior teeth, p. 98.

Principal sources: J. J. Murray 1996 *Prevention of Dental Disease*, OUP. E. A. M. Kidd 1987 *Essentials of Dental Caries: The Disease and Its Management*, Wright R. J. Elderton 1987 *Positive Dental Prevention*, Heinemann. R. J. Elderton 1990 *Clinical Dentistry in Health and Disease, Vol. 3, The Dentition and Dental Care*, Heinemann. A. Rugg-Gunn 1993 *Nutrition and Dental Health*, OUP. B. A. Burt and S. A. Eklund 2005 *Dentistry, Dental Practice, and the Community*, Elsevier Saunders.

Dental caries

Dental caries is a sugar-dependent infectious disease.[1] Acid is produced as a by-product of the metabolism of dietary carbohydrate by plaque bacteria, which results in a drop in pH at the tooth surface. In response, calcium and phosphate ions diffuse out of enamel, resulting in demineralization. This process is reversed when the pH rises again. Caries is ∴ a dynamic process characterized by episodic demineralization and remineralization occurring over time. If destruction predominates, disintegration of the mineral component will occur, leading to cavitation.

Enamel caries The initial lesion is visible as a white spot. This appearance is due to demineralization of the prisms in a subsurface layer, with the surface enamel remaining more mineralized. With continued acid attack the surface changes from being smooth to rough, and may become stained. As the lesion progresses, pitting and eventually cavitation occur. The carious process favors repair, as remineralized enamel concentrates fluoride and has larger crystals, with a ↓ surface area. Fissure caries often starts as two white spot lesions on opposing walls, which coalesce.

Dentin caries comprises demineralization followed by bacterial invasion, but differs from enamel caries in the production of secondary dentine and the proximity of the pulp. Once bacteria reach the dentinoenamel junction (DEJ), lateral spread occurs, undermining the overlying enamel.

Rate of progression of caries Although it has been suggested that the mean time that lesions remain confined radiographically to the enamel is 3–4 years,[2] there is a great deal of individual variation and lesions may even regress.[3] The rate of progression through dentine is unknown; however, it is likely to be faster than through enamel. Progression of fissure caries is usually rapid due to the morphology of the area.

Arrested caries Under favorable conditions a lesion may become inactive and even regress. Clinically, arrested dentine caries has a hard or leathery consistency and is darker in color than soft, yellow active decay. Arrested enamel caries can be stained dark brown.

Susceptible sites The sites on a tooth that are particularly prone to decay are those where plaque accumulation can occur unhindered, e.g., interproximal enamel surfaces, cervical margins, and pits and fissures. Host factors, e.g., the volume and composition of the saliva, can also affect susceptibility.

Saliva and caries Saliva acts as an intraoral antacid, due to its alkali pH at high flow-rates and buffering capacity. In addition, saliva
- ↓ plaque accumulation and aids clearance of foodstuffs;
- acts as a reservoir of calcium, phosphate, and fluoride ions, thereby favoring remineralization; and
- has an antibacterial action because of its IgA, lysozyme, lactoferritin, and lactoperoxidase content.

1 E. A. M. Kidd 1987 *Essentials of Dental Caries: The Disease and its Management*, Wright.
2 N. B. Pitts 1983 *Community Dent Oral Epidemiol* **11** 228.
3 N. B. Pitts 1991 *BDJ* **171** 313.

An appreciation of the importance of saliva can be gained by examining a patient with a dry mouth.

Some manufacturers are now promoting the remineralizing potential of chewing gum, effected by an increase in salivary production. Chewing sugar-free gum (Xylitol) regularly after meals does appear to ↓ caries, but the reduction is small.[1]

Root caries With gingival recession, root dentine is exposed to carious attack. Rx requires first control of the etiological factors, and for most patients this involves dietary advice and OHI. Topical fluoride may aid remineralization and prevent new lesions from developing. However, active lesions will require restoration with glass ionomer (GI) cement (p. 241).

Caries prevention

Classically, three main approaches are possible:
- Tooth strengthening or protection
- Reduction in the availability of microbial substrate
- Removal of plaque by physical or chemical means

In practice this means dietary advice, fluoride, fissure sealing, and regular toothbrushing (which is also important in the prevention of gingivitis). The relative value of these varies with the age of the individual.

Of equal importance in the prevention of new lesions is a preventive philosophy on the part of the dentist, so that early carious lesions are given the chance to arrest and a minimalist approach is taken to the excision of caries where primary prevention has failed.

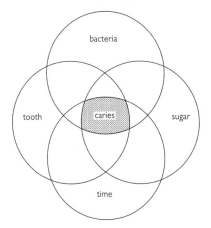

Diagram showing the factors involved in the development of caries.

Caries diagnosis

As caries can be arrested or even reversed, early diagnosis is important.

Aids to diagnosis

- Good eyesight (and a clean, dry, well-illuminated tooth). Magnification between x2 and x6 (leaning forward with the naked eye magnifies the image but you can only get so close to your patient); loupes are better!
- A blunt probe should only be used to horizontally dredge plaque away from the fissures (a sharp probe may actually damage an incipient lesion and sterile fissures may be inoculated by probing after previous contact with an infected fissure).
- Bitewing (b/w) radiographs are useful in the detection of interproximal caries. They are best approached systematically viewing the "inter-proximal–occlusal–interproximal" surface for each tooth, first in enamel then dentine, first with the naked eye and then with a viewing box (magnification and external light blackened out). The clinical situation is more advanced than the radiographic appearance. However, it is thought that the probability of cavitation is low when a lesion is confined to enamel on X-ray.
- Fiber optic transillumination (FOTI) probes with a 0.5 mm tip are useful for detecting dentinal lesions at interproximal sites. FOTI is considered to be an adjunct to bitewing radiographs.[1]
- Diagnodent is a laser-based instrument that uses fluorescent properties of the carious lesion to produce a quantitative reading of infected carious tissue, particularly dentine caries. Diagnodent should be used with care—it can produce false positives due to stain or dental materials.
- The electronic caries monitor (ECM) was designed to assess for occlusal carious lesions using site-specific electrical conductance. The reported false-positive rates and false-negative rates for ECM in diagnosing dentinal carious lesions of permanent premolar and molar teeth have been shown to range from 4% to 33% and 2% to 29%, respectively.[2]

Diagnosis and its relevance to management

- ▶ Remember: precavitated lesion—prevention
  cavitated lesion—prevention and restoration
- ▶ Counsel the patient that if the lesion is not cavitated it has the potential to arrest. This makes the preventive advice very relevant to the patient, increasing the chance that the patient will act on the advice.

Smooth surface caries is relatively straightforward to diagnose. The chances of remineralization are ↑ as it is obvious, and accessible for cleaning. Restoration is indicated if prevention has failed and the lesion is cavitated, or if the tooth is sensitive or esthetics poor.

1 1998 *Selection Criteria for Dental Radiography*, Faculty of General Dental Practitioners RCS (Eng).
2 S. Tranaeus 1993 Community Dent Oral Epidemiol **33** 265.

Pit and fissure caries is difficult to diagnose reliably, especially in the early stages. Traditional diagnostic methods, such as visual inspection, have been shown to have a low false-negative rate (high specificity) but a high false-positive rate (low sensitivity).[1]

A sharp probe is of limited value as stickiness could be due to the morphology of the fissure. The anatomy of the area also tends to favor spread of the lesion, which often occurs rapidly. As fissure caries is less amenable to fluoride and OH, fissure sealing is preferable to watching and waiting. Occlusal caries evident on b/w radiographs should not always be excised. If the tooth is fissure-sealed or restored, check the margins very carefully; if intact, monitor the lesion radiographically. If marginal integrity is not intact, investigate the area with a small, round bur. The "cavity" can be aborted if no caries is found and the surface sealed.

Interproximal caries Currently accepted practice:
- If lesion is confined to enamel on b/w, institute preventive measures and keep under review.
- If lesion has penetrated dentine radiographically, a restoration is indicated unless serial radiographs show that it is static.

If in doubt of whether an interproximal lesion has cavitated, fit an elastic orthodontic separator for 3–7 days so the surfaces can be visualized.

Recall intervals[2]

This subject has evoked considerable controversy, some arguing that regular attendance puts a patient more at risk of receiving replacement fillings, while others contend that regular and frequent checkups are necessary to monitor prevention. Primary care dental practitioners in many countries have most commonly recommended checkups every 6 months. A 2005 Cochrane Collaboration systematic review determined that currently there is insufficient evidence to support or refute the existing practice.[1]

1 S. TraNaeus 1993 Community Dent Oral Epidemiol **33** 265.
2 P. Beirne 2005 *Cochrane Database Syst Rev* **2** CD 004346.

Fluoride

The history of fluoride is covered well in other texts.[1]

Mechanisms of the action of fluoride in reducing dental decay

Enamel deposition → and calcification	Enamel maturation →	Eruption into oral environment
↑	↑	↑
Fluoride in blood	Fluoride in tissue fluid	Fluoride in saliva fluid and cervicular fluid

The concentration of fluoride in enamel ↑ with ↑ fluoride content in water supply and ↑ toward the surface of enamel.

Pre-eruptive effects Enamel formed in the presence of fluoride has
● Improved crystallinity and ↑ crystal size, and ∴ ↓ acid solubility.
● More rounded cusps and fissure pattern, but the effect is small.

Discontinuation of systemic fluoride results in an ↑ in caries, ∴ pre-eruptive effects must be limited.

Post-eruptive effects **Note:** Newly erupted teeth derive the most benefit.
● Inhibits demineralization and promotes remineralization of early caries. Fluoride enhances the degree and speed of remineralization and renders the remineralized enamel more resistant to subsequent attack.
● Decreases acid production in plaque by inhibiting glycolysis in cariogenic bacteria.
● An ↑ concentration of fluoride in plaque inhibits the synthesis of extracellular polysaccharide.
● It has been suggested that fluoride affects pellicle and plaque formation, but this is unsubstantiated.

At higher pH fluoride is bound to protein in plaque. A drop in pH results in release of free ionic fluoride, which augments these actions.

Note: Fluoride is more effective in ↓ smooth surface than pit and fissure caries.

Safety and toxicity of fluoride

Fluoride is present in all natural waters to some extent. Many simple chemicals are toxic when consumed in excess, and the same is true of fluoride.

Fluoride is absorbed rapidly mainly from the stomach. Peak blood levels occur 1 h later. It is excreted via the kidneys, but traces are found in breast milk and saliva. The placenta only allows a small amount of fluoride to cross, ∴ prenatal fluoride is relatively ineffective.

Enamel fluorosis (or mottling) occurs with a long-term excess of fluoride. It is endemic in areas with a high level of fluoride occurring naturally in the water. Clinically, it can vary from faint white opacities to severe pitting and discoloration. Histologically, it is caused by porosity in the outer third of the enamel.

1 J. J. Murray 1996. *Prevention of Oral Disease* 3rd ed, OUP.

Concentration of fluoride (ppm) in water supply	Degree of mottling
<0.9	+
0.9	+
2	++
>2	++++

Toxicity

Safely tolerated dose (STD) Dose below which symptoms of toxicity are unlikely = 1 mg/kg body weight

Potentially lethal dose (PLD) Lowest dose associated with a fatality. Patient should be hospitalized = 5 mg/kg body weight

Certainly lethal dose (CLD) Survival unlikely = 32–64 mg/kg body weight

Fluoride concentration in various products

Standard adult fluoride toothpaste 1000 ppm F (parts per million fluoride) = 1 mg F/ml, usually in the form of sodium fluoride or sodium monofluorophosphate.

Toothpaste available by prescription 1.1% NaF = 5000 ppm and for sensitive teeth 1.1% NaF + 5% potassium nitrate

Daily fluoride mouth rinse 0.05% NaF = 0.023% F = 0.23 mg F/ml
APF gel 1.23% F = 12.3 mg/ml

Fluoride varnish 5% NaF = 2.26% F = 22.6 mg/ml

To reach the 5 mg F/kg threshold (requiring hospitalization), a 5-year-old (about 42 lb) would have to ingest 95 (1 mg F) tablets, 95 ml of toothpaste, or 7.6 ml of 1.23% of APF gel.

Antidotes <5 mg F/kg body weight—large volume of milk. >5 mg F/kg body weight—refer to hospital quickly for gastric lavage. If any delay, give IV calcium gluconate and an emetic.

Musculoskeletal effects[1]

Concerns about the effect of fluoride on the musculoskeletal system stem from the fact that fluoride is readily accumulates in the crystalline structure of bone.

Skeletal fluorosis is a bone and joint condition in which bone density and growth of osteophytes is increased, resulting in joint stiffness and pain. The National Research Council determined that "more research is needed to clarify the relationship between fluoride ingestion, fluoride concentrations in bone, and stage of skeletal fluorosis before any conclusions can be drawn."

Bone fracture risk has been reported to be elevated when drinking water has moderately high levels (4 mg/l) of fluoride, according to several strong observational studies. Insufficient evidence exists to judge the effect of lower concentrations of fluoride.

---

1 National Research Council. 2006. *Fluoride in Drinking Water: A Scientific Review of EPA's Standards.*

Cancer Bone is the most probable site for fluoride-associated cancer because of its accumulation in bone and its mitogenic effects on bone cells *in vitro*. Claims of an association between fluoride and bone cancer have been controversial. According to the National Research Council "the evidence of the potential of fluoride to initiate or promote cancers is tentative and mixed".

▶ Advice about managing fluoride overdose can be sought from the American Association of Poison Control Centers (1-800-222-1222).

Planning fluoride therapy

Many consider the most important action of fluoride to be promoting remineralization of the early carious lesion. Although fluoride incorporated within developing enamel results in a high local concentration following acid attack, the maximum benefit appears to be derived from frequent low-concentration topical administration.[1] Fluoridated water is the most effective method, as it provides both a systemic and topical effect.

Systemic fluoride

▶ To minimize the risk of mottling, only one systemic measure should be used at a time.

Water fluoridation Hexafluorosilicic acid (H_2SiF_6) and its sodium salt (Na_2SiF_6) are the most common forms of fluoride used in fluoridation of water supplies in the United States. A concentration of 1 ppm (1 mg F per liter) results in a caries reduction of 50%. The two main advantages of this measure are that it benefits all people in the community and it is low in cost. In 2000, it was estimated that approximately 57% of the total U.S. population had artificially fluoridated water. In some countries school water has been fluoridated, but a concentration of 5 ppm is required to offset the less frequent intake.

Fluoride drops and tablets Recommended regimen (mg F/day) depends on drinking water content (see table). However, calls have been made for a reevaluation of their use among children less than 7 years of age because evidence to support a pre-eruptive anticariogenic effect is weak, supplements have been identified as a risk factor for dental fluorosis, and the prevalence of caries continues to decline.

Milk with 2.5–7 ppm F has been tried successfully.

Salt fluoridation is an alternative to water fluoridation and can be used when water fluoridation is not feasible.

Topical fluoride

Professionally applied fluorides A wide variety of solutions, gels, and application protocols are available. Overall, caries reductions of 20–40% are reported. If these are applied in trays without adequate suction the systemic dosage can be high ∴ it is better to apply to a few, well-isolated teeth at a time. Fluoride varnish (e.g., Duraphat) is useful for applying directly to individual lesions to aid arrest, and regular site-specific application has been shown to be effective at reducing caries incidence. However, care is required and it should be applied sparingly, especially in young children, as it contains 23,000 ppm fluoride.

Rinsing solutions Mouth rinses are contraindicated (C/I) in children <7 years. The concentration prescribed depends on the frequency of use: 0.2% weekly or 0.05% daily. Daily use is the most beneficial. Caries reductions on the order of 16–50% have been reported with rinsing alone. The most widely used solution is sodium fluoride.

Toothpastes aid tooth cleaning and polishing but, most importantly, act as a vehicle for fluoride delivery. Toothpastes contain abrasives, detergents,

1 E. A. M. Kidd 1987 *Essentials of Dental Caries: The Disease and Its Management,*, Wright.

humectants, flavoring, binding agents, preservatives, and active agents, including the following:

- Fluoride. Most toothpastes contain sodium monofluorophosphate and/or sodium fluoride, in concentrations of 1000–1100 ppm (i.e., 1–1.1 mg per 1 cm paste). Caries reductions of 15% (in fluoridated areas) to 30% (in non-fluoridated areas) are reported. Low-dose formulations for children <7 years containing <500 ppm are available, to ↓ risk of mottling. Fluoride-free toothpaste is also available.
- Anticalculus agents, e.g., sodium pyrophosphate, can ↓ supragingival calculus formation by 50%
- Desensitizing agents, e.g., 10% strontium or potassium chloride or 5% potassium nitrate
- Antibacterial agents, e.g., triclosan, which have been shown to reduce existing plaque and gingivitis

Recommended daily fluoride supplementation (mg F)[1,2]

For children considered at high risk of caries and who live in areas with suboptimal fluoride in the water supplies:

	Concentration of F in water (ppm)		
Age	<0.3	0.3–0.7	>0.7
6 months to 3 years	0.25	—	—
3 to 6 years	0.5	0.25	—
>6 years	1.0	0.50	—

Suggested guidelines for children (CDC)
Oral hygiene and toothpaste

- As soon as the first tooth appears, begin wiping it with a clean, damp cloth every day. When more teeth come in, switch to a soft, small toothbrush.
- In general, begin using toothpaste with fluoride when the child is 2 years of age, unless the clinical situation warrants earlier use.
- Parents should brush the teeth twice a day until the child has the skill to brush his or her own teeth. They should continue to supervise brushing up to at least 7 years of age to ensure adequate plaque removal and to avoid overingestion of toothpaste.
- Children under 6 years of age should use a "smear," or no more than a small pea-sized blob (<0.3 ml) of toothpaste.
- Children should spit out well and rinse after brushing.

Fluoride supplement (drops and tablets)

This may be prescribed for children deemed at risk of developing caries who live in areas with less than optimal fluoride in the water supply. Fluoridation of water still remains the most cost-effective method.

Recommended fluoride concentration of toothpaste for children		
Age (years)	**Concentration of fluoride (ppm)**	
	Low caries risk	High caries risk
0.5–5	<600	1000
6+	1000	1500

1 American Dental Association 1994 ADA News 25 14.
2 R. Holt 1996 Int J Paediatr Dent 6 139.

Bacterial plaque and dental decay

Evidence for role of bacteria in dental caries

- *In vitro*. Incubating teeth with plaque and sugar in saliva results in caries.
- Animal experiments—e.g., germ-free rodents fed a cariogenic diet do not develop caries, but following the introduction of *Streptococcus mutans* caries occurs.
- Epidemiological evidence showing that a supply of bacterial substrate results in caries.
- Clinical experiments—e.g., stringent removal of plaque ↓ decay.

A correlation has been found between the presence of *Strep. mutans* and caries. This is not surprising, because this organism is acidophilic, can synthesize acid rapidly from sugar, and produces a sticky extracellular polysaccharide that helps bind it to the tooth. However, caries can develop in the absence of *Strep. mutans*, and its presence does not inevitably lead to decay; e.g., root caries has been associated with *Strep. salivarius* and *Actinomyces* species. *Lactobacilli* are also acidophilic and have been implicated in fissure caries. In addition, plaque prevents acid diffusion away from the enamel and hinders the neutralizing effect of salivary buffers.

Methods of preventing caries by bacterial control

Physical removal of plaque

- By a professional. If sufficiently frequent it can ↓ caries.[1]
- By the individual. Unfortunately, at the standard employed by most of the general public, toothbrushing per se is not an effective method of caries control. However, brushing with a fluoridated toothpaste provides regular topical fluoride. It also ↓ gingivitis.

Chemical removal of plaque

To achieve more than a transitory effect, an antiseptic needs to be retained in the mouth. The only chemical capable of this at present is chlorhexidine, a positively charged bactericidal and fungicidal antiseptic, which is attracted to the negatively charged proteins on the surface of teeth and oral mucosa, and in saliva from where it gradually leaches out. It is available in the United States as Peridex and PerioGard, both of which contain 0.12% chlorhexidine gluconate. Although the main application of chlorhexidine is in the management of gingivitis, it has been shown to be effective at ↓ caries when used regularly.[2] While its widespread use for this purpose is not practical, it can be helpful in the management of handicapped patients or those with ↓ salivary flow. Unwanted effects include staining, disturbance of taste, and parotid swelling (which is reversible). It is less effective in the presence of a large buildup of plaque and is inactivated by commercial toothpastes.

---

1 J. Lindhe 1975 *Community Dent Oral Epidemiol* **3** 150.
2 H. Loe 1972 *Scand J Dent Res* **80** 1.

A variety of pre-brushing rinses are now available. Research suggests that these do have a small beneficial effect if used in conjunction with toothbrushing.[1]

Immunization against caries As no vaccine is completely safe, the ethics of vaccinating against caries, an avoidable nonlethal disease, have been hotly debated.[2] Yet despite considerable research, efforts to produce a viable vaccine have been unsuccessful due to a number of problems:

- Which species of *Strep. mutans* to target, and whether pathogenicity would then shift to another species.
- Differing modes of action in monkeys and rodents, ∴ ? relevance of experiments to humans.
- Cross-reactivity with heart muscle in animal experiments.
- Duration of effect and acceptance by public. Some patients may prefer caries to repeated injections of a vaccine.

1 H. V. Worthington 1993 *BDJ* **175** 322.
2 W. Sims 1985 *Community Dent Health* **2** 129.

Fissure sealants

Pits and fissures in teeth provide a sheltered niche for bacterial proliferation. Toothbrush bristles are too wide to fit into these areas, making complete plaque removal impossible. A fissure sealant is a material that provides an impervious barrier to the fissure system to prevent the development of caries.

Historical Several approaches to ↓ fissure caries have been tried:
- Chemical Rx of the enamel, e.g., with silver nitrate
- Prophylactic odontotomy. This involved restoring the fissure with amalgam (hardly a preventive approach!).
- Sealing of the fissures. Several materials have been tried, including black copper cement (not retained), cyanoacrylate (toxic), polyurethane, and GI cement. The most common type of fissure sealant (f/s) is a composite resin used with an acid-etch technique.

Is there a need for sealants? Although developed countries have enjoyed a reduction in dental decay in recent years, this has not been uniform for all tooth surfaces. Given that part of this reduction is thought to be due to an increased availability of fluoride, it is not surprising that there has been a greater reduction in interproximal, rather than in pit and fissure, caries. Fluoride works on smooth-surface caries, not pits and fissures. If decay is to be eliminated, then the need for a method of occlusal caries is even more pressing.

Are sealants effective? To be effective, sealants need to be carefully applied to susceptible teeth. Unfortunately, those situations in which they are most valuable (recently erupted first molars) are often where moisture control is the most difficult; ∴ sealants should be monitored, and replaced if lost. For maximum benefit, teeth should be sealed as soon as practicable after eruption and certainly within 2 years. Guidelines for placement of f/s have been described.[1]

A 2004 Cochrane Collaboration systematic review[1] found that the placement of second-generation resin sealants on permanent first molars in 5- to 10-year-olds was associated with a reduction in carious lesions ranging from 86% at 12 months and 57% at 48 to 54 months. Significant reductions were also seen in 12- to 13-year-olds followed for 24 months. There was insufficient information to make conclusions about the effectiveness of GI sealants. The authors concluded that sealing is recommended to prevent caries of the occlusal surfaces of permanent molars, though the carious lesion prevalence of both individuals and the population should be taken into account.

Patient selection f/s should be provided for permanent first molars in
- children with impairments; and
- those with extensive caries in the primary dentition (decayed, missing, filled [dmf] is 2 or more).

Children with caries-free primary dentitions do not need routine f/s of permanent first molars but should be monitored regularly.

---

1 J. H.Nunn 2000 *Int J Paediatr Dent* **10** 174.
2 A. Ahovuo-Saloranta 2004 *Cochrane Database Syst Rev* **3** CD001830.

Tooth selection

For children who fulfill the criteria above:

- All susceptible fissures of permanent teeth should be sealed—occlusal, fissures and cingulum, buccal, and palatal pits. Teeth should be sealed as soon as sufficiently erupted for adequate moisture control.
- Where occlusal caries affects one first molar, the remaining caries-free permanent molars (first and second) should be f/s.
- f/s of primary molars is not normally recommended.

If there is doubt about a stained fissure, a b/w radiograph should be taken. If the lesion is in enamel, f/s and monitor clinically and radiographically. If in doubt, carry out an enamel biopsy. If the lesion extends to dentine place a preventive resin restoration (PRR), providing the cavity does not extend to more than one-third of the occlusal surface, in which case a conventional restoration is required. It should be noted that the clinician need not fear placing a sealant over incipient decay, as well-placed sealants have been shown to arrest these lesions.

The accepted figures for composite resin-based sealant retention are >85% after 1 yr and >50% after 5 yr.[1]

Discussion of the cost-effectiveness of sealants compared to resto-ration has been well aired over the years, which is surprising given that the end results are not comparable. However, recent studies indicating that amalgam restorations have a more finite life than was once assumed (p. 244) have deflated this debate.

Types of fissure sealant Sealants can be classified by polymerization method (light- or self-cure), resin system (Bis-GMA or urethane diacrylate), color (clear or tinted), and whether they are filled or unfilled. The choice is one of personal preference; however, it has been pointed out that colored and opaque sealants are more readily obvious to the patient. The retention rates of the different types are similar: success depends on maintaining an absolutely dry field during application.

GI sealants do release fluoride but have poorer retention than resin sealants. They are useful for high caries-risk children as a temporary sealant where adequate isolation for successful placement of resin-based sealants is not possible, e.g., for partially erupted teeth when there is poor cooperation.

Fissure sealant technique

- Prophylaxis (this may be omitted if the tooth is already relatively free from plaque)
- Isolate and dry the tooth.
- Etch for the time recommended by the manufacturer (usually 20–40 sec) with 30–50% phosphoric acid.
- Wash thoroughly, re-isolate, and dry very, very well. If salivary contamination occurs, re-etch.
- Apply f/s (method depends on delivery system).
- After polymerization try to remove the sealant. If satisfactory, occlusal adjustment is usually not required unless a large volume has inadvertently been applied or a filled resin is used.

Follow-up f/s should be monitored clinically and, where appropriate, radiographically (b/w). Defective sealants should be replenished to maintain their marginal integrity.

1 National Institutes of Health 1984 *J Am Dent Assoc* **108** 233.

Sugar

The term *sugar* is commonly used to refer to the mono- and disaccharide members of the carbohydrate family. Monosaccharides include glucose (dextrose or corn sugar), fructose (fruit sugar), galactose, and mannose. Disaccharides include lactose (in milk), maltose, and sucrose (cane or beet sugar). Polysaccharides (starch) are composed of chains of glucose molecules and are not readily broken down by the oral flora. Dietary sugars have been classified as intrinsic when they are part of the cells in a food (vegetables and fruit) or extrinsic (milk sugar or, the really bad one, non-milk extrinsic sugar, e.g., table sugar). Both intrinsic and extrinsic sugars may cause decay, although non-milk extrinsic sugars are generally considered to be the most cariogenic.

Evidence for the role of sugar in dental caries[1]
- Epidemiological evidence:
  - Worldwide comparison of sugar consumption and caries levels
  - Low caries experience of people on low-sugar diet, e.g., wartime diet; patients with hereditary fructose intolerance
  - ↑ caries experience following ↑ availability of sugar, e.g., among Inuits
  - Cross-sectional studies relating caries experience to sugar intake
- Clinical studies, e.g., Vipeholm study, Turku sugar study (Xylitol)
- Plaque pH studies, *in vivo* and *in vitro*. See Stephan curve below.
- Animal experiments, e.g., rats fed by stomach tube do not develop caries

Sucrose is considered a major culprit, in part because it is the most commonly available sugar, but also because of its ability to facilitate production of extracellular polysaccharide in plaque. However, other sugars can also cause caries. For example, frequent consumption of fruit-based drinks is known to be a key factor in the development of early childhood caries (ECC). In ↓ cariogenicity:
- Sucrose, glucose, fructose, maltose (honey)
- Galactose, lactose
- Complex carbohydrate (e.g., starch in rice, bread, potatoes)

The frequency of sugary intakes and the interval between them, the total amount of sugar eaten in the diet, and the concentration of sugar and stickiness of a food were shown to be important in the Vipeholm (1946–1952) study. However, some studies indicate that frequency of consumption of sugars may play a smaller cariogenic role in today's low-caries environment.[2]

Sugar and health In 1989 the Committee on Medical Aspects of Food Policy (COMA) panel on Dietary Sugars and Human Disease reported that dental decay is positively associated with the frequency and amount of non-milk extrinsic sugar consumption. However, while sugar may contribute to the excess calorific intake that causes obesity and predisposes toward diabetes or coronary heart disease, there is no direct evidence linking sugar intake and these medical conditions.[2]

1 A. Rugg-Gunn 1993 In *Nutrition and Dental Health*, OUP.
2 B. A. Burt and S. A. Eklund 2005 *Dentistry, Dental Practice, and the Community*, Elsievier Saunders.
2 COMA 1989 *Dietary Sugars and Human Disease*, HMSO.

Prevention of caries by ↓ the availability of microbial substrate

The following aims take into account the modern habit of snacking (also known as "grazing"):

- Remove sugar from selected foods.
- Substitute with non-cariogenic sweeteners.
- Modify sugar-containing foods so that they are less cariogenic.

Modification of only a restricted number of snack foods would probably have a significant effect.

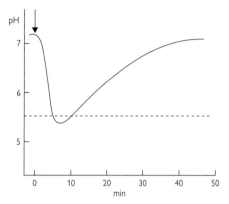

Diagram of a Stephan curve showing the pH drop that occurs after a sugary drink is consumed (shown by arrow). The dashed line indicates the critical pH; below this pH demineralization will occur. The shape of the curve is affected by a number of factors, including the type of sugary food, buffering potential of the saliva, and foods or drinks ingested after the sugary challenge.

Alternative sweeteners (sweetness of sucrose = 1)

Sweetener	Type	Sweetness	Cariogenicity	Comments
Sorbitol	Bulk sweetener	0.5	Low	Isocalorific to sugar
Mannitol	Bulk sweetener	0.7	Low	
Xylitol	Bulk sweetener	1	None	Diarrhea
Isomalt	Bulk sweetener	0.5	Low	
Lycasin*	Bulk sweetener	0.75	Low	
Acesulfame	Intense	130	None	
Aspartame	Intense	200	None	C/I in phenyl-ketonuria
Saccharin	Intense	500	None	Bitter aftertaste
Thaumatin	Intense	4000	None	

* Lycasin is the trade name for hydrogenated glucose syrup.

The bulk sweeteners (largely polyols) can cause osmotic diarrhea if consumed in large amounts and are ∴ C/I in small children. However, it is probably wise for preschool children to avoid all artificial sweeteners. The bulk sweeteners are isocalorific with sucrose, whereas the intense sweeteners are low calorie.

Recommendations for ↓ the risk of caries
- Reduce frequency of consumption of sugar-containing foods and drinks, especially between meals.
- Reduce frequency of consumption of fruit-based drinks, even those labeled "no added sugar."
- A few snack foods are "safe" (e.g., nuts and cheese), but foods containing artificial sweeteners may be less decay producing.
- Foods containing starch and sugar in combination (e.g., cakes, biscuits) and carbonated sugary drinks are especially decay producing.

Dietary analysis and advice

Diet can affect teeth:

Pre-eruptively Fluoride is the most important. The effect of calcium, phosphate, vitamins, and sugar is unclear, but is unlikely to be great.

Post-eruptively Again, fluoride is important, as is sugar. Acidic foods or drinks can cause erosion (p. 276).

Dietary analysis

Aim To ↓ the time when teeth are at risk of demineralization and increase the potential remineralization period.

Indications **1** high caries activity, **2** unusual caries pattern, **3** suspected dietary erosion.

Dietary advice should be tailored to the individual. This is most easily done after analyzing the patient's present eating pattern.

Method A consecutive 3- or 4-day analysis (including at least one weekend day) is the most widely used, with the patient recording the time, content, and quantity of food and drink consumed. In addition, toothbrushing and bedtime should be indicated. When the form is returned the entries should be checked with the patient.

Analysis

- Circle the main meals. If in any doubt, identify those snacks that contain complex carbohydrate. Assess nutritional value of meals.
- Underline all sugar intakes in red.
- Identify between-meal snacks and note any associations, e.g., following insubstantial meals or at school.
- Decide on a maximum of three recommendations.

Dietary advice should include an explanation of the effect of between-meals eating and sugary drinks. It must also be personal, practical, and positive! The suggestion that a child should select chips when friends are buying sweets is more likely to be followed than total abstinence.
Some helpful hints:

- Suggest saving sweets to be eaten on one day, e.g., Saturday dinnertime, or to be eaten at the end of a meal.
- All-in-one chocolate bars are preferable to packets of individual sweets.
- Foods that stimulate salivary flow (e.g., cheese, sugar-free chewing gum) can help to reverse the pH drop due to sugar, if eaten afterwards.
- Honey and fruit (especially fruit juice) are cariogenic.
- Artificial sweeteners should be avoided among preschool children.
- Fibrous foods, e.g., apples, are preferable to a sucrose snack, but they can still cause decay, and there is no evidence that they can clean teeth.

Where the nutritional content of meals is inadequate, considerable tact is necessary. It may be possible to suggest that larger meals would reduce the temptation to eat snacks. For children who are "picky" eaters, snacks and sweets saved until the end of a meal can act as an encouragement to consume more food at mealtimes.

BUT remember that while cheese, peanuts, and chips may constitute a safe snack in dental terms, they are all high in fat, and peanuts can be inhaled by small children. Also, "diet" cola is sugar-free, but can still cause erosion if large quantities are drunk.

Therefore, dental dietary advice should be given in the wider context of the general health of the individual, i.e., ↓ consumption of sugars and fats, and ↑ consumption of fiber-rich starchy foods, fresh fruit, and vegetables. Meals provide a better nutritional balance than snacks. Hence the combination of good eating and drinking at mealtimes and ↓ in-between meals snacking is healthy.

Dental health education

What is it? The objective of dental health education is to influence the attitude and behavior of the individual to maintain oral health for life and prevent oral disease.

Primary prevention seeks to prevent the initial occurrence of a disease or disorder and is aimed at healthy individuals.

Secondary prevention aims to arrest disease through early detection and Rx.

Tertiary prevention helps individuals to deal with the effects of the disease and to prevent further recurrence.

Who should give it? All health professionals. In practice, many patients relate better to advice from a hygienist or nurse.

What information should be given? It is important that the information given is factual and that different sources do not give conflicting advice. The Center for Disease Control and Prevention's (CDC) Oral Health for Adults fact sheet at http://www.cdc.gov/OralHealth/factsheets/index.htm gives the following recommendations:

• Drink fluoridated water and use a fluoride toothpaste.
• Take care of your teeth and gums by thoroughly brushing and flossing.
• Avoid tobacco.
• Limit alcohol.
• Avoid sugars and starches when snacking and limit the number of snacks.
• Visit the dentist regularly.
• Diabetic patients should work to maintain control of their disease.
• Medications that produce a dry mouth should be substituted, when possible.
• Have an oral health check-up before beginning cancer treatment.

How? The way in which the advice is imparted is as important as its content. There are three main routes for dental health education:

• The mass media. This is an expensive alternative and, while commercial advertisers tempt the consumer, the success of a dental health education exhorting the public to stop doing something they find pleasurable is not guaranteed.
• Community programs. These need to be carefully planned, targeted, and monitored.[1]
• One-to-one in the clinical environment. This is usually the most successful approach, because the message can be tailored to the individual and reinforcement is facilitated. However, it is expensive in terms of manpower.

Individual dental health education

Because many patients find the dental operatory threatening, it may be better to choose a more neutral environment, e.g., a dental health or preventive unit. It is important that the information be given by someone the patient trusts and can relate to—this is not always the dentist! It is important also to have adequate time, as a hurried approach is of dubious value, and to choose words that the patient will understand.

1 Notes on Dental Health Education, Scottish Health Education Group, Woodburn House, Canaan Lane, Edinburgh.

The following approach has been used successfully:
- Define the problem and its etiology. For example, poor OH that has resulted in periodontal disease—is it because the patient lacks motivation or the appropriate skills? This stage includes questioning the patient to discover how often and for how long they brush.
- Set realistic objectives. It is better to start with trying to motivate the patient to brush well once a day rather than teaching them how to floss.
- Demonstrate on the patient, as this makes the advice more relevant, and more likely to be remembered.
- Monitor by comparing plaque scores before and after. This not only enables you to monitor improvement but also allows improvements in the patient's OH behavior to be reinforced.
- Remember that everyone responds well to praise, so if a patient is doing well, tell him.

Keys to successful dental health education
- Make it relevant to the individual, their lifestyle, and problems.[1]
- Keep the message simple. Too much information may be counter-productive.
- Repeat the message.
- Use positive reinforcement.

Effectiveness of dental health education
A systematic review[2] found that educational programs
- Effectively enhance knowledge
- Have a positive but temporary effect on plaque levels
- Have no discernible effect on caries experience.

Where to go for help or information
Advice on preparing a talk on dental health education, setting up a preventive unit, or even a health program can be obtained from:
- Local health education (or promotion) service or group. These groups will be happy to provide leaflets, educational packs, slides, videos, or just advice.
- Centers for Disease Control and Prevention (CDC). Contact information: CDC, National Center for Chronic Disease Prevention and Health Promotion, 4770 Buford Highway NE, Mail Stop F-10, Atlanta, GA 30341-3717; Tel: (770) 488-6054; E-mail: ccdinfo@cdc.gov; Web: http://www.cdc.gov/oralhealth.
- State dental director. You can get contact information for your state dental director through the Association of State and Territorial Dental Directors, Tel: (252) 637-6333; Web: http://www.astdd.org.
- The nearest postgraduate dental public health education program. You can find the location of these programs through the American Association of Public Health Dentistry, Tel: (217) 391-0218; Web: http://www.aaphd.org.

1 A. S. Blinkhorn *BDJ* 1998 **184** 58.
2 E. J. Kay 1996 *Community Dent Oral Epidemiol* **24** 231.

Delivery of dental care

Private dental practice

Dental care in the United States has overwhelmingly been delivered through either solo or group private practices. While this approach offers flexibility to both patients and providers, private practice cannot meet the dental demands of all patients.

Franchised practices

The concept of franchises is common in the United States, but it has not enjoyed great success in the field of dentistry.

Hospital dentistry

Only a small proportion of dental care is provided in a hospital setting, but it plays an important role for some patients. Dental care provided in hospitals is for those patients who require general anesthesia or other resources of a hospital, such as very young children with rampant caries or patients who suffer from serious systemic illness.

Public programs

Major federal dental services include the United States Public Health Service (USPHS); the dental corps of the Air Force, Army, and Navy (which also serves the Marine Corps); and the Department of Veterans Affairs (VA). The USPHS provides clinical care primarily to residents of federal prisons, the Coast Guard, merchant seamen, American Indians, and Alaska Natives; it also provides grants through the Community and Migrant Health program. Another program to attract dentists to under-served areas is the National Health Service Corps.

State, county, and city dental care programs vary widely and have mostly been aimed at delivering care for people eligible to receive public assistance, and prevention programs for school children.

Access to dental care

Most of the U.S. population has routine access to dental care, but there is a significant subset of the population who has difficulties accessing care. The primary reasons for access problems are limited financial, physical, and personnel resources.

The scope of the access problem can be assessed by the inadequacy of the existing, largely government-subsidized safety net system. In 2002, health centers subsidized by this system were able to provide dental care to 1.6 million people, while nearly 45 million people were enrolled in Medicaid and the State Children's Health Insurance Program.

An inadequate supply of dentists has intermittently been considered a potential cause of the access problem. Some factors favor a shortage of dentists:

- Increased demand due to good economic times
- Increased demand due to high expectation for oral health
- Decrease in edentulism
- Growing utilization
- Aging of the baby boomers, who have high carious lesion experience
- Decline in the dentist/population ratio

Other factors favor a *surplus of dentists*:

- Falling disease levels
- Smaller birth cohorts since the early 1960s with low carious lesion experience
- Slower economic times
- Expanded roles for auxiliary personnel

In fact, access problems may be limited to certain populations because of the following:

- Availability and accessibility of dental services. Research shows that a greater proportion of the public visits the dentist regularly where the dentist-to-population ratio is high. This ratio tends to follow a geo-demographic pattern.
- Social class, which affects both the incidence of dental disease and the uptake of dental care. Interestingly, the differences in caries experience between the social classes are much lower in fluoridated regions.

Strategies to solve the access problem

- Expanding and strengthening the safety net system
- Providing adequate reimbursement for both safety net providers and private practitioners
- Optimizing the role of allied dental personnel
- Having adequate arrangements for special populations such as the elderly and disabled
- Developing cultural competency
- Commitment of the profession to solving the access problem

Dentistry for the disabled

A disabled person is someone with a physical or mental impairment that has a substantial and long-term adverse effect on his or her ability to carry out normal day-to-day activities. Over 50 million Americans have one or more physical or mental disabilities.

Intellectual impairment (mental handicap, learning difficulty) is classified as mild (IQ 50–70) or severe (IQ <50). Many cases lack well-defined etiology, but there are some subgroups where the/Δ cause is known:
- Down syndrome; Fragile–X syndrome
- Cerebral palsy, birth anoxia
- Meningitis, rubella
- Autism, microcephaly

Physical impairment Most common is cerebral palsy, which is the motor manifestation of cerebral damage. Many patients with cerebral palsy have normal IQs, but ↑ muscle tone and hyperactive reflexes can make Rx difficult. Many individuals can be treated by the general or pediatric dentist, provided there is wheelchair access.

Medical impairment 1% of children have either heart disease, bleeding disorders, diabetes, or kidney disease.

Sensory impairment i.e., blindness, deafness.

Many individuals have more than one type of impairment.

The above groups are general disabilities. We also need to consider those who are orally disabled, i.e., have a gross oral problem or deficit that necessitates special dental Rx (e.g., cleft lip and/or palate).

Americans with Disabilities Act (ADA) of 1990 prohibits disability-based discrimination in the areas of employment, public services provided by state and local governments, public services operated by private entities, transportation, and telecommunications. The Act requires the following:
- Employers must not discriminate against a qualified individual with a disability.
- Service providers (including dentists) must remove "physical barriers" that are "readily achievable" following the ADA Standards for Accessible Design. Requirements for facilities built before 1993 are less strict than for those built after early 1993. The requirements apply whether you own, operate, lease, or lease to a business that serves the public.

Problems

It is difficult to generalize, but usually mental disability provides the biggest challenge. Difficulties ↑ in patients with more than one impairment.
- Delivery of care. This has three aspects: **1** demand, due to low priority placed on dental health; **2** lack of provision made to provide the necessary care; **3** practical difficulties in carrying out dental work.
- In general, disabled patients have plaque control and ∴↑ periodontal problems.
- Although caries incidence is not significantly ↑ compared to the normal population, the amount of untreated caries is.

- Long-term sugared medications
- Prevalence of hepatitis in institutionalized patients
- Dentures may be impractical ∴ extractions are not a realistic solution to the problems of providing dental Rx.
- Consent (see p. 649).

Management

Again, it is difficult to generalize. Patients with less severe disabilities can be treated by general or pediatric dentist along with other members of the family. Those with severe medical and/or mental impairments may be better managed by a specialist who will have greater access to facilities.

Rx planning An initial plan should be formulated ignoring the disability. This can then be discussed with the patient, parent, or caregiver and modified for the individual. It is advisable to start with OHI and prevention then reassess Rx requirements in light of the response. For those patients for whom a satisfactory standard of OH is not possible, restorative Rx should aim to ↓ plaque accumulation.

OHI Those patients who can brush their own teeth should be encouraged to do so. Modification of toothbrush handles or purchase of an electric one may be helpful. When patients are unable to brush their teeth, instruction should be given to their caregiver. The best method is to stand behind the patient and cradle the head with one arm, leaving the other free to brush. If possible, this should be supplemented with regular professional cleaning. Chemical control of plaque with chlorhexidine may be helpful.

Restorative care Under some circumstances, there may be no alternative to restraint—ideally, get the patient's caregiver to help. A mouth prop may be needed. It may be easier to use intraligamentary LA technique. Sedation may help reduce the spontaneous movements of cerebral palsy. In some cases there is no alternative but to carry out examination and Rx under GA. In addition, for those patients who can tolerate outpatient Rx, but only a little at a time, it may be kinder to clear a backlog under GA, thus allowing concentration on prevention subsequently. However, this approach requires special facilities and no medical C/I.

Down syndrome See p. 681.

Resources can be found at the Special Care Dentistry Association (http://www.scdonline.org), the National Foundation of Dentistry for the Handicapped (http://www.nfdh.org), the ADA Information Line (1-800-514-0301) and Web site (http://www.usdoj.gov/crt/ada/adahom1.htm), and through the National Institute of Dental and Craniofacial Research (Developmental Disabilities and Oral Health, http://www.nidcr.nih.gov/HealthInformation/DiseasesAndCondtions/DevelopmentalDisabilitiesAndOralHealth/default.htm).

Professions complementary to dentistry (PCD)

Dental auxiliary personnel (or professions complementary to dentistry) are becoming increasingly important as the skill mix of the dental team changes. Delegation of repetitive duties to trained PCDs allows the dentist to concentrate on Rx planning and management.

The World Health Organization (WHO) classifies dental auxiliary personnel as follows:
- Non-operating auxiliaries: Type I, dental technician; Type II, dental nurse; Type III, dental preventive worker.
- Operating auxiliaries: Type IV, hygienist; Type V, dental therapist.

Hygienists' functions in the United States vary because each state has its own regulations regarding the dental hygienists' responsibilities. Nevertheless, their most fundamental general duties can be said to concern the preventive aspects of dental care:
- Scaling and polishing
- Application of topical fluoride and other preventive agents
- OHI and preventive advice, e.g., diet

Expanded duties have been developed in some states, with a few states even permitting some independent practice of dental hygiene (Colorado, New Mexico, California).

Additional information about the practice of dental hygiene may be obtained through the American Dental Hygienist's Association (Web site: http://www.adha.org/; tel: (312) 440-8900).

Dental assistants are the most numerous of all dental personnel groups in the United States. Like hygienists, their roles also vary by state, due to dramatic differences in regulations. More information can be obtained through the American Dental Assistants Association (Web site: http://www.dentalassistant.org/; tel: (312) 541-1550).

Expanded-function dental auxiliaries have been a source of long-standing controversy in the United States, with the American Dental Association most recently discouraging any further expansion of the roles of dental auxiliaries. Again, the duties that can be performed vary by state. Some examples include the following:
- Applying topical fluorides
- Applying desensitizing agents
- Applying pit and fissure sealants
- Placing, carving, and polishing amalgam restorations
- Placing and finishing composite restorations
- Placing and removing matrix bands
- Placing and removing rubber dams
- Monitoring nitrous oxide use
- Taking impressions
- Exposing and developing radiographs
- Removing sutures
- Removing and replacing ligature wires on orthodontic appliances

Dental laboratory technicians fabricate crowns, bridges, dentures, and orthodontic and other appliances upon the prescription of a dentist. Most technicians today are employed by independent commercial laboratories. Recently, there have been significant drops in enrollments in technician training programs, raising the concern that there will be a shortage.

Denturists are dental laboratory technicians that treat the public directly for the fabrication of dentures. Denturists are now legally recognized in most Canadian provinces and a few states (Arizona, Idaho, Washington, Maine, Montana, and Oregon).

Orthodontic auxiliaries This type of auxiliary is widely employed in many countries, including the United States and Scandinavia. Their work includes placement of fixed appliances, changing archwires, and taking impressions.

The future—a dental team

With increasing demand for dental Rx and restraints on health care costs, there are clear advantages to delegating more routine tasks to dental auxiliaries. Nevertheless, as previously mentioned, this subject has been a source of long-standing controversy in the United States. Studies have shown that both hygienists and dental assistants are capable of performing a broad spectrum of expanded duties at a high level of quality when they are adequately trained.[1] However, in addition to dentists' worries about the economic impact of expanded-function dental auxiliaries on the dental profession, there has been some concern that the requirements for expanded functions in many states are not rigorous or selective enough.[2]

With the introduction of more auxiliaries, the role of the dentist will inevitably change, to become more centered on diagnosis and Rx planning, and more complex Rx, with team leadership skills becoming increasingly important.

1 J. Abramowitz and L. E. Berg 1973 *J Am Dent Assoc* **87** 623; J. Bader 1983 *J Am Dent Assoc* **106** 338; E. M. Boyer 1996 *J Dent Hyg* **70** 35; P. E. Hammons 1971 *J Am Dent Assoc* **122** 155.
2 E. M. Boyer 1996 *J Dent Hyg* **70** 35.

Lies, damn lies, and statistics

Sugar

- The average consumption of all sugars in the United States was 146.1 pounds in 2002,[1] one of the highest levels in the world.
- In 2002, the average soft drink consumption in the United States was 54.2 gallons per person.[2]

Fluoride

- In 2000 the CDC estimated that 66% of people using community water systems (approximately 162 million people) had access to fluoridated water.
- Water fluoridation ↓ caries experience by about 50%.
- Water and other beverages provide 75% of flouride intake for most people, whether or not the drinking water is fluoridated. For example, Gatorade was found to contain 0.85 ppm.[3]

Caries

- A reduction of 10–60% in caries experience in developed countries has been widely reported. This is thought to be due to a variety of factors, including fluoride toothpaste, increased public awareness, changes in infant feeding practices, ↓ sugar consumption, and antibiotics in the food chain.
- In addition, there has been a change in the pattern of carious attack, with a greater ↓ in smooth surface than fissure caries (perhaps reflecting the influence of fluoride).
- Small occlusal lesions appear to be becoming the predominant type of lesion.[3]
- **BUT** there is uneven distribution of caries in the United States: 60% of all affected teeth are found in about 20% of the children.[4] The higher socioeconomic groups have experienced the sharpest decline in caries experience.[5]

Adult dental health in persons age 20+[6]

	1988–94	1999–2002
% of adults edentulous	11%	7.7%
Average number of teeth	23	24
Average condition of teeth		
• Missing	• 4.7 teeth	• 3.58 teeth
• Decayed	• 0.8 teeth	• 0.7 teeth
• Filled	• 8.2 teeth	• 7.3 teeth

1 U.S. Dept of Agriculture Economic Research Service. Per Capita Consumption of Sugars in the United States 1972–2002.

2 Beverage Marketing Corporation. 2003. Soft Drink Top 10 Review.

3 D. T. Y. Pang 1992 *J Dent Res* **71** 382.

4 U.S. Department of Health and Human Services National Center for Health Statistics. Third National Health and Nutrition Examination Survey 1988–1994.

5 R. C. Graves 1986 *J Public Health Dent.* **46** 23.

6 E. D. Beltran-Aguilar *et al* 2005 MMRW **54** 1.

Child dental health[6]

- The prevalence of dental caries in primary teeth among children aged 2–11 years was essentially unchanged from 1988–1994 (40%) to 1999–2002 (41%). The prevalences of untreated tooth decay in primary teeth in this group were 23% and 21%, respectively.
- Reductions in levels of dental caries among children in the US were substantially greater in the permanent dentition than those found in primary dentition. The 1988–94 prevalence of dental caries in the permanent teeth among children and adolescents aged 6–19 years was 49%, and in 1999–2002, it was 42%. The prevalences of untreated tooth decay in this group were 15% and 14%, respectively.
- Sealant prevalences in were 20% in 1988–1994 and 32% in 1999–2002.

Indices

DMFT   decayed, missing, and filled permanent teeth.
dmft   decayed, missing, and filled deciduous teeth.
deft   decayed, exfoliated, and filled deciduous teeth.
dft   decayed and filled deciduous teeth.
DMFS   decayed, missing, and filled surfaces in permanent teeth.

Periodontal disease

- Over 70% of adults in all parts of the world have some degree of gingivitis or periodontitis.[7]
- Only a small proportion of people (5–15%) exhibited severe periodontitis, where tooth loss occurs or is threatened.[8]

Oral Cancer

- In 2004 there were approximately 28,300 new oral cancer cases in the United States and 7,200 deaths from oral cancer.[9]
- Oral cancer is twice as prevalent in males than in females.
- Survival rates are far better for whites than for African Americans, even when controlling for stage of metastatic spread.[10]

6 E. D. Beltran-Aguilar 2005 *MMWR Morb Mortal Wkly Rep* **54** 1.
7 D. E. Barmes 1977 *J Clin Periodontol.* **4** 80.
8 B. A. Burt and S. A. Eklund 2005 *Dentistry, Dental Practice, and the Community*, Elsievier Saunders.
9 E. Silverberg and J. A. Lubera 1988 *Cancer J Clin* **38** 5.
10 U.S. Public Health Service National Cancer Institute. SEER Program; A. Burt and S. A. Eklund 2005 *Dentistry, Dental Practice, and the Community*, Elsievier Saunders.

Resources in Spanish for dentists

After English, Spanish is by far the most commonly spoken language in the United States. In 2000, the Census Bureau estimated that there were 262,375,152 people in the U.S. (300 million in 2006) 28,101,052 of these people spoke Spanish at home, of whom 2,801,448 did not know how to speak English at all. Most of these people lived in the South and the West of the country. As most practicing dentists in the United States are English-speaking, this can pose a barrier to dental care. Thus, a number of Spanish translations of patient education information have been produced by the American Dental Association (http://www.ada.org/public/espanol/index.asp), the Colgate-Palmolive Company (www.colgate-professional.com), Proctor & Gamble (www.dentalcare.com), and the National Oral Health Information Clearinghouse (http://www.nohic.nidcr.nih.gov/cgi-bin/ohpubgen_new). Additional information can be found through the Hispanic Dental Association (website: http://www.hdassoc.org/; tel: (217)-793-0035).

There are books published for members of the dental team who want to expand their working knowledge of Spanish. Two such resources are *Spanish Terminology for the Dental Team*, published by Mosby, and *Spanish for Dental Professionals: A Step by Step Handbook*, published by the University of New Mexico Press.

Pediatric dentistry

Principal sources: J. R. Pinkham 2005 *Pediatric Dentistry: Infancy Through Adolescence* 4th ed., Elsevier Saunders. R. Andlaw 1996 *A Manual of Paedodontics*, Churchill Livingstone. J. O. Andreasen 1981 *Traumatic Injuries of the Teeth*, Munksgaard. J. O. Andreasen 1992 *Atlas of Replantation and Transplantation of Teeth*, Mediglobe. G. J. Roberts and P. Longhurst 1996 *Oral and Dental Trauma in Children and Adolescents*, OUP. R. R. Welbury 2001 *Paediatric Dentistry*, 2nd ed., OUP. M. E. J. Curzon 1999 *Handbook of Dental Trauma*, Wright. M. S. Duggal et al. 2002 *Restorative Techniques in Paediatric Dentistry*, Dunitz.

The child patient

▶ Treat the patient, not the tooth.

Principal aims of treatment
- Freedom from pain and infection
- A happy and cooperative patient
- Prevention
- Development and maintenance of healthy and attractive primary and permanent dentitions

Points to remember
- Praise good behavior (reinforcement, p. 60), discourage bad.
- Involve parents (they determine whether the child will return).
- Do not offer choice where there is none. Avoid rhetorical questions (Would you like to get into my chair?).
- Children have short attention spans (with age).
- Children have decreased sensory acuity (they may confuse pressure with pain, sensitivity tests are less reliable).
- Children have decreased manual dexterity, therefore they need help with tooth brushing <7 years.
- Formulate a comprehensive treatment plan, which should address both operative and preventive care, at an early stage.
- Start with easy procedures (e.g., OHI) and progress, at the child's pace, to more complicated treatment.
- Set attainable targets for each visit and attain them.

The first visit
- Children should first visit a dentist as soon as they have teeth (i.e., about 6 months of age). For young children, watching other members of the family receive treatment prior to their turn may be preferable.
- Let parent accompany child: check medical history and reason for dental visit.
- Talk to the child: communication is the key to success!
- Show patient the chair, mirror, and light, and explain purpose (tell, show, do, p. 60).
- Count the patient's teeth.
- If there is good progress, polish a few teeth, but don't tire child by attempting too much.
- Show parent the child's teeth and what has been done that visit.
- If child is in pain, the source of this needs to be determined and dealt with as quickly as possible.
- Younger children can be more successfully examined if parent sits with the child facing dentist and then lowers child back onto his or her arm or the dentist's lap (knee-to-knee technique).

Treatment planning for children

Diagnosis Dental caries is often a rapidly progressing condition in children. It is essential to accurately diagnosis disease prior to development of a treatment plan. This is achieved by taking a history, doing an examination, and, where possible, taking bitewing radiographs.

Bitewings are essential for an accurate diagnosis unless all surfaces of the primary molars can be visualized (i.e., the dentition is spaced).

Treatment plan The ultimate aim in dentistry for children is for the child to reach adulthood with good dental status and a positive attitude toward dental health and dental care. The final treatment plan will take into account the following considerations:

- Behavior management (p. 60)
- Prevention (Chapter 2)
- Restorative treatment (p. 80)
- Developing occlusion

Remember to consider the developing occlusion:

- Long-term prognosis for first permanent molars (p. 140)
- Palpate for maxillary permanent canines at age 9–10 years (p. 144)
- Be aware of disturbances in eruption sequence (p. 65) and asymmetry
- Early referral to specialist for skeletal discrepancies and for any abnormal findings

The treatment plan is drawn up visit by visit. Each visit has both a preventive and operative component (delivering one preventive message per visit).

Since it is considered easier to administer LA for maxillary teeth, these teeth are usually treated before mandibular teeth.

Restorative care (i.e., repair) without prevention is of limited value.

Dental caries is treated by "preventive" measures; restoration purely repairs the damage caused by the carious process.

Children with caries in primary molars treated by prevention alone are likely to experience toothache or infection, especially if the child is young when the caries is first diagnosed. A combination of prevention and restoration and extraction is indicated for most children with caries in the primary dentition.

Other considerations

Pain or evidence of infection may alter the order of the treatment plan.

Temporization of open cavities at the start of treatment

- gives a good introduction to dentistry;
- helps to minimize the risk of pain before treatment is completed;
- improves comfort (e.g., during brushing and eating);
- reduces salivary *Streptococcus mutans* count;
- produces a preliminary coronal seal, enhancing the chances of pulpal recovery and survival; and
- may provide slow release of fluoride in the short term if a GI cement is used.

Delivery of care

Once the treatment plan has been decided upon, discuss appropriate delivery of care with the parent and child:

- Council parent and patient about the treatment options.
- LA/sedation/GA—consider and discuss risks vs. benefits of each (p. 61).
- Plan operative care at a pace appropriate to the child's ability to cope.
- Be prepared to reconsider method of delivery of care (e.g., sedation or GA) if patient proves unable to accept treatment using original delivery strategy.

Look out for any signs of underlying medical or social problems that may modify the treatment plan:

- Small stature
- Failure to thrive
- Systemic disease
- Non-accidental injury (NAI; p. 100).

The anxious child

Techniques for behavior management

Most of these are fancy terms to describe techniques that come with experience of treating children over a period of time. However, for the student they may prove useful for answering essay questions as well as for handling their first few child patients.

General principles
- Show interest in the child as a person.
- Touch > facial expression > tone of the voice > what is said.
- Don't deny the patient's fear.
- Explain—why, how, when.
- Reward good behavior, discourage bad.
- Get the child involved in treatment, e.g., holding saliva ejector.
- Giving the child some control over the situation will also help them to relax, e.g., raising their hand if they want you to stop for any reason.

Tell, show, do This is self-explanatory, but use language the child will understand.

Desensitization Used for children with preexisting fears or phobias, this involves helping the patient to relax in the dental environment, then constructing a hierarchy of fearful stimuli for that patient. These are introduced to the child gradually, with progression to the next stimulus only when the child is able to cope with the previous situation.

Modeling is useful for children with little previous dental experience who are apprehensive. Encourage the child to watch other children of similar age or siblings receiving dental treatment happily.

Behavior shaping The aim of this is to guide and modify the child's responses, selectively reinforcing appropriate behavior, while discouraging/ignoring inappropriate behavior.

Reinforcement is the strengthening of patterns of behavior, usually by rewarding good behavior with approval and praise. If a child protests and is uncooperative during treatment, do not immediately abandon the session and return them to the consolation of their parent, as this could inadvertently reinforce the undesirable behavior. It is better to try and ensure that some phase of the treatment is completed, e.g., placing a dressing.

Should parent accompany child into the operatory? This is essential on first visit, thereafter it depends on child's age. If in doubt, ask for the child's preference. However, if the parent is dental phobic, their anxiety in the dental environment may adversely affect child, so in these cases it is probably wiser to have the parent remain in the waiting room. Some children will play up to an overprotective parent to gain sympathy or rewards, and may prove more cooperative by themselves. However, many parents wish to be involved in and informed about their child's treatment. Ideally parents should be motivated positively and instructed implicitly to act in the role of the "silent helper". Any device used to restrain the child such as Papoose boards requires prior parental consent.

Sedation

Indicated for the genuinely anxious child who wishes to cooperate with treatment.

Oral Drugs such as midazolam and chloral hydrate can be used, although specialized knowledge and skills are required.

Intramuscular Rarely used in children.

Intravenous Rarely used in children.

Per rectum Popular in some Scandinavian countries.

Inhalation A nitrous oxide/oxygen mixture is used to produce relative analgesia (RA) and is the most popular technique for use with children. It is effective for reducing anxiety and increasing tolerance of invasive procedures in children who wish to cooperate but are too anxious to do so without help. For technique, see p. 578. It is a good idea not to carry out any treatment during the visit when the child is introduced to "happy air." Let the child position the nosepiece him- or herself.

Hypnosis

Hypnosis produces a state of altered consciousness and relaxation, though it cannot be used to make subjects do anything they do not wish to do. Although many good books[1] and articles are available on the subject, attendance of a course is necessary to gain experience with susceptible subjects, so the operator has confidence in their ability. It can be described as either a way of helping the child to relax or as a special kind of sleep.

General anesthesia

GA allows dental rehabilitation and/or dental extractions to be achieved at one visit. It should only be used for dental treatment when absolutely necessary (i.e., when other methods of management, e.g., LA or sedation, are deemed unsuitable). Alternative strategies and the risks of GA must be discussed to enable parents to make an informed decision. Legally, GA should be provided in a hospital setting.

Risks

The risk of unexpected death of a healthy person
- under GA has been estimated to be about 3 in 1 million;
- under sedation has been estimated to be about 1 in 2 million.

Other behavior problems and their management

- The questioner attempts to delay treatment by a barrage of questions. Firm but gentle handling is needed. Tell the patient that you understand their anxieties and that you will explain as you go along.
- The temper tantrum: try to establish communication. Praise good and discourage bad behavior. Set an easily achievable goal, e.g., brushing teeth, and make sure it is achieved—comment on the positive outcome, not what was not achieved.

1 J. Hartland 1982 *Medical and Dental Hypnosis*, Baillière Tindall.

The child with toothache

When faced with a child with toothache the dentist should use clinical judgment to try and determine the pulpal state of the affected tooth or teeth, as this will determine the treatment required. To that end, the following information should be obtained:

History Take a pain history (see p. 228) from the child and parent. Beware of variations in accuracy; anxious children may deny being in pain when faced with the prospect of undergoing dental treatment, whereas parents who feel guilty for delaying seeking dental care may exaggerate pain. Remember some pathology is painless, e.g., chronic periradicular periodontitis.

Examination Swelling, temperature, lymphadenopathy. Intraorally look for caries, abscesses, chronic buccal sinuses, mobile teeth (due to exfoliation or apical infection) and erupting teeth.

Percussion Can be unreliable in children. Care is needed to establish a consistent response.

Sensitivity testing Again, this is unreliable in primary teeth, but for permanent teeth a cotton roll, ethyl chloride, and considerable ingenuity may provide some useful information. In older children electric pulp testing may be helpful.

Radiographs Bitewing radiographs are most useful because they not only are less uncomfortable for small mouths than periapicals but also show the bifurcation area where most primary molar abscesses begin.

Remember, the only 100% accurate method is histological!

Diagnosis

Sharp, short pain on hot/cold/sweet stimuli = reversible pulpitis.

Longer-lasting pain on hot/cold/sweet stimuli = irreversible pulpitis.

Spontaneous pain with no initiating factor (no mobility, not tender to percussion [TTP]) = irreversible pulpitis.

Pain on biting and pressure and/or swelling and tenderness of adjacent tissues, mobility = acute periradicular periodontitis.

With an irritable child keep examination and operative intervention to a minimum, doing only what is necessary to alleviate pain and win the child's trust.

If extractions under GA in the hospital setting are required, consider carefully the long-term prognosis of remaining teeth to try and avoid a second trip to the operating room in the near future.

Other common potential causes of toothache:
- Dentoalveolar trauma (p. 98)
- Mucosal ulceration (p. 434)
- Teething (p. 65)

Diagnosis	Emergency management	Definitive management
Reversible pulpitis	LA Excavate soft caries: If exposed and vital—dress formocresol Restore temporarily with a zinc oxide/eugenol cement	Pulpotomy or extraction
Irreversible pulpitis	LA Excavate soft caries: If exposed and vital—dress formocresol Restore temporarily with a zinc oxide-eugenol cement	Pulpotomy/pulpectomy or extraction
Acute periodontitis	LA (may not be necessary if loss of vitality is certain) Excavate soft caries until pulp chamber accessed—dress pulp chamber with formocresol on cotton pellet Seal with temporary dressing	
Acute periodontitis with facial swelling If • No or mild pyrexia (<38 °C) • Localized acute erythematous tender soft tissue swelling • No significant involvement of "danger areas" (see below) • Not otherwise systemically unwell	Antibiotics and analgesics Ensure adequate fluid intake Establish drainage via tooth (and dress) if possible Review every 24 h to ensure resolution	Extraction of tooth (or pulpectomy in selected cases) once acute phase has resolved
If: • Significant pyrexia >38 °C • Poorly localized, spreading infection • Systemically unwell: dehydration, lethargy, nausea, and vomiting • Swelling involving a danger area, i.e., floor of mouth, submandibular/neck, infraorbital region	Aggressive antibiotic treatment (e.g., amoxicillin and metronidazole) Immediate referral to specialist center	Extraction of tooth and/or intra-/extraoral drainage

Abnormalities of tooth eruption and exfoliation

Natal teeth are usually members of the primary dentition, not supernumerary teeth, and so should be retained if possible. They most frequently affect the mandibular incisor region and, because of limited root development at that age, are mobile. If in danger of being inhaled or causing problems with breastfeeding, they can be removed under LA.

Teething As eruption of the primary dentition coincides with a reduction in circulating maternal antibodies, teething is often blamed for systemic symptoms. However, local discomfort, and so disturbed sleep, may accompany the actual process of eruption. A number of proprietary "teething" preparations are available, which usually contain a combination of an analgesic, an antiseptic, and anti-inflammatory agents for topical use. Having something hard to chew may help, e.g., teething ring.

Eruption cyst is caused by an accumulation of fluid or blood in the follicular space overlying an erupting tooth. The presence of blood gives a bluish hue. Most rupture spontaneously, allowing eruption to proceed. Rarely, it may be necessary to marsupialize the cyst.

Failure of/delayed eruption It must be remembered that there is a wide range of individual variation in eruption times. Developmental age is of more importance in assessing delayed eruption than chronological age.

▶ Disruption of normal eruption sequence and asymmetry in eruption times of contralateral teeth >6 months warrants further investigation.

General causes
Hereditary gingival fibromatosis, Down syndrome, Gardner syndrome, hypothyroidism, cleidocranial dysostosis, rickets.

Local causes
• Congenital absence. This is the most likely cause for failure of appearance of maxillary lateral incisor (p. 66).
• Crowding. Treatment: extractions.
• Retention of primary tooth. Treatment: extraction of primary tooth.
• Supernumerary tooth. This is the most likely reason for failure of eruption of maxillary permanent central incisor (p. 66).
• Dilaceration (p. 68)
• Dentigerous cyst
• Trauma to primary tooth leading to apical displacement of permanent incisor
• Abnormal position of crypt. Treatment: extraction or orthodontic alignment. See options for palatally displaced maxillary permanent canine (p. 144).
• Primary failure of eruption usually affects molar teeth. The etiology is not understood. Although bone resorption proceeds above the unerupted tooth, they appear to lack any eruptive potential. Treatment: keep under observation, but ultimately extraction may be necessary.

Infraoccluded (ankylosed) primary molars occur where the primary molar has failed to maintain its position relevant to the adjacent teeth in the developing dentition and is below the occlusal level of adjacent teeth. This is caused by preponderance of repair in the normal resorptive/repair cycle of exfoliation. This is usually self-correcting (if the permanent successor is present and not ectopic) and the affected tooth is exfoliated at the normal time.[1] However, where the premolar is missing or where the infraoccluded molar appears in danger of disappearing below the gingival level, extraction may be indicated.

Ectopic eruption of the upper first permanent molars resulting in impaction of the tooth against the second primary molar occurs in 2–5% of children. It is an indication of crowding. In younger patients (<8 years) it may prove self-correcting ("jump"). If still present after 4–6 months ("hold") or in older children, insertion of an orthodontic separator may allow the first permanent molar to erupt normally. More severe impactions should be kept under observation. If the second primary molar becomes abscessed or the first permanent molar is in danger of becoming carious, then the primary tooth should be extracted. The resulting space loss can be dealt with as part of the overall orthodontic treatment plan later.

Premature exfoliation The most common reason for early tooth loss is extraction for caries. Traumatic avulsion is less common. More rarely, systemic disease such as leukemia, congenital or cyclic neutropenia, diabetes, hypophosphatasia, Langerhans cell histiocytosis, Papillon-Lefevre syndrome, Chediak-Higashi syndrome, or Down syndrome may result in an abnormal periodontal attachment and thus premature tooth loss (p. 192). Alveolar bone loss in a young child is a serious finding and warrants referral.

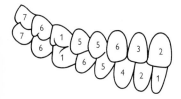

Normal sequence of eruption (permanent dentition).

1 J. Kurol 1985 *Am J Orthod* **87** 46.

Abnormalities of tooth number

Anodontia

Complete absence of all teeth. Rare. Partial anodontia is a misnomer.

Hypodontia

Absence of less than six teeth.

Oligodontia

Absence of six or more teeth.

Prevalence

Primary dentition 0.1–0.9%, permanent dentition 3.5–6.5%.[1] In Caucasians the most commonly affected teeth are third molars (25–35%), maxillary lateral incisor (2%), and maxillary and mandibular second premolars (3%). Affects F>M and is often associated with smaller than average tooth size in the remainder of dentition. Peg-shaped maxillary lateral incisor often occurs in conjunction with absence of contralateral maxillary lateral incisor **NB** canine migrates down guided by the distal aspect of maxillary lateral incisor. When maxillary lateral incisor is absent, peg shaped, or small rooted, it is important to monitor the upper canine for signs of ectopic eruption.

Etiology

Often familial—polygenic inheritance. Also associated with ectodermal dysplasia and Down syndrome.

Treatment

Primary dentition—none. Permanent dentition—depends on crowding and maloccusion.
Third molar—none.
Maxillary lateral incisor—see p. 114.
Mandibular second premolar—late development of mandibular second premolar is not unknown. If patient crowded, extraction of mandibular second primary molar, either at around 8 yrs for spontaneous space closure or later if space is to be closed as a part of orthodontic treatment. If lower arch well-aligned or spaced, consider preservation of mandibular second primary molar, and bridgework later.

Hyperdontia

Better known as supernumerary teeth.

Prevalence

Primary dentition 0.8%, permanent dentition 2%.[1] Occurs most frequently in premaxillary region. Affects M>F. Associated with cleidocranial dysostosis and cleft lip/palate (CLP). In about 50% cases supernumerary in primary dentition followed by supernumerary in permanent dentition, so inform parents.

Etiology

Theories include offshoot of dental lamina, third dentition.

1 A. H. Brooks 1974 *J Int Assoc Dent Child* **5** 32.

Classification by either		
Shape	or	**Position**
Conical (peg-shaped)		Mesiodens
Tuberculate (barrel-shaped)		Distomolar
Supplemental		Paramolar
Odontome		

Effects on dentition and treatment

- No effect. If unerupted, keep watching; if erupts, extract.
- Crowding. Treatment: extract; if supplemental, extract tooth with most displaced apex.
- Displacement. Can cause rotation and/or displacement. Treatment: extraction of supernumerary tooth and fixed appliance, but tendency to relapse.
- Failure of eruption. Most likely cause of maxillary incisor to fail to erupt. Treatment: extract supernumerary tooth and ensure sufficient space for unerupted tooth to erupt. May require extraction of primary teeth and/or permanent teeth and appliances. Then *wait*. Average time to eruption in these cases is 18 months.[1] If after 2 years unerupted tooth fails to erupt despite sufficient space may require conservative exposure and orthodontic traction.

1 D. DiBiase 1971 *Dent Pract* **22** 95.

Abnormalities of tooth structure

Disturbances in structure of enamel

Enamel usually develops in two phases, first as an organic matrix and second, mineralization. Disruption of enamel formation can manifest as the following conditions.

Hypoplasia

Caused by disturbance in matrix formation and characterized by pitted, grooved, or thinned enamel.

Hypomineralization

Hypocalcification is a disturbance of calcification. Affected enamel appears white and opaque, but post-eruptively may become discolored. Affected enamel may be weak and prone to breakdown. Most disturbances of enamel formation will produce both hypoplasia and hypomineralization, but clinically one type usually predominates.

Etiological factors (not an exhaustive list)

Localized causes Infection, trauma, irradiation, idiopathic (see enamel opacities, p. 72).

Generalized causes
1 Environmental (chronological hypoplasia)
    (a) Prenatal, e.g., rubella, syphilis
    (b) Neonatal, e.g., prolonged labor, premature birth
    (c) Postnatal, e.g., measles, congenital heart disease, fluoride, nutritional
2 Hereditary
    (a) Affecting teeth only—amelogenesis imperfecta
    (b) Accompanied by systemic disorder, e.g., Down syndrome

Chronological hypoplasia

So called because the hypoplastic enamel occurs in a distribution related to the extent of tooth formation at the time of the insult. Characteristically, because of its later formation, maxillary lateral incisor is affected nearer to its their incisal edge than maxillary central incisor or maxillary canine.

Fluorosis See p. 28.

Treatment of hypomineralization/hypoplasia

Treatment depends on extent and severity:

Posterior teeth Small areas of hypoplasia can be sealed or restored conventionally, but more severely affected teeth will require crowning. Stainless steel crowns (p. 86) can be used in children as a semipermanent measure.

Anterior teeth Small areas of hypoplasia can be restored using composites, but larger areas may require veneers (p. 258) or crowns. For treatment of fluorosis, see p. 72.

Molar incisor hypomineralization (MIH)

- Etiology unknown, but prevalence appears to have increased over the past two decades in developed countries.
- Primarily affects first permanent molars, but significant proportion of affected individuals have defects on permanent incisors.
- Affected first permanent molars have hypomineralized defects of enamel, which vary from discoloration to severe enamel dysplasia exhibiting post-

eruptive breakdown. Increased sensitivity, increased secondary caries. Defects may affect anything from one to all of the first permanent molars.

- Yellow/white opacities on buccal surface of affected incisors. Distribution is often asymmetrical. No clear chronological pattern. Incisors are less prone to enamel breakdown than the first permanent molars.

Treatment options include intracoronal restoration, stainless steel crowns, or extraction (p. 140). Opacities in anterior teeth can be improved by partial composite veneering.

Amelogenesis imperfecta

Many classifications exist, but generally these are classified by the type of enamel defect and/or the mode of inheritance.

Main types

Hypoplastic The enamel may be thin (smooth or rough) or pitted. Most commonly autosomal dominant inheritance.

Hypocalcified Enamel is dull, lusterless, opaque white, honey, or brown colored. Enamel may breakdown rapidly in severe cases. Increased sensitivity, increased calculus. May be autosomal dominant or recessive.

Hypomaturation Mottled or frosty-looking white, opacities, sometimes confined to incisal third of crown ("snow-capped teeth").

Usually both primary and permanent dentitions and all the teeth are affected. The different subgroups give rise to a wide variation in clinical presentation, ranging from discoloration to soft and/or deficient enamel. It is therefore difficult to make general recommendations, but it is wise to seek specialist advice for all but the mildest forms. Treatment in more severe cases requires stainless steel crowns, and composite resin can be used to maintain molars and permanent incisors, prior to more permanent restorations when the child is older.

Disturbances in the structure of dentine

Disturbances in dentinogenesis include dentinal dysplasias (types I and II), regional odontodysplasia, vitamin D–resistant rickets, and Ehlers–Danlos syndrome—all of which are rare. A more common defect is hereditary opalescent dentine, referred to as dentinogenesis imperfecta (II). Main types of dentinogenesis imperfecta:

I—associated with osteogenesis imperfecta

II—teeth only

Dentinogenesis imperfecta affects 1 in 8000 people. Both primary and secondary dentitions are involved, although later-formed teeth appear to be less affected. Affected teeth have an opalescent brown or blue hue, bulbous crowns, short roots, and narrow, flame-shaped pulps. The DEJ is abnormal, which results in the enamel flaking off, leading to rapid wear of the soft dentin. Treatment is along similar lines as for severe amelogenesis imperfecta.

▶ Early recognition and treatment of amelogenesis and dentinogenesis imperfecta are important to prevent rapid tooth wear.

Disturbances in the structure of cementum

Hypoplasia and aplasia of cementum are uncommon. The latter occurs in hypophosphatasia and results in premature exfoliation. Hypercementosis is relatively common and may occur in response to inflammation, mechanical stimulation, or Paget disease, or be idiopathic. Concrescence is the uniting of the roots of two teeth by cementum.

Abnormalities of tooth form[1]

Normal width maxillary central incisor = 8.5 mm, maxillary lateral incisor = 6.5 mm.

Double teeth
Gemination
This occurs by partial splitting of a tooth germ. *Fusion* occurs as a result of the fusion of two tooth germs. As fusion can take place between either two teeth of the normal series or, less commonly, with a supernumerary tooth, counting the number of teeth will not always give the correct etiology.

As the distinction is really only of academic interest, the term *double teeth* is preferred. Both primary and permanent teeth may be affected and a wide variation in presentation is seen. The prevalence in the permanent dentition is 0.1–0.2%.

Treatment for esthetics should be delayed to allow pulpal recession. If the tooth has separate pulp chambers and root canals, separation can be considered. If due to fusion with a supernumerary tooth, the supernumerary portion can be extracted. Where a single pulp chamber exists, either the tooth can be contoured to resemble two separate teeth or the bulk of the crown reduced.

Macrodontia/megadontia
Generalized macrodontia is rare, but is unilaterally associated with hemifacial hypertrophy. Isolated megadont teeth are seen in 1% of secondary dentitions.

Microdontia
Prevalence in primary dentition <0.5%. In permanent dentition overall prevalence is 2.5%. Of this figure 1–2% is accounted for by diminutive maxillary lateral incisor. Peg-shaped maxillary lateral incisors often have short roots and are thought to be a possible factor in the palatal displacement of maxillary canine (p. 143). Maxillary third molars are also commonly affected.

Dens in dente
This is really a marked palatal invagination, which gives the appearance of a tooth within a tooth. It usually affects the maxillary lateral incisor, but can also affect premolars. Where the invagination is in close proximity to the pulp, early pulp death may ensue. Fissure sealing of the invagination as soon as possible after eruption may prevent this, but is often too late. Conventional root canal treatment is difficult and extraction is usually required.

1 A. H. Brooks 1974 *J Int Assoc Dent Child* **5** 32.

Dilaceration

This term describes a tooth with a distorted crown or root, usually affecting the maxillary central incisor. Two types seen, depending on etiology.

Developmental[1]	Traumatic
Crown turned upward and labially	Crown turned palatally
Regular enamel and dentin	Disturbed enamel and dentin formation seen
Usually no other affected teeth	
Affects females > males	

The traumatically induced type is caused by intrusion of the primary incisor, resulting in displacement of the developing permanent incisor tooth germ. The effects depend on the developmental stage at the time of injury.

Treatment depends on severity and patient cooperation. If mild, it may be possible to expose the crown and align orthodontically provided the apex will not be positioned against the labial plate of bone at the end of the treatment, otherwise extraction is indicated.

Turner tooth

This term used to describe the effect of a disturbance of enamel and dentine formation by infection from an overlying primary tooth, therefore usually affecting premolar teeth. Treatment is the same as for hypoplasia, p. 68.

Taurodontism

This form is of academic interest only, but seems to appear on radiographs during examinations much more frequently than in clinical practice. The term means bull-like, and radiographically an elongation of the pulp chamber is seen. No treatment is required.

---

1 D. J. Stewart 1978 *BDJ* **145** 229.

Abnormalities of tooth color

Extrinsic staining By definition this is caused by extrinsic agents and can be removed by prophylaxis. Green, black, orange, or brown stains are seen and may be formed by chromogenic bacteria or be dietary in origin. Chlorhexidine mouthwash causes a brown stain by combining with dietary tannin. Where the staining is associated with poor OH, demineralization and roughening of the underlying enamel may make removal difficult. Treatment: a mixture of pumice powder and toothpaste or an abrasive prophylaxis paste together with a bristle brush should remove the stain. Give OHI to prevent recurrence.

Intrinsic staining This can be caused by the following:
- Changes in the structure or thickness of the dental hard tissues, e.g., enamel opacities
- Incorporation of pigments during tooth formation, e.g., tetracycline staining (blue/brown), porphyria (red)
- Diffusion of pigment into hard tissues after formation, e.g., pulp necrosis products (gray), root canal medicaments (gray)

Enamel opacities are localized areas of hypomineralized (or hypoplastic) enamel. Fluoride (p. 28) is only one of a considerable number of possible etiological agents.

Treatment

There are four possible approaches:

1 The acid pumice abrasion technique is used only for surface enamel defects. Hydrochloric acid technique (quicker), or phosphoric acid technique (slower but potentially safer). Preoperative photos are helpful to assess improvement

▶ Rubber dam, protective eyewear, bicarbonate of soda placed around teeth to be treated, and care are essential.

Hydrochloric acid technique A mixture of 18% hydrochloric acid and pumice is applied to the affected area using a wooden stick. The mixture is rubbed into the surface for 5 sec and then rinsed away. These two steps are repeated (max.10 times—removing <0.1 mm enamel) until the desired color change is achieved. The enamel is then polished and a fluoride solution applied.[1]

Phosphoric acid technique Etch with 30–50% orthophosphoric acid for 1 min, wash, then pumice slurry (pumice and water) on rubber prophy cup for 1 min (take care not to overheat tooth). Wash. Repeat etch and pumice stage twice more, washing between stages. Dry tooth and apply topical fluoride solution (avoid pigmented varnishes). May be repeated up to twice more, but leave at least 6 weeks before each repeat to check for improvement.

2 Bleaching, p. 282.
3 Veneers, p. 258.
4 Crowns, p. 250.

1 T. P. Croll 1986 *Quintessence Int* **17** 81.

Anatomy of primary teeth (and relevance to cavity design)

Primary teeth differ in several respects from permanent teeth, affecting both the sequelae of dental disease and its management.

Thinner enamel (1) Enamel in primary teeth is approximately 1 mm thick, which is 1/2 that of permanent teeth.

Larger pulp horns (2) The pulp chamber in primary teeth is proportionately larger, with more accentuated pulp mesiobuccal, distobuccal, and palatal. Mandibular first and second primary molars—four pulp horns mesiobuccal, mesiolingual, distobuccal, and distolingual. These features mean that caries will affect the pulp sooner and there is a greater likelihood of pulp exposure during cavity preparation. Aim for 0.5–1.0 mm penetration of dentin only.

Pulpal outline (3) follows the dentinoenamel junction more closely in primary teeth, therefore the cavity floor should follow the external contour of the tooth to avoid exposure.

Narrower occlusal table Greater convergence of the buccal and lingual walls results in a proportionately narrower occlusal table. This is more pronounced in the first primary molar than second primary molar. Therefore, overextension of an occlusal cavity or lock can lead to weakening of the cusps.

Broad contact points (4) make detection of interproximal caries more difficult, and means that in primary molars divergence of the buccal and lingual walls toward the proximal surface is necessary to ensure cavity margins are self-cleansing. Isthmus should not extend >1/2 intercuspal distance.

Bulbous crown (5) Primary molars have a more bulbous crown form than permanent molars, making matrix placement more difficult.

Inclination of the enamel prisms (6) In the cervical 1/3 of primary molars the enamel prisms are inclined in an occlusal direction so there is no need to bevel the gingival floor of a proximal box.

Cervical constriction (7) is more marked in primary molars, so if the base of the proximal box is extended too far gingivally it will be difficult to cut an adequate floor without encroaching on the pulp.

Alveolar bone permeability is increased in younger children, thus it is usually possible to achieve LA of primary mandibular molars by infiltration alone, up to 6 years of age.

Thin pulpal floor and accessory canals (8) may explain the greater incidence of interradicular involvement following pulp death.

Root form (9) Primary molars have proportionately longer roots than their permanent counterparts. They are also more flared to straddle the developing premolar tooth. The roots are flattened mesiodistally, as are canals within.

Radicular pulp (10) follows a tortuous and branching path, making complete cleansing and preparation of the root canal system almost impossible, although instrumenting canals is often easier than suggested in some texts. In addition, as the roots resorb, a different approach to RCT is needed for the 1° dentition, pure zinc oxide and eugenol being the obturation material of choice.

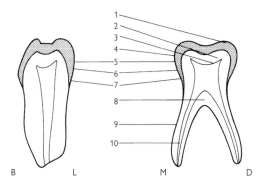

Cross sections of second primary molar showing features of anatomy of primary molars.

Extraction versus restoration of primary teeth

Despite a welcome reduction in the prevalence of dental decay, the dilemma of whether to restore or extract a primary tooth is still all too familiar. In making a decision, a number of factors should be considered:

Age This will influence the likely cooperation for restorative procedures, the expected remaining length of service of the affected tooth, and the severity of sequelae following early tooth loss (as the earlier the tooth is lost the greater the potential for space loss).

Medical history Possible sources of recurrent bacteremia should be avoided in patients with a history of cardiac disease and in those who are immunocompromised. (Hence pulp therapy is inappropriate and extractions should be carried out under antibiotic coverage). In hemophiliacs, extractions should be avoided and primary teeth preserved, if possible, until their exfoliation. Prevention is particularly important for these patients.

Motivation and cooperation of parents As it is the parents that bring the child to the surgery, we must explain to them the benefits of maintaining the primary dentition. Unfortunately, a small proportion of the population still regard a dentist that fills primary teeth with suspicion—after all, everyone knows that baby teeth fall out!

Caries rate In a child with an otherwise caries-free mouth, every attempt should be made to preserve an intact dentition. Where there is extensive caries, restoration of second primary molars and loss of first primary molars can be an acceptable compromise.

Pain If a child is suffering pain from one or more teeth, this needs to be alleviated as soon as possible. If symptom-free, then the dentist will have more time to explore the extent of the lesion(s) and the child's cooperation.

Extent of lesion(s) In primary molars destruction of the marginal ridge indicates a high probability of pulpal involvement.[1] If several primary molars require pulp therapy and cooperation or motivation is poor, serious thought should be given to extraction rather than to restoration.

Position of tooth Although early loss of primary incisors will have little effect, extraction of primary canine, primary first, or second molar teeth will, in a crowded patient, lead to localization of the crowding. Extraction of primary second molars, particularly in the upper arch, should be deferred, if possible, until the first permanent molar has erupted.

Presence/absence of permanent successor Bear in mind the amount of crowding present and the likelihood of spontaneous space closure.

Malocclusion If still undecided, it is worth considering the occlusion. In a particularly crowded case, restoration of a decayed tooth may be indicated if further space loss would mean that extraction of more than one premolar per quadrant would be required. Much has been written about

1 M. S. Duggal 2002 *Eur J Paediatr Dent* 3 112.

compensating (same tooth in opposing arch) and balancing (contralateral tooth) extractions, although this is still an area of some controversy.[1] The rationale is that a symmetrical problem is easier to deal with later, but if taken to its logical conclusion, gross caries of primary first molars and primary second molars will result in a clearance. In general, loss of primary canines or primary first molars in a crowded patient should be balanced to prevent a midline shift.

So much for the theory; in practice, it should be remembered that a happy and cooperative patient is more important over the long term. For some children this may mean that the extraction of several carious teeth at one visit is preferable to prolonged open combat in the dental chair. For most, restoration is better than running the risk of GA, which in itself may be a distressing experience. Inevitably, the wrong decision will sometimes be made, for we are all human.

1 W. P. Rock 2002 *Int J Paediatr Dent* **12** 151.

Local anesthesia for children

Although there is no scientific evidence to suggest that primary teeth are less sensitive than permanent teeth, clinically it is often possible to complete cavity preparation without LA, provided extensive dentin removal is not required. However, Walls *et al.* found that restorations placed without LA did not survive as long as those where LA was used.[1]

General principles

- Explain to the patient in terms they will understand what you are trying to do and why.
- Use flavored topical anesthesia (20% benzocaine).
- Warm anesthetic solution to room temperature only.
- Use a fine-gauge disposable needle.
- Always have a dental assistant available to help.
- Hold mucosa taut.
- Use a slow rate of injection.
- Warn about postop numbness and avoidance of self-inflicted trauma (e.g., lip chewing).

Choice of anesthetic agent

First choice: Lidocaine 2% with 1:100,000 epinephrine.
Second choice: prilocaine 4% with 1:200,000—gives less profound anesthesia.

Dosage

Lidocaine maximum dose = 7 mg/kg
Prilocaine maximum dose = 8 mg/kg

This equates to a maximum for a 15 kg (33 lb) child of 5.25 ml of 2% lidocaine with 1:100,000 epinephrine or 2.9 cartridges. The maximum for a 15 kg child is 3 ml 4% prilocaine with 1:200,000 epinephrine.

Infiltration injection

This is used for maxillary teeth, mandibular incisors, and lower primary molars before first permanent molar is erupted. After 6 years of age bone permeability is reduced and an inferior alveolar nerve block is required. Technique is as for adults (p. 574). In children, the malar buttress overlies the maxillary first permanent molar, so it is often advisable to deposit some solution over the more permeable bone mesial and distal to this tooth.

Block injection

Inferior alveolar nerve block Using thumb and forefinger, find the shortest width of ramus. Penetrate about 1 cm into lingual tissues from internal oblique ridge, on a line between the thumb and finger. An aspirating syringe is essential.

Posterior superior alveolar nerve block is rarely required in children. If necessary due to failure of infiltration for maxillary first permanent molar, the technique should be modified by depositing solution distal to the zygomatic buttress and massaging it backward toward the posterior superior alveolar foramen (maxillary molar block).[2]

1 A. W. G. Walls 1985 *BDJ* **158** 133.
2 A. K. Adatia 1976 *BDJ* **140** 87.

Alternative techniques

Intraligamentary injection These purpose-designed syringes have an ultra-short needle and a "gun" or "pen" appearance. This makes it helpful for children with a needle phobia, or as a more acceptable alternative or adjunct to an inferior alveolar nerve block. In addition, as the lips and tongue are not anesthetized it is useful for young or disabled children, in whom there is a greater risk of postoperative soft tissue trauma.

Computer-controlled delivery (e.g., The Wand) Allows carefully controlled, slow delivery via a line and needle resembling an IV giving set. This technique is especially useful for direct palatal anesthesia.

Restoration of carious primary teeth

Making an accurate preoperative diagnosis (including appropriate radiographs) and treatment plan is essential, so that treatment can be provided as efficiently as possible (p. 58)

Local anesthesia See p. 78.

Isolation Ideally, a rubber dam should be used routinely for all restorative procedures. It not only protects the airway but also improves moisture control and visibility and aids in patient management. It is essential for all root canal and pulp therapy for permanent teeth, and is advisable for restoration of primary teeth. If placement of a rubber dam is not possible, plastic disposable salivary ejectors are better tolerated than the metal flange type.

Instruments

Burs High-speed: pear-shaped bur numbers 330 and 525, and fissure bur number 245. Slow-speed: a selection of pear-shaped and round burs are most useful. For access use a small bur, and for caries removal use the largest round bur that fits into the cavity.

Handpiece A miniature-head handpiece is invaluable. Some children are apprehensive of the aspirator tip, making use of a high-speed, water-cooled handpiece difficult; others find the vibration of the slow-speed handpiece distressing, and may confuse it with pain. In these cases a vivid imagination and considerable ingenuity help. It is possible, but time consuming, to complete cavity preparation with hand instruments.

Material selection for intracoronal restorations

Amalgam In spite of concerns about toxicity and environmental pollution, this still remains an acceptable and durable material for Class I and II restorations in primary molars.

GI cement has the advantages of adhesion and fluoride release, but is more technique sensitive than amalgam and less wear resistant. It is most useful in non-load-bearing Class III and V cavities, temporization of primary teeth in young, pre-cooperative children, or teeth within a year or so of exfoliation.

Compomer A modified composite-type material with some of the properties of GI cement. It is more technique and moisture sensitive than amalgam, but studies suggest similar longevity.

Composite resin Early studies suggested poor performance in primary teeth, but modern materials placed with good isolation (i.e., rubber dam) should perform similarly to compomers, although little recent data on performance in primary molars exist.

▶ Plastic, intracoronal restorations perform best in primary molars with small Class I and II cavities. Stainless steel crowns (p. 86) give superior longevity where lesions are more extensive.

Principles of cavity design

Outline form should include any undermined enamel. Extension for prevention is now outmoded, but any suspect adjacent fissures should be included. Do not cross transverse marginal ridges unless they are undermined.

Caries removal Caries should be excavated from the dentinoenamel first. If necessary, you may need to reestablish outline form to improve access to ensure that the dentinoenamel is caries free. Then progress to carefully removing caries from floor.

Resistance form/retention form The completed restoration must be able to adequately resist dislodgement. Usually a 90° cavosurface angle and caries removal suffice.

Reasons for failure of restorations in primary teeth

- Recurrent caries, often due to failure to adequately complete caries removal because of flagging patient cooperation or failure to use adequate LA. If unable to finish completing a cavity, it is better to place a temporary dressing and try again at another visit.
- Cavity preparation does not satisfy the mechanical requirements of the filling material.
- Inadequate moisture control, especially true of GI cements, compomers, and composites
- Presence of occlusal high spot

There are many others, but these are the most common.

Useful tips

- Let child participate by "looking after" the saliva ejector or cotton roll.
- If the child is nervous, give them some control by asking them to signal, e.g., by raising their hand, if they want you to stop.
- If the child's cooperation runs out before the cavity is completed, try and ensure that all caries is removed from the DEJ and place a dressing of either zinc oxide or GI cement. This can then be left for several visits, until you are ready to try again.
- Vibration is less of a problem with lower teeth; therefore, if possible, start with a lower tooth.
- However, giving LA is easier in the maxilla.
- Don't try to do too much at one visit; quadrant conservation is not really feasible in an 8-year-old!

Communication

▶ It is important to explain to the child what you are trying to do, and why, in terms they can understand. It may be helpful to describe some of the instruments we use in ways that can make them seem less threatening to a child, such as the following:

slow-speed handpiece	Mr Buzz/buzzy bee/bumble bee
high-speed handpiece	Mr Spray/wizzy brush/tooth tickler
handpiece and prophylaxis cup	electric toothbrush/tooth polisher
aspirator tip	vacuum cleaner/Hoover
rubber dam	tooth raincoat
saliva ejector	straw
	curly-wurly (coiled type only)
air from 3-in-1	wind
fissure sealant	plastic coating
etchant solution	tooth shampoo/cleaner
	lemon juice
cotton roll	snowman
dental light	the sun/car light

Class I in primary molars

See p. 74 for anatomy of 1° molars and effect on cavity design. Have all necessary instruments and filling materials ready so that the appointment is kept as short as possible.

- Explain and show child (and parent) what you are trying to do.
- Use LA if required (p. 78).
- To gain access to a small cavity you can use a high-speed handpiece and pear-shaped bur. The outline can then be established and caries removed.
- In larger cavities an excavator or large round bur can be used to start caries removal from the walls. Any undermined enamel should be cut back.
- If caries is deep, stop and reassess whether pulpotomy (p. 92) is required.
- Check retention and that walls are caries free.
- Wash and dry cavity.
- Line with hard-setting calcium hydroxide if using amalgam.
- Place amalgam incrementally. GI or composite are also acceptable.
- Check occlusion.
- This is usually a good opportunity to reinforce any preventive advice, but keep it brief.

▶ Praise child, and if bribery has not been used, don't forget the sticker/ badge/toothbrush.

Polishing of amalgam restorations in primary molars is unnecessary.

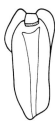

Cross-sectional view of Class I restoration (buccolingually).

Class II in primary molars—amalgam

See p. 74 for anatomy of primary molars and effect on cavity preparation. Class II cavities are designed for treatment of interproximal caries and consist of three parts.

Occlusal key is designed to retain the restoration and eliminate any occlusal caries. This should be prepared first and is identical to Class I cavity preparation, p. 82. This component is essential for Class II amalgam restorations, but can be omitted for minimal cavities restored with adhesive materials.

Isthmus joins the occlusal key with the interproximal box. It is the part of the filling most prone to fracture. Dimensions of the isthmus are a balance between:

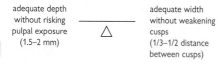

adequate depth without risking pulpal exposure (1.5–2 mm) ⟶ △ ⟶ adequate width without weakening cusps (1/3–1/2 distance between cusps)

Proximal box is to allow access for caries removal. Ideally this should just extend into embrasures and walls should converge occlusally.

Minimal caries with marginal ridge intact (usually diagnosed on preoperative bitewing radiographs).
• Follow steps for small occlusal cavity.
• When occlusal cavity (key) is complete, extend it toward proximal surface. Most texts advise retaining some enamel interproximally to protect adjacent tooth, but this is often easier said than done.
• Establish floor of box, taking care not to extend beyond maximum bulbosity of tooth.
• Fracture away remaining proximal enamel with hand instruments.
• Complete preparation of box following external contours of tooth and 90° cavosurface angle.
• Remove all caries. If exposure, then do pulp treatment.
• Check retention.
• If amalgam, place hard-setting lining; if adhesive material, no lining is needed.
• Position narrow matrix band and wedge.
• Place material and shape/carve with matrix in place. Use light cure if necessary.
• Check occlusion.

More advanced proximal caries (marginal ridge broken down—likelihood of pulpal involvement). Plastic restorations work best in Class I and small Class II cavities. In extensive cavities and/or where pulp treatment is necessary, stainless steel crowns provide a more durable restoration.

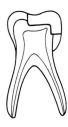

Cross section of lower right primary first molar MO restoration (mesiodistally).

Stainless steel (SS) crowns

▶ SS crowns are the most durable restoration for primary molars with extensive caries, caries on three or more surfaces, and those where pulp treatment has been performed.
▶ Although made of stainless steel, SS crowns do contain small traces of nickel and are therefore not suitable for patients with a known nickel allergy.

Indications
• Badly broken down primary molar
• After pulp therapy in primary molars
• As interim measure for permanent molars, where crowns are required but the patient is too young
• Temporary coverage during preparation of cast crown for premolar or permanent molar
• Developmental anomalies
• Severe tooth loss due to bruxism or erosion.

Instruments High-speed tapered diamond bur (e.g., 582) and diamond occlusal wheel. Straight handpiece and a stone. Slow-speed handpiece and burs as required. Crown scissors, dividers, selection of suitable crowns, utility or Howe's pliers. Contouring pliers and crimping pliers are also useful for making accurate adjustments.

Technique
For retention, SS crowns rely only on a tight adaptation at the gingival margin of the preparation, therefore, taper of preparation walls is not critical.
• Use LA and, if possible, rubber dam.
• Measure M–D length with dividers to aid crown selection.
• Remove caries.
• Perform occlusal reduction (approximately 1 mm) with occlusal wheel, roughly following cuspal planes.
• Perform proximal reduction (approximately 20° from vertical) using tapered diamond, without producing a ledge at gingival margin.
• Remove buccal and lingual bulbosities only enough to set crown (often little or no reduction is required).
• Select crown. Correct size will be a "click" fit (like a press-stud).
• Check height and occlusion. Minor prematurity is not a problem. If extensive blanching of surrounding tissues or overextended, trim crown. With modern crowns this step will usually not be necessary.
• Use contouring and crimping pliers to adapt contact points to crimp margins, and smooth trimmed margins with stone.
• Cement with zinc polycarboxylate or GI cement.

The technique for permanent molars is similar but more careful adjustment is necessary.

Success rates
A number of studies have demonstrated that SS crowns have a far superior longevity to that of other types of restoration in primary molars.

Further reading

J. R. Pinkham 2005 *Pediatric Dentistry: Infancy Through Adolescence*, 4th ed., Elsevier Saunders, Stainless steel crowns. RCS clinical guideline. *Int J Paediatr Dent* 1999 **9** 311. M. S. Duggal et al. 2002 *Restorative Techniques in Paediatric Dentistry*, Dunnitz.

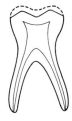

Occlusal reduction

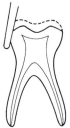

Mesial (and distal) reduction

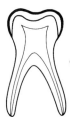

Completed crown

Preparation for stainless steel crown.

Classes III, IV, and V in primary teeth

Carious primary incisors and canines are seen less frequently than molars and are therefore indicative of a high caries rate (see Severe Early Childhood Caries, p. 89).

Management Objectives are relief of pain and prevention. Aesthetics are less important.

Treatment options include the following:
- Extraction
- Topical fluoride (2% sodium fluoride) and observation. Intervene if caries progresses.
- Discing (safer to use flat fissure No. 1 bur, than disc) plus topical fluoride
- Restoration; usually there is insufficient hard tissue for adequate retention, therefore adhesive materials are preferable.

Class III restoration Similar technique to that used for permanent incisors, but omit incisal retention groove.

Class IV restoration If restoration is essential, the greater strength of composite is required. Polycarboxylate (strip) crowns are advocated by some pediatric dentists, for the well-motivated child.

Class V restoration Remove caries with inverted cone and restore with GI cement.

Composite strip crowns Cellulose acetate crown forms for primary incisors. Enable restoration of primary incisors using composite resin.

Severe early childhood caries

Etiology Frequent ingestion of sugar and/or reduced salivary flow.

Nursing caries or bottle caries is associated with frequent consumption of a sugar-containing drink, especially from a feeding bottle. It is also attributed to prolonged on-demand breastfeeding, especially at night, from the lactose in breast milk.[1] Characteristically, caries starts with the maxillary primary incisors, but in more severe cases the first primary molars are also involved. The mandibular incisors are relatively protected by the tongue and saliva.

Rampant caries A term often used to describe extensive, rapidly progressing caries affecting many teeth in the primary and/or permanent dentition.

Severe early childhood caries may also be caused by the prolonged and frequent intake of sugar-based medications; however, both pharmaceutical companies and doctors are more aware of the problem and the number of alternative sugar-free preparations is increasing. See p. 118 for a list of such preparations.

Management
- Removal of etiological factors (education, artificial saliva)
- Fluoride rinses for older age groups (daily 0.05%)
- Primary dentition—may need to extract teeth of poor prognosis and concentrate on prevention for permanent dentition
- Permanent dentition—need assessment of long-term prognosis for teeth. Final treatment plan should be drawn up in consultation with orthodontist.

1 G. J. Roberts 1982 *J Dent* **10** 346.

Primary molar pulp therapy

Note where primary molar roots resorb.

Where the carious process has jeopardized pulp vitality there are two alternatives: (1) extraction and (2) pulp therapy.

Indication and contraindications See Extraction versus Restoration, p. 76.

▶ Any medical condition where a focus of infection is potentially dangerous (e.g., congenital heart disease, rheumatic fever) is an absolute contraindication to pulp therapy. Extraction under antibiotic coverage as advised by the child's physician is necessary.

Pulp therapy is preferable to extraction in children with bleeding disorders. The tooth must be restorable following pulp therapy.

Diagnosis of pulpal state can be difficult, as not only is a child's perception of pain less precise than an adult's, but the clinical picture may also be complicated by death of one root canal while the other(s) remains vital.

Indicators of possible pulpal involvement
- Breakdown of marginal ridge
- Symptoms
- Tenderness to percussion, increased mobility, buccal swelling/sinus
- Interradicular radiolucency seen radiographically

Definitions
Pulpotomy: Removal of coronal pulp and treatment of radicular pulp.

Pulpectomy: Removal of entire coronal and radicular pulp.

Principles of treatment Attempting to retain the vitality of the pulp in primary molars is not recommended because (1) pulpal involvement is more likely, (2) it is difficult to accurately determine the likely condition of the pulp, and (3) calcium hydroxide frequently leads to internal resorption. Therefore, direct pulp capping is only advisable for small traumatic exposures. Pulpotomy remains the treatment of choice for primary molars:

               one-visit pulpotomy (procedure of choice)

VITAL PULP ⟨

               two-visit pulpotomy or (only used when
                  one visit not possible)

             non-vital pulpotomy

NON-VITAL PULP ⟨

             pulpectomy

Materials
Among the more commonly used medicaments is *formocreosol* (for one-visit pulpotomy).

▶ This material is caustic, therefore use cautiously.

Success rates vary from 50% for non-vital teeth to over 90% for vital pulps.[1]

Because of concerns about the potential toxicity of formocresol, numerous other medicaments have been tried. The most promising is 15.5% ferric sulfate (Astringident–Optident), which appears to have a similar success rate to that of formocresol. Other potentially viable alternatives include calcium hydroxide (difficult to use successfully) and mineral trioxide aggregate (MTA; very expensive).

1 M. E. J. Curzon 1986 *Dental Advertiser* **51** 14.

Pulpotomy techniques for vital pulps

In primary molars the relatively larger pulps result in earlier pulpal involvement; therefore, devitalization and fixation of the pulpal tissues gives more consistent results than techniques that attempt to retain vitality, e.g., indirect pulp capping. There are two alternative approaches:

- one-visit formocresol pulpotomy; and
- two-visit devitalization pulpotomy.

The choice of technique depends on the status of the pulp and cooperation of the child. The generally accepted pulpotomy treatment for primary molars is the one-visit formocresol pulpotomy.

One-visit formocresol pulpotomy

This method fixes most of the radicular pulp, but the apical part may be unaffected by the medicament.

- Give local anesthetics and place rubber dam.
- Complete cavity preparation and excavate caries.
- Remove roof of pulp chamber.
- Amputate coronal pulp with a large excavator or sterile round bur.
- Wash chamber and arrest bleeding with damp cotton pellet.
- Place cotton pellet dampened with formocresol on exposed pulp stumps for 5 min, then remove.
- Apply dressing of reinforced ZOE cement.
- Restore tooth, usually with a stainless steel crown.

Problems

Inadequate local anesthesia Repeat local anesthesia or use a two-visit technique.

Necrotic pulp Proceed with non-vital technique.

Profuse hemorrhage indicates more serious inflammation of the radicular pulp. Formocresol can be sealed in the canal for 1 week, then continue the procedure as above.

Alternative medicaments Ferric sulfate.

Two-visit devitalization pulpotomy

Sometimes there are occasions where it is not possible to obtain anesthesia of a vital pulp, or cooperation is difficult and a two-visit devitalization technique may be justified. Devitalizing paste is applied to the exposure on cotton pellet and sealed tightly in place for 2 weeks. On re-opening the pulp should be non-vital and treatment can proceed as for a non-vital tooth.

Non-vital pulp techniques

There are two methods used for treatment of the non-vital pulp.

Pulpotomy

This method removes infected coronal pulp and disinfects radicular pulp, thus allowing normal root resorption to proceed. It is still practiced in some centers, but carries a relatively low success rate (50%).

First visit
- LA is required as part of pulp could still be vital.
- Complete cavity preparation and removal of caries.
- Remove roof of pulp chamber and excavate pulpal debris.
- Place cotton pellet moistened with beechwood creosote or formocresol in pulp chamber.
- Seal with temporary dressing (GI or zinc oxide-eugenol [ZOE]).
- Arrange next appointment for 1–2 weeks later.

Second visit
- Check for symptoms; if there are none, proceed.
- Remove temporary dressing and cotton pellet.
- Place antiseptic dressing (50:50 formocresol and eugenol mixed with zinc oxide powder) and press down into root canals.
- Restore tooth.

Problems

Vital and/or sensitive tissue encountered Place devitalizing paste and seal for 1–2 weeks before proceeding with non-vital pulpotomy.

Abscess formation during treatment Either repeat (consider whether you need to incise abscess), carry out pulpectomy, or extract tooth.

Alternative medicaments Formocresol, and "Kri" liquid have been suggested.

Technique for abscessed teeth Acute abscesses require drainage to relieve symptoms. This can be achieved by either leaving the tooth on open drainage for 1 week before proceeding as above (this is more applicable to upper teeth) or incising the abscess under topical LA. Chronic abscess drainage may be occurring through a sinus; if so, proceed straight to first-visit technique. If drainage is occurring through an occlusal cavity, placement of a seal may lead to exacerbation in symptoms; therefore, always warn parents to return if there are any problems.

Pulpectomy

A pulpectomy is often considered difficult in primary molars because of the complexity of ribbon-shaped canals (although instrumentation is often easier than some texts might suggest). The risk of damage to the permanent successor also needs to be considered, but if conditions are favorable it is the treatment of choice for non-vital pulps.[1] The technique can be carried out in one or two visits.

---

1 M. .D. Duggal 1989 *Dental Update* **16** 26.

- Use LA and rubber dam.
- Remove the necrotic pulp, locate and file canals.
- A radiograph to show position of files is desirable but not essential.
- Fill canal with plain ZOE paste with a spiral filler.
- Restore with SS crown.

If there is evidence of any infection or there is bleeding from the radicular pulp, a two-stage treatment is recommended, leaving formocresol on a cotton pellet in the canal for 1–2 weeks prior to filling.

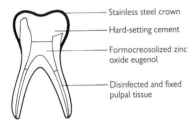

Stainless steel crown

Hard-setting cement

Formocreosolized zinc oxide eugenol

Disinfected and fixed pulpal tissue

Non-vital pulpotomy.

Pulp therapy for primary anterior teeth

The usual treatment is extraction, as first and second maxillary primary molars are exfoliated before the patient is able to cooperate satisfactorily with more complicated treatment. However, the maxillary primary canine is exfoliated later and unilateral loss may result in midline shift, thus pulp treatment is indicated for some patients. The root canal morphology is amenable to pulpectomy and the canal should be cleaned using files, with care (remember underlying successor). A resorbable filling material, e.g., calcium hydroxide or ZOE, should be used.

Dental trauma

▶ If there is evidence of head injury, transfer the patient to a hospital emergency room immediately.

Note
- By 15 years of age 33% of children have experienced at least one episode of dental trauma.[1]
- Prognosis is good with immediate treatment, so see patient as soon as possible.
- Avulsed permanent teeth should be replanted immediately.
- The child and parent may be upset, therefore handle accordingly and defer any non-urgent treatment.
- Take good notes for future reference and medicolegal purposes.
- If the crown fractures this will have dissipated most of the energy of impact, making root fractures less likely.

History
Take a detailed history. A complete history is important for medicolegal purposes.

▶ Loss of consciousness? Concussion/headache (p. 398)? Immediately refer to hospital emergency room for evaluation.

- Accompanied by? Parent/teacher? Consider consent issues.
- When? Time interval between injury and fractures affects prognosis.
- Where? Does patient need a tetanus booster? If so, refer to pediatrician or primary care physician.
- How? Be alert to the possibilities of other injuries and non-accidental injuries.
- Tooth fragments? These may have been inhaled or embedded in soft tissues (e.g., lip). If fragment or tooth is not accounted for and/or there is loss of consciousness, a chest X-ray (CXR) is mandatory.
- Past dental history? Previous trauma may affect prognosis, cooperation in the dental setting.
- Past medical history? Risk of infective endocarditis, bleeding disorder, or allergy to penicillin.

Aims of Treatment

Primary dentition (1) preserve integrity of permanent successor; (2) preserve primary tooth if cooperation is good and is compatible with first aim.

Permanent dentition (1) preserve vitality of the tooth to allow maturation of the root; (2) restore the crown to prevent drifting, tilting, and overeruption.

---

1 J. E. Todd 1985 *Children's Dental Health in the UK*, HMSO.

Principles of Treatment

Emergency treatment
- Elimination of pain
- Protection of pulp
- Reduction and immobilization of mobile teeth
- Suturing of soft tissue lacerations (intraoral—3/0 resorbable suture (gut, chromic gut Vicryl); extraoral —refer to hospital).
- ? antibiotics, ? tetanus, ? analgesics, ? chlorhexidine mouthwash

Intermediate treatment
- Pulp therapy
- Consider orthodontic requirements and long-term prognosis of damaged teeth
- Semipermanent restorations
- Keep under review, usually every 1 month, 3 months, and then 6 months for 2 years.

Permanent treatment
- Usually deferred until >16 years (to allow pulpal and gingival recession and decrease likelihood of further trauma), e.g., porcelain crown, post and core crown.

Classification of tooth injuries

Several exist; some use roman numerals, others describe the injuries sustained (WHO system):
Complicated fracture—pulp is exposed.
Uncomplicated fracture —pulp is intact.

Prevention

- Prevalence increases as the overjet increases (>9 mm prevalence doubles), therefore ? early orthodontics.

Mouth guard for sports (vacuum-formed thermoplastic vinyl is best, triple thickness).

▶ Be alert for evidence of non-accidental injury (p. 100).

Non-accidental injury (NAI)

All professionals involved with children need to be alert to the possibility of NAI (a term now favored over *child abuse*).

The following signs are associated with NAI:

- Usually younger children are involved.
- The presenting injuries may not match the parent's account of how they were sustained.
- Attendance at a surgery or clinic for treatment of the injury is often delayed.
- Bruises of different stages are found on examination.
- Ear pinches and frenal tears in children <1 year old are highly suspicious.
- 50% of abused children will have signs on the head and/or neck.

Management

In most areas local guidelines have been drawn up. These can usually be obtained from social services or the pediatric department at the local hospital. A copy of these should be kept in every practice.

If an NAI is suspected, the practitioner should refer to the local protocol, or contact either a local pediatrician or the duty social worker at the local services department for advice. If the referral is made to the social services department this will need to be confirmed in writing. The child's medical practitioner should also be informed. If a child presents with serious injuries that are suspicious, they should be referred to the nearest emergency room (ER) and the ER staff informed of the situation before the child's arrival.

Tact is required in dealing with the patient's family. It is better to concentrate on treating the patient's injuries, referring them to the experts who will fully evaluate the case, before making a diagnosis of NAI.

Injuries to primary teeth

Eight percent of 5-year-olds have experienced dental trauma,[1] mainly at toddler stage. As alveolar bone is more elastic in the younger the child, the most common injuries are loosening and/or displacement. Crown and root fractures are rare.

Management

If radiographs are required, you may have to get the parent to hold the child to film. Alternatively, try placing a periapical film between the teeth (like an occlusal view) and angle the beam at 45°.

You need to consider the effect of any proposed treatment on the permanent successor. Splinting of primary incisors is exceedingly difficult and not indicated. When in doubt, extract the primary tooth! (For definitions, see p. 108.)

Concussion Reassurance and soft diet.

Subluxation If tooth is close to exfoliation, extract. Otherwise, soft diet is indicated (for about 1 week). The tooth may become non-vital, therefore keep under observation.

Luxation Extraction is indicated unless the crown is displaced palatally (away from permanent tooth), the tooth is not in danger of being inhaled, and it does not interfere with occlusion. If the crown is displaced labially, there is risk of damage to underlying permanent incisor.

Intrusion is the most common injury (>60%).[2] If X-ray confirms that the tooth has been forced into follicle of the underlying permanent tooth, extract the primary incisor. Otherwise, leave the tooth and wait to see if spontaneous eruption occurs (between 1 and 6 months). Unfortunately, pulpal necrosis often follows, necessitating either pulp treatment (p. 94) or extraction. Should the tooth fail to erupt, extraction is indicated. It is prudent to warn parents about possible damage to the underlying permanent tooth.

Extrusion If >1–2 mm, extract, as it is difficult to splint and will probably become non-vital.

Avulsion Do not replant primary teeth.

Crown fracture Rare. Minimal fracture can be smoothed and left under observation.

Larger fracture Either restore with composite and/or root canal treatment if pulp is involved, or extract.

Root fracture Provided not displaced and little mobility, advise soft diet and keep under review. If coronal fragment displaced or mobile, extract, but leave apical portion as it will usually resorb.

1 J. E. Todd 1985 *Children's Dental Health in the UK,* HMSO.
2 J. O. Andreasen 1981 *Traumatic Injuries of the Teeth,,* Munksgaard.

Sequelae of trauma

Primary dentition

Discoloration If tooth becomes gray in the early post-trauma period, pulp may be vital and discoloration reversible. Graying later indicates pulp necrosis. Yellowing of tooth is suggestive of calcification of pulp—no treatment is required.

Ankylosis treatment Extraction to prevent displacement of permanent incisor.

Pulp death treatment Root canal treatment or extraction.

Permanent dentition

In about 60% of children <4 years of age, trauma to primary tooth affects underlying developing successor.[1] The effect depends on the stage of development, type of injury and severity, treatment, and pulpal sequelae. Such trauma can cause hypomineralization, hypoplasia (likelihood <4 years and more severe injury), dilaceration, severe malformation, and arrest of development.

1 G. Roberts 1996 *Oral and Dental Trauma in Children and Adolescents*, OUP.

Injuries to permanent teeth—crown fractures

Prevalence: 26–76% of injuries.

Enamel only

For small enamel fracture, smooth with white stone.

Enamel and dentin

You need to protect the exposed dentine, preferably with hard-setting calcium hydroxide cement and acid-etch retained composite. If time permits, this can be done with a crown former to restore tooth contour. Keep under review. Veneer or porcelain jacket crown can be considered later. If fracture is near pulp, treat as for pulp involvement.

Acid-etch composite tip technique

- Place rubber dam, if possible.
- Place hard-setting calcium hydroxide on exposed dentine. There is no need to bevel enamel.
- Using contralateral tooth as a guide, select a cellulose acetate crown former.
- Trim crown former to within 1–2 mm of fracture line.
- Etch enamel for 20sec, wash, and dry.
- Place bonding resin and cure.
- Put sufficient composite and a little extra into crown former and position.
- Allow to cure and remove crown former.
- Trim, using Soflex discs. Shofu points are useful for palatal aspect.
- Check occlusion.

Enamel, dentin, and pulp

Treatment depends on size of exposure, state of root development (maxillary permanent central incisor root is radiographically complete by age 10–11 years, histologically by 14–15 years), time since injury, and other injuries (e.g., root fracture). If apex is open with blood supply to pulp, there is a reduced likelihood of pulp death. This is advantageous, as treatment should be directed toward retaining vitality of radicular pulp to allow root closure to continue. If pulp is non-vital, see p. 112. Otherwise, treatment alternatives are as follows.

Pulp cap with non-setting calcium hydroxide (mixed with water) followed by hard-setting calcium hydroxide (e.g., Dycal), and place composite tip. Review vitality.

Partial (Cvek) pulpotomy

Indications Exposure >1 mm; up to 4 days old; complete or incomplete root development.

- Use LA and rubber dam.
- Slightly enlarge access at site of exposure with high speed and amputate pulp to a depth of 2–4 mm into healthy pulp tissue.

- Arrest bleeding with sterile, moist cotton pellet (this usually takes several minutes).
- Cover amputation site with non-setting calcium hydroxide.
- Seal with glass ionomer cement.
- Restore crown.

Full coronal pulpotomy

Indications Large, contaminated exposures; long duration; incomplete root development.
- Use LA and rubber dam.
- Open up pulp chamber and amputate coronal pulp to cervical construction with sterile bur or sharp excavator.
- Wash with sterile water.
- Place non-setting calcium hydroxide and restore tooth with GI cement and composite.
- Leave 6–8 weeks, then review symptoms and vitality. Investigation of the presence of a calcified barrier is not necessary.
- If tooth becomes non-vital, see p. 112.

All pulpotomized teeth should be kept under long-term follow-up as pulp necrosis and calcification are common sequelae. Success rates of 72% for cervical pulpotomies and 96% for minimal pulpotomies have been reported.[1]

1 M. E. J. Curzon 1999 *Handbook of Dental Trauma*, Wright.

Root fractures

Prevalence: <10% of injuries to permanent dentition.

Where root fracture is suspected, two radiographic views at different angulations in the vertical plane are advisable to improve chances of visualizing the fracture line.

The prognosis for this type of injury depends on whether the fracture line communicates with the gingival crevice. Actual treatment depends on position of the fracture.

Apical 1/3 Usually no treatment is required unless mobility increases significantly. However, the tooth should be kept under observation, as death of coronal 2/3 of pulp may occur. You only need to prepare canal to fracture line as apical 1/3 usually retains vitality. Prognosis is good. If extraction is required, the apical 1/3 can be left in situ to preserve bone.

Middle 1/3 In most cases the tooth is loosened, therefore, to achieve repair of the fracture line with hard-tissue union, the tooth should be splinted rigidly for 8–12 weeks. If the coronal part is not displaced, loss of vitality is unlikely. Where the coronal fragment is displaced, reposition, splint, and, if loss of vitality occurs, perform root canal treatment to fracture line. Calcium hydroxide should be used as an interim dressing to limit inflammation and resorption. Delay in treatment diminishes good prognosis. If extraction is required, consider leaving apical portion in situ.

Coronal 1/3 By definition, fractures in this group communicate with the gingival crevice, allowing ingress of bacteria into pulp. Emergency treatment consists of a choice between either extraction of both parts of the tooth or, preferably, removal of the coronal fragment, root canal treatment of the remainder, and then placement of a dressing that will prevent gingival tissues overgrowing the root surface. This can be achieved by placing a temporary post-retained crown, although replacement of the coronal fragment using a dentin-bonding agent has been described. For permanent treatment, place a post and core crown. However, if fracture extends below the alveolar crest, you need improved access for crown fabrication; there are two alternatives:

Ostectomy/gingivectomy	*Orthodontic extrusion*
Gives quicker result	Cervical circumference of crown
Needs post	smaller compared to
Tend to get perio pocket	contralateral tooth
Leads to reduced gingival width	Better crown/root ratio
	Maintain attached gingiva

Orthodontic extrusion can be accomplished, using a maxillary removable appliance with a buccal arm that engages either an attachment bonded onto the labial surface of the temporary post and core crown or any available enamel. Forces of 50–100g should be used. When sufficient extrusion has been achieved, retain for at least 3–6 months before fabricating a permanent restoration.

If the tooth is extracted, a maxillary partial denture will need to be fabricated (p. 302).

Oblique Provided fracture extends <4 mm below alveolar crest, it can be treated as a coronal fracture. Otherwise, if possible, extract coronal portion only, leaving apical portion in situ to preserve bone.

Vertical Extract.

Luxation, subluxation, intrusion, and extrusion

Prevalence: 15–40% of injuries.

Definitions

Concussion Injury to supporting tissues of tooth, without displacement.

Luxation Displacement of tooth (laterally, labially, or palatally).

Subluxation Actually means partial displacement, but commonly used to describe loosening of a tooth without displacement.

Intrusion Displacement of tooth into its socket. Often accompanied by fracture of alveolar bone.

Extrusion Partial displacement of tooth from its socket.

Treatment

Concussion Reassurance and soft diet.

Luxation You need to reposition the tooth as soon as possible. Give LA and use fingers to push back into place. Then tooth should be splinted flexibly for 2–3 weeks. If there has been a delay of more than 24 h since the injury, manual reduction is unlikely to be successful. In these cases the tooth can be repositioned orthodontically. If the displaced tooth is interfering with the occlusion, an upper removable appliance (URA), with buccal capping, should be fitted as soon as possible. If root development is complete, loss of vitality is a common sequela following luxation, leading to inflammatory resorption (p. 112). Teeth with immature apices have a much better chance of pulp survival. External or internal resorption and pulp canal obliteration may also occur, therefore, keep under observation.

Subluxation If minor, treatment other than advising a soft diet is necessary. If mobile, splint for 1–2 weeks and watch vitality.

Intrusion[1] Teeth with immature roots are likely to erupt and therefore no immediate treatment is required, although consideration should be given to surgical repositioning if displacement is severe (i.e. >6 mm intrusion). However, teeth with closed apices have a limited potential for re-eruption and will need orthodontic extrusion. This should be started as soon as possible to facilitate access for root canal treatment. Again, surgical repositioning may be indicated when intrusion is severe. Surgically repositioned teeth require flexible splinting for 1–2 weeks. Pulp death and/or root resorption can ensue rapidly after injury and early pulp extirpation, and placement of the calcium hydroxide dressing is advisable. In immature teeth the increased blood supply means that loss of vitality is less likely, but not impossible.

Extrusion The affected tooth should be repositioned under LA with digital pressure and splinted for 1–2 weeks. Again, loss of vitality is a common sequela, so the tooth should be observed for any signs of resorption or pulp death.

If any of the above occurs in conjunction with fracture of the alveolar bone, the splinting period should be increased to 3–4 weeks to aid bony healing. If, however, the socket is comminuted, splinting needs to be extended to 6–8 weeks.

1 M. J. Kinirons 1998 *Int J Paediatr Dent* **8** 165.

Splinting

Indications

- To stabilize a loosened tooth to promote periodontal healing and improve patient comfort. To encourage fibrous rather than bony healing (ankylosis), a short splinting time with a flexible splint is recommended (avulsion = 7–10 days; luxation = <3 weeks).
- To stabilize a root fracture and encourage healing with calcified tissue. Rigid splinting for 12 weeks is generally indicated.

Methods

Direct Constructed on patient. An almost infinite variety of methods have been described, but the following are the most popular:

- Acid-etch splint with composite resin and/or wire/orthodontic attachments
- Lone standing teeth can be supported by sling suture.
- Interdental wiring is of historical interest.

Indirect This type of splint is removable, allowing an assessment of mobility or firmness, which is valuable in cases of reimplantation. The more common types are the following:

- Upper removable appliance with cribs on maxillary first permanent molars and occlusal coverage
- Vacuum-formed thermoplastic polyvinylacetatepolyethylene (!) "Vaccuform" type

However, this approach requires an impression of traumatized mouth and involves some delay (a few hours/days) before the splint can be fitted, so in practice direct splinting is usually preferred.

Factors affecting choice of splint

- Type of injury and therefore length of time splint required. For example, root fracture will need 8–12 weeks of splinting, therefore composite and wire splint is advisable. For a replanted tooth prolonged splinting should be avoided as it may lead to ankylosis.
- Dental status of patient, e.g., in mixed dentition and when both maxillary central incisors are traumatized, a full-coverage acrylic splint is needed.
- Facilities and time available
- Number of teeth injured and availability of uninjured adjacent teeth
- Luxated or replanted teeth can be held in place with sling sutures if there are no adjacent teeth to splint to.

Management of the avulsed tooth

Exarticulation = avulsion. Prevalence: 0–16% of injuries.

Factors affecting prognosis Success depends on reestablishment of a normal periodontium.

- *Time from loss to reimplantation*. As periodontal ligament cells rarely survive >60 min extraorally, immediate replacement (by whoever is available at the scene) is the treatment of choice.
- *Storage medium*. Prognosis saliva > milk > water > air. (Dry storage rapidly damages periodontal cells.)
- *Splinting time* 7–10 days for flexible splinting. Prolonged splinting will promote ankylosis.
- *Viability of pulp*. Seepage of pulp breakdown products into periodontal ligament will contribute to development of inflammatory resorption. Although revascularization is possible in a tooth with an open apex that is replanted within 30 min, those teeth with closed apices and longer extra-alveolar times should be considered non-vital.

Immediate treatment (if avulsed tooth not already replaced)
- Avoid handling root surface. If tooth is contaminated, hold crown and agitate gently in saline.
- Place tooth in socket. If it does not readily seat, get patient to bite on gauze for 15–20 min.
- Compress buccal and lingual alveolar plates.
- Splint a curved piece of light wire (a light twist-flex type wire is ideal) to acid-etched enamel of affected and adjacent teeth using temporary crown material, as this is less traumatic to remove than composite.
- Prescribe antibiotics and chlorhexidine mouthwash, and arrange tetanus booster if necessary.

Intermediate treatment (7–10 days later)
- Review splinting. Stop if tooth appears firm. Continue for another week if still mobile. (If still mobile after 2 weeks, check that nothing has been overlooked, e.g., root fracture or loss of vitality—in these cases prognosis is poor.)
- If apex is closed (or tooth has open apex, but extra-alveolar period >30 min) extirpate pulp, clean canal, and place an initial intracanal dressing of calcium hydroxide. An intermediate dressing of polyantibiotic/steroid paste may be placed for 1–2 weeks prior to placement of calcium hydroxide.
- Keep teeth with open apices under close observation, so that at the first sign of pulp death root canal treatment can be instituted. Waiting for radiographic evidence of inflammatory resorption is too late.
- Keep tooth under observation. If calcium hydroxide is placed in canal, this should be renewed every 3 months until apical barrier is formed and then GP filling placed.

Prognosis If the above procedure is followed, medium-term survival is relatively good:[1]
- Incomplete root formation: 66% survive 5 years.
- Complete root formation: 90% survive 5 years.

1 J. O. Andreasen 1992 *Atlas of Replantation and Transplantation of Teeth*, Mediglobe.

Long-term survival is closely related to extra-alveolar dry-storage time. Teeth stored dry for >30 min have a very poor long-term prognosis, but replantation may still be worthwhile, as failure is usually by replacement resorption, which is slow (i.e., tooth may last several years) and maintains bulk of alveolus (facilitates future prosthetic replacement).

Where prognosis is deemed poor, premolar transplant can be considered at 10–12 years old.

Sequelae

Surface resorption occurs as a result of minor trauma to periodontal ligament cells. Usually this is self-limiting and affected areas are repaired by cementum. No treatment is required.

Replacement resorption (ankylosis) is caused by damage to periodontal ligament cells during the extra-alveolar period and is promoted by prolonged splinting. It appears that the absence of vital periodontal ligament allows resorption of the root and replacement by bone. In a growing child this results in infra-occlusion of the affected tooth. Once started, it is usually progressive, resulting in eventual loss of the tooth.

Inflammatory resorption Development of inflammatory resorption is dependent on both damage to the periodontal ligament and breakdown products from pulp necrosis diffusing through the dentinal tubules to the periodontal ligament. This occurs rapidly, as soon as 1–2 weeks after injury. Once evident radiographically prognosis is poor, as it is progressive and treatment is not always successful. Inflammatory resorption can be prevented by extirpation of the pulp as soon as is practicable after injury and placement of non-setting calcium hydroxide. If resorption is halted a GP root filling can be placed.

Delayed presentation Where viability of periodontal ligament cells is doubtful, Andreasen has suggested chemical treatment of the root surface with fluoride to limit resorption.[1] Following root canal treatment with GP, the tooth is immersed in 2.4 % sodium fluoride solution for 20 min. Then tooth is replanted and splinted for 6 weeks. As some replacement resorption is inevitable, this procedure is perhaps best limited to adults. If the extra-alveolar period is > 24 h, leave and consider instead whether the resulting space should be maintained with a partial denture (p. 304).

Pulpal sequelae following trauma

Damage to the pulp can occur as a result of disruption of the apical vessels or exposure of the pulp by a crown or root fracture, or be caused by hemorrhage and inflammation of coronal pulp, resulting in strangulation.

Pulp death Remember that no response to vitality testing indicates damage to the nerve supply of a tooth, but not necessarily to the blood supply. Therefore, following trauma, you should assess vitality in light of symptoms, tooth color, mobility, presence of buccal swelling, and radiographic evidence. Except where a tooth has been replanted, it is best to adopt a wait-and-see approach if in doubt about vitality. When pulp death has occurred, subsequent treatment depends on whether the apex is closed (p. 104) or open.

Root canal treatment of teeth with immature apices As achievement of an apical seal is difficult in a tooth with an open apex, the aim of treatment should be to allow apexification to continue. Under a rubber dam, the necrotic pulp should be extirpated. The working length is set 1–2 mm short of the radiographic apex (unless vital pulp tissue is encountered earlier) and narrow files are used to negotiate any undercuts. The canal should then be filled with a radiopaque non-setting calcium hydroxide, e.g., Reogan (alternatively, use the catalyst from Dycal), to the apex and sealed. The calcium hydroxide should be replaced every 3 months until a calcific apical barrier is detectable by gentle probing with a paper point. Then the canal can be filled. Usually, because of the width of the canal, a large GP cone (a conventional point upside down) is required. This should be warmed in a flame before pressing into place and then lots of laterally condensed points used to obtain a good seal. The average time for a calcific barrier to be formed is 9 months.[1] A 5-year survival rate of 86% has been reported.[2] Clinical experience would suggest that root canal treatment of incisors in children is often complicated by intractable infection of the canal. This may be due to the patency of the dentinal tubules. Polyantibiotic pastes can be tried, but a cheaper alternative is to crush metronidazole tablets with saline and place in the canal for 1 week.

Resorption (commonly seen after avulsion, luxation, intrusion, or extrusion)

Internal resorption is associated with chronic pulpal inflammation, which results in resorption of dentin from the pulpal surface. This is progressive, therefore the pulp needs to be carefully extirpated. Dressing the tooth with calcium hydroxide appears to help arrest the resorption and, once controlled, a GP filling may be placed. If perforation has occurred the prognosis is decreased considerably. Raising a flap, removal of granulation tissue, and placement of an amalgam seal are indicated.

External resorption Three types are seen: surface, replacement, and inflammatory (p. 111).

---

1 I. C. Mackie 1988 *Dental Update* **15** 155.
2 I. C. Mackie 1993 *BDJ* **175** 99.

Calcification occurs in 6–35% of luxation-type injuries. Prophylactic endodontic treatment is not necessary as pulp necrosis occurs in only 13–16% of cases. A high rate of success (80%) has been reported for subsequent root canal treatment, despite a hairline or no root canal detectable on radiograph.

Management of missing incisors

Upper central incisor Rarely congenitally absent; usually lost following trauma or because of dilaceration.

Upper lateral incisor Congenitally absent in approximately 2% of population (with likelihood of displacement of maxillary canine) but may also be lost following trauma.

Both can occur unilaterally, bilaterally, or together.

Missing upper anterior teeth are noticed by the general public before other types of malocclusion (e.g., overjet), so the aim of treatment is to provide a full smile. Although Cary Grant did well enough with a missing upper central incisor, symmetry is usually preferable. The management of missing incisors involves either recovery or maintenance of space for a prosthetic replacement, or orthodontic space closure. Nordquist[1] found that space closure was better aesthetically and periodontally than prosthetic replacement; however, with the introduction of newer materials and techniques, this finding may be outdated. For each patient a number of factors need to be considered:

Skeletal relationship In a Class III case, space closure in the upper arch could compromise the incisor relationship, whereas in a Class II/1 it would facilitate overjet reduction. Consider also the vertical relationship, as space closure is easier in patients with increased lower facial height and vice versa in decreased lower facial height.

Crowding/spacing In a patient with no crowding, space closure is difficult and requires prolonged retention. Before opening space it is important to ensure that sufficient space will be available at the end of treatment for an aesthetic replacement (minimum width for maxillary permanent lateral incisor is 5 mm), for which a Kesling setup is useful.

Color and form of adjacent teeth Although much can be done with composite additions and grinding, if the maxillary permanent canine is significantly darker and/or caniform in shape, it will be difficult to turn it into a convincing maxillary permanent lateral incisor if space closure is planned. The maxillary permanent lateral incisor can only be used to mimic the maxillary permanent central incisor if root length and circumference at gingival margin are not significantly shorter.

Inclination of adjacent teeth This will influence the type of appliance required to open or close the space. The final axial inclination of the teeth will determine the aesthetics of the finished result.

Buccal occlusion If a good buccal interdigitation exists, this may contraindicate bringing the posterior teeth forward to close space.

Unilateral loss A symmetrical result is more pleasing, therefore maintenance or opening of space is preferable. If a maxillary permanent lateral incisor is missing and the contralateral tooth is peg shaped, thought should be given to extracting this tooth to achieve symmetry.

1 G. G. Nordquist 1975 *J Periodont* **46** 139.

Gingival level can alter with periodontal surgery.

Patient's wishes and cooperation Only after assessing the above factors can the patient be given an informed choice. If the patient refuses fixed appliances this may alter the treatment plan.

Kesling set-up requires duplicate models of both arches, including at least two of the upper arch. Using a small hacksaw, the teeth that will require orthodontic movement are removed from the model and repositioned with wax. As many alternatives as desired can be tried to find the best result.

Space closure This can be facilitated by early extraction of the primary teeth on the affected side; therefore, the earlier the decision is made to close space, the better. This almost invariably involves the use of fixed appliances, because even though spontaneous space closure may occur in a crowded mouth, overcorrection of the axial inclination is advisable. It is better to carry out any masking procedures before orthodontic treatment, e.g., contouring maxillary permanent canine to resemble maxillary permanent lateral incisor (by removal of enamel incisally, interproximally, and from the palatal aspect and/or composite addition), as this will facilitate final positioning and occlusion. Retain with a bonded retainer.

The average difference in width between the maxillary permanent canine and maxillary permanent lateral incisor is 1.2 mm, which can easily be removed mesially and distally from the maxillary permanent canine. If the lower arch is crowded, extraction of a lower premolar will allow establishment of a Class I buccal segment relationship.

Space-maintenance/opening If an incisor is selectively extracted and space maintenance is desired, a partial denture or acid-etch bridge should be fitted immediately. Where a maxillary permanent lateral incisor is congenitally missing, this will not be possible and space may need to be opened orthodontically. The inclination of teeth to be moved will determine whether fixed or removable appliances will be required. Following tooth movement, retention with a partial denture for 3–6 months is advisable to allow teeth to settle. If an acid-etch retained prosthesis is planned, ensure that there is sufficient room occlusally for the wings.

Resin bonded bridge See p. 274.

Transplantation of a lower premolar into the socket of an extracted incisor can be considered if the lower arch is crowded.

Implant can be considered when growth is complete (p. 390).

Common childhood ailments affecting the mouth

▶ Refer any patient with an ulcer that doesn't heal within 3 weeks or with any soft-tissue lesion of unknown etiology for appropriate follow-up or biopsy.

See Chapter 9 (Oral Medicine).

The most common disease is gingivitis (p. 182).

Viral

Primary herpetic gingivostomatitis Occurs >6 months of age. Symptoms: febrile, cervical lymphadenitis, vesicles that turn into ulcers on gingiva and oral mucosa. Treatment: soft diet with plenty of fluids. Self-limiting, lasts for approximately 10 days.

Secondary herpes labialis Vesicles form around the lips, and crust. Self-limiting, but 5% acyclovir cream will speed healing.

Hand, foot, and mouth disease Rash on hands and feet plus ulcers on oral mucosa and gingiva. Little systemic upset. Self-limiting.

Herpangina Febrile illness with sore throat due to ulcers on soft palate and throat. Usually lasts about 3–5 days. Treatment: soft diet.

Warts Check hands. Usually self-limiting.

Also chickenpox (vesicles that turn into ulcers), mumps (inflamed parotid duct), glandular fever (ulcers), measles.

Bacterial

Impetigo Very infectious staphylococcal (and/or streptococci) rash. Starts around mouth and may be mistaken for secondary herpes.

Streptococcal sore throat Can contract associated streptococcal gingivitis.

Localized aggressive periodontitis (LAgP) Rare <16 years (p. 192).

Fungal

Candida Commissure of the mouth, which may become pathogenic when oral environment favors its proliferation. Two types of manifestation are seen in children.

Acute pseudomembraneous candidiasis (thrush) Seen in newborn, under-nourished infants after prolonged use of antibiotics or steroids. Presents as white patches that rub off. Treatment: miconazole (25mg/ml) and correct underlying problem.

Chronic atrophic candidiasis Most commonly with upper removable appliance and poor oral hygiene and/or high sugar intake. Treatment: oral hygiene instruction for appliance and teeth. Chlorhexidine mouthwash or miconazole gel.

Miscellaneous

- Aphthous ulceration,[1] p. 434.

Common causes of oral ulceration in children (in order of frequency) Aphthous; trauma; acute herpetic gingivostomatitis; herpangina; hand, foot, and mouth disease; glandular fever. If in doubt, refer.

Common causes of soft tissue swellings in children Abscess; mucocele; eruption cyst; epulides; papilloma.

▶ Oral cancer does occur in children, therefore if in doubt, refer to biopsy.

---

1 E. A. Field 1992 *Int J Paediatr Dent* **2** 1.

Sugar-free medications

The cariogenic effect of long-term medication sweetened with sugar is now well recognized. As the U.K. Medicines Commission has instructed that liquid formulations for use in chronic conditions in children should be free of cariogenic sugars, the future looks bright, particularly as progress has been made on the reformulation of commonly used drugs. Unfortunately, there is no evidence showing that rinsing out or brushing the teeth after use of a sugar-based medicine will significantly reduce the incidence of caries. Current medical advice is that liquid medicines be given to children by disposable syringes. This approach has the advantage that an accurate dose can be directed at the back of the mouth.

Below is a list of some sugar-free medicines. It is not exhaustive and where required, reference should be made to the most current *Physicians' Desk Reference*.

Analgesics

Aspirin (>12 years)	Chewable aspirin tablets
Tylenol	Oral suspension/tablets
Tylenol and codeine	Tylenol #3 elixir
Ibuprofen	Ibuprofen oral suspension 100 mg/ml

Antacids

Aluminum and magnesium	Maalox suspension
Cimetidine	Tagamet
Ranitidine	Zantac dispersible tablets
	Zantax suspension

Anticonvulsants

Carbamazepine	Tegretol liquid
Phenobarbitone	Phenobarbitone elixir 30 mg/10 ml
Sodium valproate	Depakene tablets/elixir

Anti-infectives

Acyclovir	Zovirax suspension
Amoxicillin	Amoxil dispersible tablets SF
	Amoxil sachets SF
Nystatin	Mycostatin
	oral suspension/lozenges
Ampicillin and cloxacillin	Ampiclox neonatal suspension
Sulfamethoxazole and	Bactrim dispersible tablets/SF
trimethoprim	syrup
	Dispersible co-trimoxazole tablets
	Chewable tablets/suspension
Erythromycin	Suspension/chewable tabs

Respiratory agents

Albuterol	Ventolin syrup/INH

Calculating drug dosages

Age (years)	Average weight (kg)	Percentage of adult dose
1	10	25
3	14	33
5	18	40
7	23	50
12	37	75

Orthodontics

Relevant pages in other chapters: Surgical management of CLP, p. 414; abnormalities of eruption, p. 65; supernumerary teeth, p. 66; orthognathic surgery, p. 416.

Further reading: British Orthodontic Society 1996 *Young Practitioners Guide to Orthodontics.* M. L. Jones and R. G. Oliver 1995 *Walther and Houston's Orthodontic Notes*, Wright. F. McDonald and A. J. Ireland *Diagnosis of the Orthodontic Patient*, OUP. W. R. Proffitt 2000 *Contemporary Orthodontics*, Mosby.

It has been said that orthodontists forget to ask the patient to open wide, thus missing any dental pathology, while generalists forget to ask the patient to close together, thus missing any malocclusion. The aim of this chapter is to help ensure that neither is the case. A problem-orientated approach has been used (rather than by classification) for simplicity.

What is orthodontics?

Orthodontics is defined by the American Association of Orthodontics (AAO) as the specialty area of dentistry concerned with the diagnosis, supervision, guidance, and correction of malocclusion. The formal name of the specialty is orthodontics and dentofacial orthopedics.

Prevalence of malocclusion in American children and youths (based on Angles' classification) Normal occlusion: approx. 30%; Class I malocclusion: approx. 50–55%; Class II malocclusion: approx. 15%; Class III: <1%.

Why provide orthodontic treatment? The main indications for orthodontic Rx are aesthetics and function. Functional reasons for Rx include crossbites (as associated occlusal interferences may tend to predispose toward temporomandibular disorders), deep traumatic overbite, increased overjet (increased risk of trauma), and labial crowding of a lower incisor (as this reduces periodontal support labially). While it is accepted that severe malocclusion may have a psychologically debilitating effect, the impact of more minor anomalies and, indeed, perceived need, are influenced by social and cultural factors. The Index of Orthodontic Treatment Need (IOTN) has been developed to try to standardize and quantify this difficult issue.

It is important that patients realize that orthodontic Rx is not without its risks. Even with good oral hygiene, a small loss of periodontal attachment and root resorption are common. In susceptible patients, this may be significant. With poor oral hygiene, greater loss of periodontal support and decalcification may result. In addition, injury from orthodontic appliances is not uncommon during treatment. Therefore, the potential benefit to the patient must be sufficient to counterbalance these risks. And, most importantly, the potential risks of orthodontic treatment should be addressed with informed consent.

Who should provide orthodontic treatment? All dentists should be concerned with growth and development. Unless anomalies are detected early and any necessary steps taken at the appropriate time, provision of the best possible outcome for that patient is less likely. It is estimated that orthodontic specialists treat almost two-thirds of orthodontic patients, with pediatric dentists treating less than 4%. Slightly less than one-third of all orthodontic patients appear to receive treatment from general practitioners. However, around 75% of general dentists provide orthodontic services, with around 20% providing comprehensive orthodontic treatment.

When should we begin orthodontic treatment? This depends on the particular anomaly. The AAO suggests that all children should get an orthodontic checkup no later than age 7. In the early mixed dentition, Rx is only indicated to correct severe skeletal discrepancy, prevent trauma to dentofacial tissues, and improve psychological issues. Most orthodontic Rx is not started until the permanent dentition has erupted. Rx during the early teens is preferable because the response to orthodontic forces is more rapid, appliances are better tolerated, and, most importantly, growth may be used to help the treatment. In adults, lack of growth, greater risk of periodontal loss, worn, damaged, and missing teeth, and slower tooth movement lead to a new challenge in orthodontic Rx.

Adult orthodontic Rx is usually included in a comprehensive treatment plan involving general practitioners and various specialties. But because of the increased acceptability of appliances, more adults are seeking Rx. It is estimated, one in five orthodontic patients is an adult.

▶ If in doubt, refer a patient earlier rather than later, especially in cases with marked skeletal discrepancies.

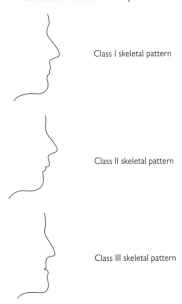

Class I skeletal pattern

Class II skeletal pattern

Class III skeletal pattern

The Index of Orthodontic Treatment Need (IOTN)

The IOTN was developed to quantify and standardize an individual patient's need for orthodontic Rx, so that the potential benefits can be weighed against the possible risks.[1] The Index consists of two components, the dental health and esthetic components.

The dental health component was developed from an index used by the Swedish Dental Health Board (which was used to determine the amount of financial help that would be given by the state toward Rx costs). The Dental Health Component of IOTN (reproduced by kind permission of VUMAN, Ltd) has five categories of Rx need, ranging from little need to very great need. A patient's grade is determined by recording the single worst feature of their malocclusion.

The esthetic component is based on a series of 10 photographs of the labial aspect of different class I or class II malocclusions, which are ranked according to their attractiveness. A patient's score is determined by the photograph, which is deemed to have an equivalent degree of esthetic impairment.

The Index of Orthodontic Treatment Need

Grade 1 (None)
1   Extremely minor malocclusions including displacements <1 mm

Grade 2 (Little)
2a   Increased overjet (o/j) 3.6–6 mm with competent lips
2b   Reverse overjet 0.1–1 mm
2c   Anterior or posterior crossbite (Xbite) with up to 1 mm discrepancy between retruded contact position and intercuspal position
2d   Displacement of teeth 1.1–2 mm
2e   Anterior or posterior openbite 1.1–2 mm
2f   Increased overbite 3.5 mm or more, without gingival contact
2g   Pre-normal or post-normal occlusions with no other anomalies. Includes up to half a unit discrepancy.

Grade 3 (Moderate)
3a   Increased overjet 3.6–6 mm with incompetent lips
3b   Reverse overjet 1.1–3.5 mm
3c   Anterior or posterior crossbites with 1.1–2 mm discrepancy
3d   Displacement of teeth 2.1–4 mm
3e   Lateral or anterior openbite 2.1–4 mm
3f   Increased and complete overbite without gingival trauma

---

1 W. C. Shaw 1991 *BDJ* **170** 107.

Grade 4 (Great)

4a Increased overjet 6.1–9 mm

4b Reversed overjet >3.5 mm with no masticatory or speech difficulties

4c Anterior or posterior crossbites with >2 mm discrepancy between retruded contact position and intercuspal position

4d Severe displacement of teeth, >4 mm

4e Extreme lateral or anterior openbites, >4 mm

4f Increased and complete overbite with gingival or palatal trauma

4h Less extensive hypodontia requiring pre-restorative orthodontic space closure to obviate the need for a prosthesis

4l Posterior lingual crossbite with no functional occlusal contact in one or both buccal segments

4m Reverse overjet 1.1–3.5 mm with recorded masticatory and speech difficulties

4t Partially erupted teeth, tipped and impacted against adjacent teeth

4x Supplemental teeth

Grade 5 (Very great)

5a Increased overjet >9 mm

5h Extensive hypodontia with restorative implications (more than one tooth missing in any quadrant) requiring pre-restorative orthodontics

5i Impeded eruption of teeth (with the exception of third molars) due to crowding, displacement, presence of supernumerary teeth, retained deciduous teeth, and any pathological cause

5m Reverse overjet >3.5 mm with reported masticatory and speech difficulties

5p Defects of cleft lip and palate

5s Submerged deciduous teeth

Definitions

Ideal occlusion Anatomically perfect arrangement of the teeth. Rare.

Normal occlusion Acceptable variation from ideal occlusion.

Competent lips Lips meet with <2 mm of interlabial gap at rest.

Incompetent lips Lips meet with >2 mm of interlabial gap at rest.

Frankfort plane Line joining porion (superior aspect of external auditory meatus) with orbitale (lowermost point of bony orbit).

Lower facial height (LFH) Clinically it is the distance from the base of the nose to the point of the chin, and in a normally proportioned face is equal to the middle facial third (eyebrow line to base of nose). Cephalometrically, it is the distance from anterior nasal spine to menton as a percentage of the total face height (from nasion to menton).

Angle's Class I malocclusion Normal relationship of molars (the mesio-buccal cusp of the upper first molar occludes in the buccal groove of the lower first molar) with incorrect line of occlusion.

Angle's Class II malocclusion The mesiobuccal cusp of the upper first molar occludes mesially to the buccal groove of the lower first molar.

   Division I the upper central incisors are upright or proclined and the overjet is increased.

   Division 2 The upper central incisors are retroclined and the overjet is usually normal.

Angle's Class III malocclusion The mesiobuccal cusp of the upper first molar occludes distally to the buccal groove of the lower first molar.

Bimaxillary proclination Both upper and lower incisors are proclined.

Overjet Distance between the upper and lower incisors in the horizontal plane.

Overbite Overlap of the incisors in the vertical plane.

Complete overbite The lower incisors contact the upper incisors or the palatal mucosa.

Incomplete overbite The lower incisors do not contact the upper incisors or the palatal mucosa.

Anterior open bite When the patient is viewed from the front and the teeth are in occlusion, a space can be seen between the upper and lower incisor edges.

Crossbite A deviation from the normal buccolingual relationship. May be anterior/posterior and/or unilateral/bilateral.

Buccal crossbite Buccal cusps of lower premolars or molars occlude buccally to the buccal cusps of the upper premolars or molars.

Lingual crossbite Buccal cusps of lower molars occlude lingually to the lingual cusps of the upper molars.

Dentoalveolar compensation The position of the teeth has compensated for by the underlying skeletal pattern, so that the occlusal relationship between the arches is less severe.

Leeway space The difference in diameter between teeth C, D, E, and teeth 3, 4, 5. Greater in lower than upper arch.

Mandibular displacement When closing from the rest position, the mandible displaces (either laterally or anteriorly) to avoid a premature contact.

Balancing extraction Extraction of the same (or adjacent) tooth on the opposite side of the arch to preserve symmetry.

Compensating extraction Extraction of the same tooth in the opposite arch.

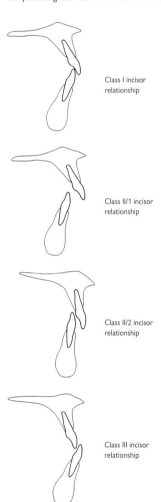

Class I incisor
relationship

Class II/1 incisor
relationship

Class II/2 incisor
relationship

Class III incisor
relationship

Orthodontic assessment

Equipment A mirror, a probe, a small ruler, and sharp eyes.

Brief screening procedure

The purpose is to ensure early detection and Rx of any abnormality, prepare the patient for any later Rx, and influence the management of any teeth of poor prognosis.

At every visit Once the permanent incisors have erupted and until permanent dentition is established (if in doubt, refer).

1 Keep the eruption sequence in mind (p. 64). Any deviations from this should be observed for a few months only and then investigated.

2 Failure of a tooth to appear >6 months after the contralateral tooth has erupted should ring alarm bells.

3 Ask child to close together and look for crossbites, reverse or increased overjet.

Consider the long-term prognosis of the first permanent molars (p. 140).

From age 9 and until they erupt, palpate for $\underline{3}$ in the buccal sulcus. A definite hollow and/or asymmetry warrants further investigation.

Detailed orthodontic examination

This should be carried out in a logical sequence so that nothing is missed.

- Who wants Rx (patient or parent) and what for?
- What complexity of Rx is patient prepared to accept? Have the patient's peers worn braces and if not, will the child make a good pioneer?
- Enquire about any previous extractions and orthodontic Rx.

Extraoral examination (with Frankfort plane horizontal)

- Assess skeletal pattern:
  1 anteroposteriorly (? convex, straight, or concave profiles);
  2 vertically (Frankfort–mandibular planes angle approx. 26°, lower 1/3 face usually 55% of total face height);
  3 transversely (? asymmetry).
- Soft tissues: Lips are only competent if they meet at rest or <2 mm opening at rest. Check the position of the lower lip relative to the incisors and how the patient achieves an oral seal (? lip to lip, lip to tongue, or by the lower lip being drawn up behind the incisors). Note also the length of the upper lip, the amount of incisors seen, and lip tonicity.
- Check rest position of mandible and for any displacement on closure.
- Habits? Does patient suck a thumb/finger, bite fingernails, or brux?

Intraoral examination

- Record OH, gingival condition, and teeth present. Any of poor prognosis?
- Lower anterior teeth: Inclination to mandibular base, crowding/spacing, displaced teeth, angulation of $\overline{3|3}$.
- Upper labial segment (ULS): Inclination to maxillary base, crowding/spacing, rotations, displaced teeth, presence and angulation of $\underline{3|3}$.

- Measure o/j (mm), o/b (increase or decrease, complete or incomplete). Check dental midline lines coincident and correct within face.
- Buccal segments: crowding/spacing, displaced teeth.
- Check molar and canine relationship. Any Xbites?

X-rays Usually require a panoramic radiograph and, if not clearly visible on the panoramic radiograph, an intraoral of the incisors. A lateral skull view is indicated if the patient has a skeletal discrepancy or anteroposterior (AP) movement of the incisors is anticipated.

- Look for unerupted, missing, or supernumerary teeth, root resorption, or other pathology.
- Cephalometric analysis, p. 130.

Summary should include a description of the patient's incisor relationship and skeletal pattern, and the main points of the malocclusion, e.g., crowding, Xbites. This gives a "problem list" from which the aims of Rx can be derived (p. 134).

Study models are not obligatory for orthodontic Rx, but they certainly help. Taking models allows you to mull over the possibilities at leisure and more accurately assess space requirements. Unless the malocclusion deteriorates, if no Rx is planned, give the models to the patient, who will usually guard them well.

▶ It is important to take models before and after orthodontic Rx so that progress can be monitored as well as for medicolegal purposes.

Overjet   Overbite

Cephalometrics

Cephalometric analysis is the interpretation of lateral skull radiographs. It is not obligatory for orthodontic Rx. Where no AP change in incisor position is planned, the X-ray exposure is not justified for the information gained. However, where AP movement is required, a lateral skull radiograph will back up the clinical assessment of skeletal pattern and help to determine the degree of difficulty and type of appliance indicated. Serial lateral skulls allow assessment of growth.

Tracing

Tracing paper (secured to the film with masking tape), a sharp pencil (a 0.5 mm mechanical pencil is ideal), and good background illumination are essential. Spotting orthodontic landmarks is infinitely easier if carried out in a darkened room. If a point is hard to see, block off the rest of the film so that only that area is illuminated. If this fails, try holding film up to a bright spotlight, but if still not clear, make a guesstimate! Due to the slight magnification (7–8%), two images of the mandibular border are usually seen. Both should be traced and an average taken for gonion. The most prominent image should be traced, i.e., the most anterior in the face so that the difficulty of Rx is not underestimated.

Pitfalls

- Consider the cephalometric values for a particular patient in conjunction with the clinical assessment, as variation from the normal in a measurement may be compensated for elsewhere in the face or cranial base.
- Angle ANB varies with the relative prominence of nasion and the lower face. If SNA angle is significantly increased or decreased, this could be due to the position of nasion, in which case an additional analysis should be used, e.g., Wits analysis.
- For landmarks that are bilateral (unless superimposed exactly) the midpoint between the two should be taken to correspond with those reference points in the midline.
- Tracing errors—with careful technique these should be of the order of ± 0.5° and 0.5 mm. Errors are compounded when comparing tracings, therefore, changes of 1° or 2° should be interpreted with caution.

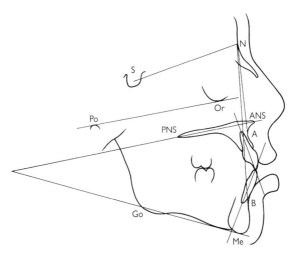

Most commonly used cephalometric points:

S = Sella: midpoint of sella turcica
N = Nasion: most anterior point on frontonasal suture
Or = Orbitale: most inferior anterior point on margin of orbit (take average of two images)
Po = Porion: uppermost outermost point on bony external auditory meatus
ANS = Anterior nasal spine
PNS = Posterior nasal spine
Go = Gonion: most posterior inferior point on angle of mandible
Me = Menton: lowermost point on the mandibular symphysis
A = A point: position of deepest concavity on anterior profile of maxilla
B = B point: position of deepest concavity on anterior profile of mandibular symphysis

Frankfort plane = Po–Or.
Maxillary plane = PNS–ANS.
Mandibular plane = Go–Me.

More cephalometrics

Analysis and interpretation

The analysis of lateral skull tracings is carried out by comparing a number of angular measurements and proportions with average values for the population as a whole. Normal values for Caucasians (Steiner analysis[1] as an example), standard deviations in parentheses, are as follows:

SNA	= 82° (±3.9°)
SNB	= 80° (±3.6°)
ANB	= 2° (±1.8°)
1-NA	= 22°; 4 mm
1-NB	= 25°; 4 mm
Interincisal angle	= 131° (±9.2°)

If SNA or SNB are more than 3 standard deviations from the normal, check your tracing! However, the ANB difference is not an infallible assessment of skeletal pattern as it assumes (incorrectly in some cases) that there is no discrepancy in the cranial base and that A and B are indicative of basal bone position. When a cephalometric tracing seems at odds with your clinical impression, it is worth doing another analysis that avoids reliance on the cranial base, such as a Wits analysis.

Before deciding on a Rx plan, it is helpful to consider what factors have contributed to a particular malocclusion, e.g., in a patient with a Class II/1 incisor relationship on a Class I skeletal pattern, the prognosis for Rx is much better if the increased o/j is due to proclination of the upper rather than retroclination of the lower incisors. The relative contribution of the maxilla and mandible to the skeletal pattern may indicate possible lines of Rx; e.g., if an increased o/j is due to a retrusive mandible, a better aesthetic result may be achieved by use of a functional appliance.

As a rough guide, assume that there is 2.5° of angular movement for every millimeter of linear movement of the incisor edge.

---

1 C. C. Steiner 1953 *Am J Orthod* **39** 729.

Wits analysis

This is used to assess AP skeletal pattern.

Method

- Construct the functional occlusal plane (FOP) by drawing a line through the cusp tips of the molars and premolars or deciduous molars.
- Drop perpendiculars to the FOP from A point (to give AO) and B point (to give BO).
- Measure the distance from AO to BO.

In Class I AP relationship

Males: BO is 1 mm (±1.9 mm) ahead of AO; females: BO = AO (±1.77 mm).

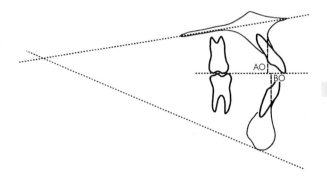

Treatment planning

Problem list Following the assessment of the patient a summary should be made of the main features of the malocclusion (p. 128). The problem list can then be drawn up—e.g.,

1 Crowding
2 Posterior crossbite
3 Increased overjet

Aims of Rx This is derived from the above problem list—e.g.,

1 Relieve crowding
2 Correct crossbite
3 Align arches
4 Maintain overbite
5 Reduce overjet

Plan lower arch The lower arch lies in a zone of stability between the lips, cheeks, and tongue; thus, it is safer to consider it as immutable. This gives a starting point around which to plan Rx. The first step is to decide if the lower arch is sufficiently crowded to warrant extractions. If the crowding is likely to increase (patient in early teens, $\overline{8/8}$ present), then extractions may be indicated (p. 138). In Class II/2 cases it may be advisable to accept a little crowding (p. 149). If in doubt, refer for advice.

Plan upper arch In most cases planning will be to a Class I incisor and buccal segment relationship. Thus, it may be helpful, in the mind's eye, to correct the upper canine into a Class I relationship with $\overline{3}$ (in corrected position if lower anterior teeth are crowded). This will give an indication of the space required and the amount and type of movement necessary. In the upper arch space for retraction of $\underline{3}$ can be gained by (1) extractions, (2) expansion (only indicated if Xbite exists), (3) distal movement of the upper buccal segments (p. 141), (4) a combination of these. Should extractions be indicated in both arches, mechanics are often easier if the same tooth is extracted in the upper as in the lower arch. However, in Class II cases it may be advantageous to extract further forward in the upper arch and vice versa in Class III.

Final Rx plan The next step is to plan what tooth movements need to be carried out, including which appliances are to be used and in what sequence. For example, if distal movement is to be carried out it may be wise to fit the headgear first and reassess before embarking on extractions. Retention of the final result also needs to be included in the Rx plan, especially when the Rx is being explained to the patient and consent sought.

The practicalities of providing Rx also warrant consideration. In some cases more than one Rx plan can be offered to the patient, with a hierarchy of complexity and finished result. If a compromise plan is chosen by the patient this should be noted in their records.

The final plan for the example above may be:
- Quad helix appliance to expand upper arch
- Extraction of all four first premolars
- Lower fixed appliance

- Upper fixed appliance once crossbite corrected
- Reduce overjet.
- Retain corrected tooth movements.

Prognosis Will the proposed Rx be stable? Beware of o/j change in a patient with grossly incompetent lips, or proclination of upper incisors in a Class III where there is no o/b to hold the corrected position.

Consent The risks and benefits of the proposed plan should be carefully explained to the patient and parent. It is advisable to get written consent, including for specific details of the Rx.

▶ *Beware* if the malocclusion under consideration contains one of the following features:

- Marked skeletal discrepancy, anteroposteriorly (II or III), or vertically
- If the o/j is increased and the upper incisors are upright
- If the o/j is reversed and there is no o/b to retain correction of the incisor relationship
- Severe Class II/2 malocclusions
- Class II/I incisor relationship, with molars a full unit Class II and a crowded lower arch

Rx planning is the most important, and most difficult, part of orthodontics.

Management of the developing dentition

See also delayed eruption, p. 65.

The way in which mixed dentition problems are approached will often affect the ease or difficulty of subsequent Rx.

Normal development of dentition The deciduous incisors are usually upright and spaced. If there is no spacing warn the parents that the permanent incisors will probably be crowded. Overbite reduces throughout the deciduous dentition until the incisors are edge to edge. All permanent incisors develop lingual to their predecessors, erupt into a wider arc, and are more proclined. It is normal for 1|1 to erupt with a median diastema that reduces as 2|2 erupt. Later, pressure from the developing canines on the roots of 2|2 results in their being tilted distally and spaced. This has been called the "ugly duckling stage," but it is better to describe it as normal development to parents. As the 3 erupts the 2 becomes upright and the spaces usually close.

Most Es erupt so that their distal edges are flush. The transition to the normal stepped (Class I) molar relationship usually occurs during the deciduous dentition as a result of greater mandibular growth and/or the leeway space.

Development of dental arches In the average child, the size of the dental arch is more or less established once the deciduous dentition has erupted, except for an increase in intercanine width (2–3 mm up to age 9), which results in a modification of arch shape.

Retained deciduous teeth If deflecting eruption of permanent tooth, extract.

Submerging deciduous molars Prevalence: 8–14%. Provided there is a successor, a submerged deciduous molar will probably be exfoliated at the same time as the contralateral tooth.[1] Extraction is only indicated if there is no successor or the submerged tooth is likely to disappear below the gingival margin.

Impacted upper first permanent molars Prevalence: 2–6%. This is indicative of crowding. Spontaneous disimpaction is rare after 8 years. Attempt to dislodge 6 by tightening a piece of brass wire around the contact point with E over several visits. Otherwise, just observe, extracting E if unavoidable and dealing with resultant space loss in the permanent dentition.

Habits Effects produced depend on duration of habit and intensity. It is best not to make a great fuss of a finger-sucking habit. If parents are concerned, reassure them (in presence of the child) not to worry, as only little girls and boys suck their fingers. Appliances to break the habit may help, but most children will stop when they are ready. However, this is no reason to delay the start of Rx for other aspects of the malocclusion.

1 J. Kurol 1985 *Am J Orthod* **87** 46.

Effects of premature loss of deciduous teeth

Unfortunately, when a child presents with a toothache, in the rush to relieve pain it is all too easy to extract the offending tooth without consideration of the consequences. The major effect of early deciduous tooth loss is localization of crowding in crowded mouths. The extent to which this occurs depends on the patient's age, degree of crowding, and the site. In a crowded mouth the adjacent teeth will move around into the extraction space, thus, unilateral loss of a C (and, to a lesser degree, a D) will result in a center-line shift. This is also seen when a C is prematurely exfoliated by an erupting 2. As correction of a center-line discrepancy often involves fixed appliances, prevention is better than cure, so loss of Cs should always be balanced. If Es are lost the 6 will migrate forward. This is particularly marked if it occurs before eruption of the permanent tooth, so if extraction of an E is unavoidable, try to defer until after the 6s are in occlusion and do not balance or compensate. The effect of early loss of deciduous teeth on the eruption of the permanent successor is variable.

Timely loss of Cs is indicated for

- $\underline{2}$ erupting palatally due to crowding. Extraction of $\underline{C|C}$ as the $\underline{2}$ erupting may allow the tooth to escape labially and prevent a Xbite.
- Extraction of $\overline{C|C}$ when a lower incisor is being crowded labially will help to reduce loss of periodontal support.

Extractions

In orthodontics, teeth are extracted to either relieve crowding or provide space to compensate for a skeletal discrepancy.

▶ Before planning the extraction of any permanent teeth a thorough orthodontic and radiographic examination should be carried out.

▶ In a Class I or II, the extraction should be at least as far forward in the upper arch as the lower; vice versa in a Class III.

Lower incisors Following the extraction of an incisor, the lower anterior teeth tend to tilt lingually followed by the upper anterior teeth. In addition, it is difficult to arrange 6 upper anterior teeth around 5 lower anterior teeth. However, if indicated, they will need fixed appliances.

Upper incisors are never the teeth of choice for extraction, but if traumatized or dilacerated, there may be no alternative (p. 114).

Lower canines should only be extracted if severely displaced, as the resulting contact between $\overline{2}\,\overline{4}$ is unsatisfactory.

Upper canines See p. 143.

First premolars are the most popular choice, because of their position in the arch and a good contact point between the canine and second premolar is more likely. For maximum spontaneous improvement, 4s should be extracted just as the 3s are appearing, but if appliance therapy is planned, defer until the canines have erupted.

Second premolars are preferred in cases with mild crowding, as their extraction alters the anchorage balance, favoring space closure by forward movement of the molars. Fixed appliances are required, especially in the lower arch. If 5s are hypoplastic or missing there may be no choice. Early loss of an E will often lead to forward movement of the 6 and lack of space for 5s. In the upper arch this results in $\underline{5}$ being displaced palatally, and provided $\underline{4}$ is in a satisfactory position, extraction of $\underline{5}$ on eruption may reduce the need for appliance therapy. In the lower arch 5s are usually crowded lingually. Extraction of $\overline{2}$ is easier and will give $\overline{5}$ space to grow upright spontaneously.

First permanent molars See p. 140.

Second permanent molars Extraction of $\overline{7}$ will not alleviate incisor crowding but may relieve mild lower premolar crowding and avoid difficult extraction of impacted $\overline{8}$.

To increase the likelihood of $\overline{8}$ erupting successfully to replace $\overline{7}$, posterior crowding is needed and $\overline{8}$ formed to bifurcation and at an angle of between 15° and 30° to long axis $\overline{6}$. Even so, appliance therapy may still be required to align $\overline{8}$ on eruption.

In the upper arch extraction of $\underline{7}$ is often limited to facilitating distal movement of the upper buccal segments.

Third permanent molars Early extraction of these teeth used to be advocated to prevent lower anterior teeth from crowding, but as crowding can occur even in their absence, wisdom teeth are only a part of the etiology. In addition, extraction of symptomless $\overline{8}$ is not advisable.

Space can also be provided in selected cases by
1 expansion (only in upper arch with a Xbite, otherwise not stable);
2 distal movement of the upper buccal segment (p. 141);
3 reducing the width of the teeth interproximally (usually limited to lower anterior teeth in selected cases).

Extraction of the first permanent molars

First permanent molars are never the first choice for extraction, as even if they are removed at the optimal time, a good spontaneous alignment of the remaining teeth is unlikely. However, when a two-surface (or more) restoration is required in a molar tooth for a child, the long-term prognosis should be considered. A well-timed extraction may be better for the child than heroic attempts to restore hopeless molars. Equally good is placing a dressing and maintaining a poor-quality 6 until the 7 has erupted and the extraction can be incorporated into an orthodontics plan. Points to note are the following:

- Check to see that the remaining teeth are present and in a good position. If not, avoid extraction of 6 in affected quadrant.
- In the lower arch good spontaneous alignment is more likely following extraction 6̄ if **1** 7̄|7̄ development has reached bifurcation; **2** angulation between crypt 7̄ and 6̄ is <30°; **3** 7̄|7̄ crypts overlap 6̄|6̄ roots.
- There is a greater tendency for mesial drift in the maxilla, thus, the timing of loss of 6̲ is less critical.
- Assess the prognosis for remaining 6s. If they are all restored then extraction of all four is probably indicated. If there is only one poor 6̲, do not extract the corresponding lower tooth. If 6̄ has a poor prognosis, it is advisable to extract the opposing 6̲ as otherwise this tooth will overerupt and prevent 7̄ from moving forward. Balancing extraction with a corresponding sound 6̄ is inadvisable; it is better to deal with the other side of the arch on its own merit.
- In Class I with anterior crowding and Class II, 6|6 should, if possible, be preserved until 7|7 have erupted, and can be held back by an appliance and the extraction space utilized.
- In Class III, if 6̲|6̲ has a poor prognosis, try to preserve it until incisor relationship is corrected (to provide retention for appliance). In cases with poor-quality 6̲|6̲, extract at optimal time to aid space closure.
- If the dentition is not crowded, avoid extraction of 6s, as space closure will be difficult.
- Extraction of 6s will relieve buccal segment crowding, but will have little effect on labial segment crowding. Impaction of 8s is less likely but not impossible.

▶ In a child with poor-quality 6s, remember that the premolars may well be in a similar condition 6 years later unless the caries rate is stabilized.

Distal movement of the upper buccal segments

This is usually thought of as an alternative to extraction, but in practice often results in the crowding being shifted distally, requiring the loss of 7̱ or 8̱. It is only applicable to the upper arch in the following situations:

- Either Class I with mild upper-arch crowding, or Class II/1 with well-aligned lower arch and molars <1 unit Class II.
- Where extraction of 4|4 does not provide sufficient space to align upper arch.

It can be achieved either by a mini-implant, or more often by headgear directly to molar bands on 6|6. As 6|6 move distally, they will need some expansion. There will be a greater chance of success with a growing child. A 1/2 unit change can be expected in 3–4 months with good cooperation. If unilateral distal movement is necessary, extraction of 7̱ on that side can be considered (provided 8̱ is in good position).

Headgear safety

There have been a number of cases where damage to the eye from wearing headgear has resulted in loss of vision. For this reason, headgear should only be used by those who have received training to avoid injury to the face. It should only be used in conjunction with safety mechanisms that prevent displacement and/or recoil of the facebow. If eye injury should occur, immediate referral to an ophthalmologist is required.

Spacing

Generalized spacing is due to either hypodontia or small teeth and/or large jaws. Note that hypodontia is associated with small teeth (p. 60). Rx of spacing is problematic; a purely orthodontic approach is liable to relapse and requires prolonged retention. In milder cases try and encourage the patient to accept the situation. In more severe cases a combined restorative/orthodontic approach will be required. This may involve composite additions or veneers to increase the width of the teeth and/or orthodontics to localize the space for provision of a prosthesis.

Median diastema

Prevalence 6-yr-olds = 98%, 11-yr-olds = 49%, 12- to 18-yr-olds = 7%.

Etiology Small teeth in large jaws; absent or peg-shaped 2|2; midline super-numerary; proclination of ULS; physiological (caused by pressure of developing teeth on upper incisor roots that resolves as 3 erupts); or a frenum.

The upper incisive frenum is attached to the incisive papilla at birth. As 1|1 erupt the frenum recedes, but this is less likely if the arch is spaced. A frenum contributes to a diastema in a small number of cases and is associated with the following features:
• Blanching of incisive papilla may occur when frenum is put under tension.
• Radiographically there is a V-shaped notch in the interdental bone between 1|1, indicating the attachment of the frenum.
• Anterior teeth may be crowded.

Management Always take a periapical X-ray to exclude presence of a supernumerary.
• Before 3 has erupted: if diastema <3 mm—review after eruption of canines, as it will probably resolve unaided. If >3 mm—may need to approximate incisors to provide space for canines to erupt, but care is required not to resorb roots of 2|2 against crowns of 3|3. Usually requires fixed appliance and prolonged retention.
• After 3 has erupted: orthodontic closure will require prolonged reten-tion as there is a high tendency to relapse. If frenum is undoubtedly a major etiological factor, perform a frenectomy during closure, but retention is still wise. Alternatively, measure width of 1 2, and if they are narrower than average (1 = 8.5 mm, 2 = 6.5 mm), consider composite additions or veneers to close space. If teeth are of normal width and no other orthodontic Rx is required, try talking patient into accepting their diastema.

Buccally displaced maxillary canines

▶ Width $\underline{3}$ > width $\underline{4}$ > width $\underline{C}$.

$\underline{3}$ is usually the last tooth to erupt anterior to $\underline{6}$. If the upper arch is crowded, $\underline{3}$ may be squeezed buccal to its normal position, in which case space needs to be created for its alignment. Usually $\underline{4}$ is the tooth of choice for extraction and, if so, this should be carried out just as $\underline{3}$ is about to erupt. If there is plenty of space it is sufficient to keep the patient under review, otherwise, fit a space-maintainer.

Where $\underline{2}$ and $\underline{4}$ are in contact, extraction of $\underline{4}$ alone will not provide sufficient space to accommodate the canine, and thought should be given to extracting $\underline{3}$.

Less commonly, a canine may develop well forward over the root of $\underline{2}$. In this case orthodontic Rx to align $\underline{3}$ will be prolonged. If the arch is crowded it may be simpler to extract $\underline{3}$ and align remaining teeth.

Alignment of mesially inclined, buccally displaced canines can, if they are the only Rx required, be accomplished by upper removable appliance, otherwise use fixed appliance.

Transposition almost exclusively involves a canine tooth. In the maxilla $\underline{3}$ is usually transposed with $\underline{4}$ and in the mandible the lateral incisor is more commonly involved. Rx options include alignment of teeth in transposed position, extraction of the most displaced tooth, or correction if transposition is not complete.

Palatally displaced maxillary canines

▶ Early detection is essential.
▶ Width $\underline{3}$ > width $\underline{4}$ > width $\underline{C}$.

Prevalence Up to 2%. Occurs bilaterally in 17–25% of cases. F > M.

Etiology In normal development the maxillary canine develops palatal to $\underline{C}$ and then migrates labially to erupt down the distal aspect of $\underline{2}$ root. The etiology of palatal displacement is not fully understood, but some suggest that a lack of guidance is the reason behind the association with missing or short-rooted $\underline{2}$.[1] Others argue that it is an inherited polygenic trait and that the link with missing or short-rooted $\underline{2}$ is part of an association with other dental anomalies including microdontia and hypodontia.[2]

Prevention Early detection may allow corrective interceptive Rx, therefore, when examining any child >9 years, palpate for unerupted $\underline{3}$. If there is a definite hollow and/or asymmetry between sides, further investigation is warranted. Extraction of $\underline{C}$ may result in improvement of a displaced $\underline{3}$,[3] but this eliminates the possibility of maintaining $\underline{C}$ should sufficient improvement in the position of $\underline{3}$ not materialize. Thus, confine extraction to those cases where the $\underline{3}$ is not too far displaced. More markedly displaced 3 should be referred to a specialist.

Assessment Clinically by palpation and from inclination of $\underline{2}$ and by X-rays. A panoramic radiograph and an intraoral view or two intraoral views with tube shift can be used to assess the position of the canine by parallax (p. 17 remember your precision apex locator [PAL] goes with you!). Consider also the position and prognosis of adjacent teeth (including $\underline{C}$), the malocclusion, and available space.

Management If the canine is only very slightly palatally displaced or impacted between $\underline{2}$ and $\underline{4}$, provision of space should result in eruption. Most palatally displaced canines, however, do not erupt spontaneously, so hopeful watching and waiting may only result in an older patient who is less willing to undergo the prolonged Rx required to align the displaced tooth. Rx alternatives available include the following:
1 Interceptive extraction of $\underline{C}$ in mixed dentition (see above).
2 Maintain $\underline{C}$ and keep unerupted canine under radiographic review. Provided there is no evidence of cystic change or resorption, removal of $\underline{3}$ can be left until GA required, e.g., for extraction of 8s. The patient must understand that $\underline{C}$ will eventually be lost, necessitating a prosthesis.
3 No Rx, if $\underline{2}$ and $\underline{4}$ are in contact and appearance is satisfactory, or if patient refuses other options. Again, $\underline{3}$ will require removal in due course.

1 A. Becker 1981 *Angle Orthodontist* **51** 24.
2 S. Peck 1994 *Angle Orthodontist* **64** 249.
3 S. Ericson 1988 *Eur J Orthod* **10** 283.

4 Exposure and orthodontic alignment is only feasible if (a) canine is in a favorable position for orthodontic alignment; (b) there is sufficient space available for 3, or space can be created; (c) the patient is willing to undergo surgery and prolonged orthodontic Rx (usually 2+ yr). The sequence is to arrange exposure and allow tooth to erupt for 3 months, and then commence orthodontic traction to move tooth toward arch. Fixed appliances are required.

5 Transplantation is not an instant solution, as space is needed to accommodate 3, which may involve appliances and/or extractions. Poor long-term results have been reported, e.g., only 1/3 still functional after 10 yr.[1] However, shorter splinting times (1–2 weeks) and root canal treatment for teeth with closed apices within 3 weeks of transplantation may improve prognosis.

Resorption Unerupted and impacted canines can cause resorption of incisor roots. For this to occur, a "head-on" collision between the two seems to be required. If detected on X-ray, a specialist opinion should be sought, and quickly. Extraction of the canine may be necessary to limit resorption, but if extensive, removal of the affected incisor may be preferable, thus allowing the canine to erupt.

1 J. P. Moss 1975 *Br J Oral Surg* **12** 268.

Increased overjet

When is an o/j increased? This is really a matter of opinion, but provided the arches are well-aligned, an o/j <6 mm is acceptable. If Rx is required for other reasons, consider reduction of o/j >4 mm.

Etiology

Skeletal pattern Increased o/j can occur in association with Class I, II, or even III skeletal patterns. If Class II, it is often due to a normally sized mandible being positioned posteriorly on the cranial base. Be wary of patients with vertical proportions at either extreme of the range, as they are difficult to treat.

Soft tissues The effects of the soft tissues are usually determined by the skeletal pattern, as the greater the discrepancy the less likely it is that the patient will have competent lips. Where the lips are incompetent, the way an anterior oral seal is achieved will influence incisor position—e.g., if the lower lip is drawn up behind the upper incisors this may have contributed to the increased o/j, but if the incisors can be retracted within control of the lower lip at the end of Rx the prognosis for stable o/j reduction is good. This is less likely if the LFH is increased and the lower lip lies beneath the upper incisors, as it will be less likely to control their position following o/j reduction. The soft tissues can also help to compensate for the skeletal pattern by proclining the lower and/or retroclining the upper incisors.

Dental crowding may contribute to an increased o/j, therefore, relief of crowding may aid stability. Digit-sucking can cause proclination of the upper and retroclination of the lower incisors, but in a growing child this will resolve once the habit is stopped unless maintained by adverse soft-tissue activity.

In most cases the skeletal pattern will determine ease of Rx, but the soft tissues will influence the stability of the end result.

Stability of overjet reduction

Provided the incisors have been retracted to a position of balance within the lower lip, this should not be a problem. Nevertheless, a period of retention is usually necessary to allow for periodontal-fiber and soft-tissue adaptation. However, prolonged retention will not make stable an inherently unstable position. A common mistake is to stop Rx before o/j reduction is complete and the lips are competent. If the patient returns to retracting the lower lip behind the upper anterior teeth to achieve an anterior oral seal, the o/j is likely to increase.

Management of increased overjet

(See also Functional appliances, p. 166.)

Principles
1 Provision of space for o/j reduction and/or relief of crowding
2 Reduce o/b before o/j reduction (p. 149)
3 Appliance is required to reduce o/j
4 Consider stability of treated result and plan retention.

Class I or mild Class II skeletal pattern

Stability of o/j reduction increases with age as the lips mature and are held together by the patient, therefore, early Rx is likely to require prolonged retention. Unless a functional appliance is indicated, it is advisable to await the permanent dentition before embarking on Rx to reduce an o/j. If the o/j is <6 mm and orthodontic Rx not indicated for other reasons, consideration should be given to accepting the position of the incisors, particularly if the incisors are not proclined, or stability following o/j reduction is questionable. In a small proportion of cases with proclined incisors, where space to retract the o/j is available or can be created by the extraction of first premolars, an URA can be used. However, most patients in this category are managed using fixed and/or functional appliances. A functional appliance (p. 166) can be used to reduce an increased o/j in a growing child, either as the sole appliance if the arches are well aligned, or as the first phase of Rx to reduce the o/j before fixed appliances and/or extractions are used to complete alignment.

Moderate to severe Class II skeletal pattern

Approaches available are as follows:
1 Modification of growth—either by restraint of maxillary growth with headgear, or by encouraging mandibular growth with a functional appliance
2 Orthodontic camouflage—by extractions in upper arch and bodily movement of incisors and fixed appliances
3 Surgical correction

Because mandibular growth predominates during the teens, a greater proportion of Class II than Class III skeletal problems is amenable to orthodontic correction. Research would suggest that the amount of growth modification that can be achieved is limited, but every little bit helps, and in practice most growing children in this category are treated by a combination of approaches **1** and **2**. This usually takes the form of an initial phase of functional appliance therapy, followed by fixed appliances and/or extractions. Adults whose skeletal pattern is not too severe may be treated by orthodontic camouflage, but in cases with a more severe skeletal problem and/or an increased o/b, a surgical correction may be the only option.

Increased overbite

Normal o/b is between 1/3 and 1/2 overlap of the lower incisors. It is more practical to record o/b in terms of whether it is increased, decreased, or normal, rather than to try to measure it with a ruler. Increased o/b is associated with Class II/2 incisor relationship, where typically 1|1 are retroclined and 2|2 are proclined, reflecting their relationship to the lower lip. But the o/b can also be increased in Class III and II/1 malocclusions. Increased o/b per se is not an indication for Rx, unless it is traumatic, which is relatively rare, but reduction of o/b may be necessary before correction of other anomalies. In Class III cases an increased o/b is advantageous as this will help to retain the corrected incisor position.

Etiology Increased o/b occurs because the incisors are able to erupt past each other due to a combination of some or all of the following interrelated factors: decreased LFH, high lower lip line, retroclined incisors, and increased interincisal angle. Normal interincisal angle is 131°. Highest acceptable angle is 145°. Above this value the tendency for the lower incisors to erupt may be inadequately resisted.

Approaches to reducing overbite

1 *Extrusion/eruption of molars.* Passive eruption of lower molars occurs when an upper removable appliance incorporating a biteplane is worn. Active extrusion of molars in either arch is possible using fixed appliances. However, unless the patient grows vertically to accommodate this increased dimension, the molars will re-intrude under the forces of occlusion once appliances are withdrawn. This approach is of limited value in adults.

2 *Intrusion of incisors.* This is difficult and requires fixed appliances, and in most cases the major effect is extrusion of the buccal segments. More successful in growing patients.

3 *Proclination of lower incisors.* This will only be stable if the lower anterior teeth have been trapped behind the upper anterior teeth, in which case provision of a removable biteplane may allow the lower incisors to spontaneously procline. Active proclination should only be attempted by the experienced orthodontist, who will be better able to judge those cases where this is indicated.

4 *Surgery.* Indicated in severe cases especially if associated with AP skeletal discrepancy, and in adults.

Stability of overbite reduction depends on eliminating or reducing the etiological factors, but decreased LFH and high lower lip line can only be altered if growth is favorable. Reduction of the interincisal angle is necessary to provide a "stop" to the incisors re-erupting, but requires fixed appliances to move incisor apices lingually.

Management of increased overbite

Class II/2 It is often prudent to avoid extractions when the lower arch is mildly crowded in a Class II/2, as extractions may be followed by lingual tipping of the lower incisors resulting in a further increase of the o/b. Cases with sufficient crowding to warrant premolar extractions in the lower arch and moderately to severely increased overbite are best treated with fixed appliances to close space by forward movement of the buccal segments and to correct incisor relationship.

Where o/b reduction is required, the interincisal angle will need to be reduced to achieve a stable result. Usually this necessitates fixed appliances, but in growing patients with a skeletal II pattern and no or mild crowding an alternative approach is to procline incisors with an upper removable appliance and then use a functional appliance to reduce the resultant o/j, or use a Twin Block functional, as a spring can be added to the upper block to procline incisors.

Class II/1 o/b reduction is required before o/j reduction. If a functional appliance is indicated for AP correction then some o/b reduction can often be achieved during this phase by trimming the appliance in the buccal segments. If headgear is being used, it may be helpful to commence o/b by using a URA clipped over the bands on the upper molars. Rx of most II/I will need fixed appliances either as the sole Rx or following a functional appliance or headgear. Including $\overline{7}$ in the fixed appliances will aid intrusion of the lower anterior teeth, but inevitably some extrusion of the molars will occur.

Class III (p. 152) Avoid reducing o/b, as it will aid retention of the corrected incisor position.

Retention Reducing the interincisal angle will aid stability. Following fixed-appliance Rx, incorporation of a flat anterior biteplane into the upper retainer may be helpful. Where the incisal relationship has been changed, retention ideally should be continued until growth is complete. In some patients this is not practicable.

Anterior open bite (AOB)

Vertical overlap of incisors (o/b)

↑o/b   normal o/b   incomplete o/b   AOB

AOB can occur in Class I, II, and III malocclusions.

Etiology Either *skeletal*—vertical > horizontal growth (increased LFH and/or increased maxillary mandibular planes angle [MMPA]), or *environmental*—habits, tongue thrust, iatrogenic, or a combination thereof. If the distance between maxilla and mandible is sufficiently increased such that even if incisors develop to their full potential they do not meet, an AOB will result. This is often associated with incompetent lips and a lip-to-tongue anterior oral seal, which may exacerbate the AOB. Tongue thrusts are usually adaptive and can maintain an AOB due to a habit even after the habit has stopped. Localized failure of maxillary dentoalveolar development resulting in an open bite is seen in CLP.

Treatment is generally difficult except where AOB is due mainly to a habit, thus it is wise to refer patient to a specialist for advice.

Skeletal In milder cases align arches and advise patient to accept, or try to restrain vertical development of the maxilla and/or upper molars with headgear and/or a functional appliance with posterior bite blocks. Extrusion of the incisors is unstable. For more severe cases the only alternative is surgery, but even this is not straightforward and is liable to relapse.

Habits It is better to await natural cessation of the habit, but not if that means deferring Rx for other aspects of malocclusion. Once habit stops o/b should reestablish within 3 yr, unless perpetuated by soft tissues or because it is skeletal in origin.

Tongue thrust None.

Hints for cases with increased vertical dimensions and reduced o/b or AOB:
- Avoid extruding molars, e.g., cervical pull headgear to 6|6, an upper removable appliance with a biteplane.
- Avoid upper arch expansion as this will tip down the palatal cusps of buccal segment teeth, reducing o/b.
- Extraction of molars will not "close down bite."
- Space closure is said to occur more readily in patients with increased LFH and increased MMPA.

Reverse overjet

This will include only those cases with more than 2 teeth in linguo-occlusion, i.e., Class III cases. For management of one or two teeth in crossbite, see p. 154.

Etiology

Skeletal Reverse overjets are usually associated with an underlying Class III skeletal pattern. This is most commonly due to either a large mandible and/or a retrusive maxilla. Class III malocclusions occur in association with the whole range of vertical patterns. Crossbites are a common feature, due either to a large mandible or the anterior position of the mandible relative to the maxilla.

Soft tissues A patient's efforts to achieve an anterior oral seal often result in dentoalveolar compensation, i.e., retroclination of the lower and pro-clination of the upper incisors. Thus, the incisor relationship is often less severe than underlying skeletal pattern.

Dental crowding This is usually greater in the upper than the lower arch.

Assessment (p. 128) Consider also the following:
- Patient's opinion about their facial appearance (be tactful!)
- Severity of skeletal discrepancy
- Amount of dentoalveolar compensation. If upper incisors are already markedly proclined, further proclination is undesirable.
- Amount of overbite. Remember that proclination of upper anterior teeth will reduce o/b and retroclination of lower anterior teeth will increase o/b.
- Can patient achieve an edge-to-edge contact of the incisors? If not, simple Rx is C/I.

Rx planning See p. 134.
▶ Class III malocclusions tend to become worse with growth.
▶ In severe cases seek a specialist's opinion before embarking on Rx or extractions. If surgery is necessary, decompensation (i.e., correcting the position of the incisors to their normal inclination) will probably involve the reverse of orthodontic camouflage.

Major factors determining the Rx approach are skeletal discrepancy and overbite:

Skeletal pattern	Normal or increased o/b	Reduced o/b
Mild to normal	Procline upper anterior teeth	Accept
Moderate	Fixed appliances to procline upper anterior teeth and retrocline lower anterior teeth	Accept or fixed appliances to retrocline lower anterior teeth and/or procline upper anterior teeth
Severe	Surgery	Align and accept if possible, or surgery

If child is on borderline between groups, assume more severe condition as growth will probably prove you right.

Management of reverse overjet

Relief of crowding Extractions in the upper arch alone may run the risk of worsening the incisor relationship, thus it is advisable to extract at least as far forward in the lower arch as in the upper.

Moderate crowding responds best to extraction of premolars. Extraction of 5|5 will maintain 4|4 to support the upper anterior teeth, but often crowding in the upper arch necessitates extraction of 4|4. Proclination of upper anterior teeth, if indicated, will provide some space for relief of crowding. If using fixed appliances to retrocline lower anterior teeth, space will be required in the lower arch to accomplish this. Distal movement of the upper buccal segments is C/I in Class III, as restraint of maxillary growth is undesirable.

Practical treatment

Accept This may be the wisest option for those patients with increased LFH and reduced o/b, with Rx directed toward achieving alignment within the arches only.

Proclination of upper anterior teeth only This is only suitable for milder, well-aligned cases where upper anterior teeth are not already proclined and where sufficient o/b will be present to retain the corrected incisor position. This is best carried out in the mixed dentition, provided 3|3 are not sitting labial to the roots of 2|2. If extraction of C|C is necessary for space, it is advisable to match this with loss of to avoid compromising the incisor relationship. Provided there is sufficient o/b, stability is not usually a problem, but if an upper removable appliance has been used it is advisable to retain for 3 months nights-only wear. Often there is adequate o/b for the 1|1, but not 2|2; if so, a bonded retainer is advisable, but remember that further eruption will be limited.

Retroclination of lower anterior teeth and/or proclination of upper anterior teeth requires fixed appliances. By interchanging the position of the incisors within the neutral zone, stability is not compromised. Class III elastic traction from the back of the upper arch to the $\overline{3}$ region helps to retrocline lower anterior teeth. However, in addition to extruding the incisors, which is desirable, this also results in extrusion of the upper molars, which reduces o/b. Therefore, these cases should be managed by a skilled operator.

Orthodontics and orthognathic surgery See p. 170.

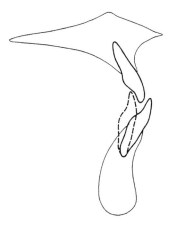

Correction of a Class III incisor relationship by retroclination of the lower incisors increases overbite.

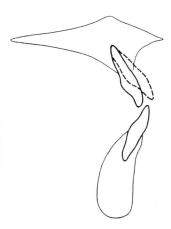

Correction of a Class III incisor relationship by proclination of the upper incisors alone reduces overbite.

Crossbites (Xbites)

By convention the lower teeth should be described relative to the upper (p. 126). Crossbites can be anterior or posterior (unilateral/bilateral), with displacement, or with no displacement.

Etiology Xbites can be skeletal and/or dental in origin. For posterior Xbites, the skeletal component is usually the major factor. Antero-posterior discrepancies obviously play a part in anterior Xbites, but can also result in posterior Xbites in Class II (lingual Xbite) and Class III (buccal Xbite) skeletal patterns.

Displacement may occur when a premature or deflecting cuspal contact is encountered on closure and the mandible is postured either anteriorly or laterally to achieve better interdigitation. This new path of closure becomes learned and the patient closes straight into interdigitation. To help detect displacement on closure, try to get the patient to close on a hinge axis by asking them to curl their tongue back to touch the back of the palate and then close together slowly, while guiding the mandible back via the chin. In addition, look for other clues like a center-line shift (of lower in direction of displacement) in association with a posterior unilateral Xbite. Evidence suggests that displacing contacts may predispose to temporomandibular dysfunction.

Anterior crossbites

Class III malocclusions are considered on p. 151. These should be treated early, especially if associated with a displacement, provided sufficient o/b exists to retain the result. If not, it is probably best to defer Rx until the permanent dentition and use fixed appliances. Correction of one or two teeth with reverse o/j and a positive overbite can be accomplished using an upper removable appliance; however, there must be enough space to accommodate the tooth in the arch (or create space with extractions). Application of force to procline the upper anterior teeth results in an upper removable appliance being unseated anteriorly; thus, good anterior retention is usually required. In mixed dentition, the morphology of the primary teeth makes this difficult. A screw appliance has the advantage that the teeth to be moved can also be clasped. Buccal capping should be added to free the tooth to be moved from contact with the lower arch. Upper lateral incisors displaced bodily and palatally due to lack of space are not amenable to simple proclination. Refer patient to a specialist.

Posterior crossbites[1]

Unilateral Generally, the greater the number of teeth involved, the greater the skeletal contribution to the etiology. If there are only one or two teeth, movement of opposing teeth in opposite directions for correction may be required. This can be achieved by cross-elastics attached to attachments on the affected teeth. 5s are often crowded palatally, but are easily aligned using a T-spring on an upper removable appliance. Unilateral Xbite from the canine region distally is usually associated with a displacement, as true skeletal asymmetry is rare. If the arches are of a

1 R. W. Wassell 1989 *J Dent* **17** 101.

similar width, displacement to the right or left will give better interdigitation. In these cases Rx should be directed toward expanding the upper arch so that it fits around the lower, provided the upper teeth are not already buccally tilted.

Bilateral buccal crossbite This suggests a greater underlying transverse skeletal discrepancy. Less commonly, this is associated with displacement. Correction of a bilateral Xbite should be approached with caution, because partial relapse may result in the teeth occluding cusp to cusp and development of a unilateral Xbite with displacement.

Bilateral lingual crossbite (or scissor bite) occurs from either a narrow mandible or a wide maxilla. In milder cases only 4|4 may be involved, and if these teeth are extracted to relieve crowding or for retraction of 3|3, so much the better. Where all of the buccal segments are involved, Rx will probably involve expansion of the lower and/or contraction of the upper; thus, refer patient to a specialist.

Rapid maxillary expansion

This involves a screw appliance comprising bands attached to 64|64 and connected to a midline screw. The object is to expand the maxilla by opening the midline suture; this is more successful in younger patients. Large forces are required to accomplish this. The screw is turned 0.5 mm a day (0.25 mm per quarter turn). Overexpansion is necessary as the teeth relapse about one-third to 50% under soft-tissue pressure. This is not to be attempted by the inexperienced!

Quad helix appliance

This is a very efficient fixed, slow expansion appliance, suitable for mixed or permanent dentition. It attaches to upper teeth by bands on 6 and is W shaped.

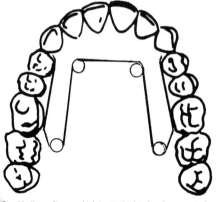

Quad helix appliance, which is attached to bands, cemented onto the upper first molar teeth.

Anchorage

Anchorage is defined as the source of resistance to the reaction from the active component(s) in an appliance. In practice, it is the balance between the applied force and the available space. For example, in a case where 3|3 are being retracted following extraction of 4|4, an equal but opposite force will also be acting on 65|56. The amount of forward movement of these anchor teeth will depend largely on their root surface area and the force used.

Anchorage loss can be minimized by limiting the number of teeth being moved at any one time, applying the correct force for the movement required, and increase the resistance of the anchor teeth (e.g., by permitting only bodily movement). In some situations, movement of the anchor teeth is desirable, e.g., in a Class III where space is being opened up for an unerupted 5. However, it is important to assess the anchorage requirements of a particular malocclusion before embarking on treatment. If no or little movement of the anchor teeth is desirable, then anchorage should be reinforced from the start.

Reinforcing anchorage

Intramaxillary (teeth in same arch) This is done by including the maximum number of teeth in the anchorage unit. It is applicable to both fixed and removable appliances.

Intermaxillary (teeth in opposing arch) This is achieved by running elastics from one arch to the other. It is mainly applicable to fixed appliances, as a URA will be dislodged. The direction of elastic pull is described according to the type of malocclusion to which it is applicable.

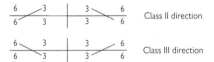

Class II direction

Class III direction

Increased mucosal coverage By virtue of its palatal coverage, an upper removable appliance has more potential anchorage than a fixed appliance.

Extraoral anchorage is transmitted to the appliance by elastic or spring force from a head or neck strap. This involves a face-bow, which engages tubes soldered on to molar Adams cribs (upper removable appliance) or bands (fixed appliance). The direction of pull can be selected according to the malocclusion with an overall direction of pull above the occlusal plane for patients with increased vertical proportions (high pull) and vice versa for patients with reduced vertical proportions (cervical pull). For extraoral anchorage, 250 g for 10 h/day should suffice. For extraoral traction (i.e., using the headgear force to achieve movement rather than just resist it) forces in the region of 500 g for 14–16 h/day are necessary.

Following reports of a number of cases where eye damage (including blindness) occurred from headgear use, the use of at least two safety mechanisms is imperative. Better still, avoid headgear if possible.

Anchorage loss

This may occur because of 1 failure to fully appreciate anchorage requirements at Rx planning stage; 2 active force exceeding available anchorage (often due to overactivation or too many teeth being moved at a time); 3 poor patient compliance.

Removable appliances—scope and limitations

Removable appliances are single-arch appliances that can be taken out of the mouth by the patient. They are only capable of tilting movements of individual teeth, but can be used for moving blocks of teeth. In addition, they can be used to allow differential eruption of teeth via biteplanes or buccal capping.

Advantages of removables	Disadvantages of removables
Easier to clean than fixed appliances	Patient can leave appliance out
Easy to adjust, thus reducing chair time	Only tipping movement possible
Contact with mucosa increases anchorage	Affects speech
Can be used for o/b reduction	Good technician required
Can transmit forces to blocks of teeth	Intermaxillary traction not possible
	Lower removable appliances are difficult to tolerate
	Inefficient for multiple tooth movements

Indications

Active
- Where only simple tipping movement of an individual tooth is required
- Movement of blocks of teeth, e.g., correction of a buccal crossbite by expansion of upper arch
- As an interceptive Rx in the mixed dentition, e.g., correction of an upper incisor in crossbite
- Overbite reduction
- In conjunction with other appliance, e.g., to facilitate distal movement of upper molar(s) with headgear; to free occlusion to allow movement of a tooth over the bite during fixed appliance Rx

Passive
- Space maintainer, e.g., following loss of an upper central incisor due to trauma
- Retaining appliance, e.g., following fixed appliance Rx

Correction of unilateral posterior crossbites

Removable appliances are useful in the correction of unilateral posterior crossbites, particularly in the mixed dentition where mobile primary teeth may make placement of a fixed appliance problematic. Usually the design involves a midline screw that works by reciprocal anchorage, i.e., each side of the arch moves equally in opposite directions.

Interestingly, a recent Cochrane systematic review indicated that for cases with a posterior crossbite in the mixed dentition, active intervention was indicated to prevent perpetuation of the crossbite in the permanent dentition.[1] The most effective Rx was grinding of the primary teeth responsible for causing the premature contact. If this was not successful then use of an upper removable appliance to expand the upper arch was effective.

1 J. Harrison 2001 *Cochrane Database Syst Rev* **1** CD000979.

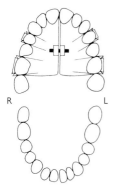

Upper removable appliance to expand upper arch with midline screw.
Adams cribs 6|6 0.028 (diameter in inch) stainless steel wire
4|4 0.024 (diameter in inch) stainless steel wire

Removable appliances—design

Four components need to be considered for every appliance.

Active component

This exerts force required for desired movement.

Springs

Springs are the most commonly used active component because they are versatile and cheap to construct.

The relationship between the distance (*d*) that an orthodontic spring is deflected on activation, the length of the spring (*l*), the diameter or radius (*r*) of the wire it is composed of, and the force generated is:

$$F \propto \frac{dr^4}{l^3}$$

In practice this means that for two identical springs of the same length, one made in 0.020 (diameter in inch) wire and one in 0.028 (diameter in inch) wire, to deliver the same amount of force, the spring of 0.020 wire would be activated about 3 mm, whereas the spring of 0.028 wire spring requires only 1 mm activation.

Palatal finger springs are the most commonly used active components for mesial or distal movement along the arch. They are fabricated in 0.020 wire and are easy to adjust and activate. If boxed out from the acrylic and made with a guard wire they are more stable in the vertical plane than a buccal spring and, thus, should be used in preference.

For details of other types of spring, the reader should consult a specialist text.

Elastics

These are less commonly used today, but are useful for aligning displaced teeth, e.g., palatal canine, using an attachment bonded onto the tooth surface, to which an elastic is applied by the patient to a hook soldered on to a labial bow or Adams crib.

Screws

The Hyrax type of screw design is used almost exclusively. This type of screw is opened (or closed) by means of a key, a quarter turn of which separates the two halves by 0.25 mm. A screw appliance is useful when the teeth to be moved need to be clasped for retention (e.g., expanding the upper arch in the mixed dentition). It is advisable to start patients turning the screw only once a week, progressing on to a maximum of two turns per week. If worn intermittently, a screw appliance will become progressively ill-fitting. Remember that these screws have about 18 activations and if considerable movement is necessary a second appliance may be required.

Retention

This is the means by which the appliance is retained in the mouth. The best retention posteriorly is provided by the Adams cribs, which is made in SS in either 0.030 (diameter in inch) (for permanent molars) or 0.028 (diameter in inch) (for premolars and primary molars) wire. These clasps are very technician sensitive and no amount of adjustment will compensate for a badly made one. They should engage about 1 mm of undercut, which on a child's molar may be at, or just under, the gingival margin and in an adult may only be partway down the clinical crown. The versatility of the cribs can be increased by soldering tubes for extraoral anchorage or traction, labial bows, or buccal springs onto the bridge of the clasp.

Anterior retention can be gained by a labial bow or either an Adams or Southend clasp. All these components are usually constructed in 0.7 mm wire.

Anchorage

This resists force generated by active component(s); see p. 156.

Baseplate

This not only holds other elements together but may also itself be active. Heat-cure acrylic is more robust than self-cure.

- A flat anterior biteplane should only be prescribed if o/b reduction is required. In case your technician isn't telepathic, it is wise to specify the height (e.g., half the height of 1/1) and how far back the biteplane should extend (e.g., o/j = 3 mm). To increase the likelihood of the URA being worn, the molars should only be separated by 1–2 mm by the biteplane, therefore, self-cure acrylic should be added during Rx to continue o/b reduction.
- Buccal capping frees the occlusion on the tooth being moved and allows further relative eruption of the incisors (thus is C/I if o/b is already increased). It should be trimmed so that the teeth to be moved are separated only by 1–2 mm.

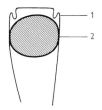

Adjustment of Adams crib.
1 Arrowhead moves horizontally toward tooth.
2 Arrowed moves toward tooth and also vertically toward gingival crevice.

▶ The easier it is for the patient to insert and wear their upper removable appliances, the more likely it is that Rx will be successful, so keep the design simple.

Clear vacuum-formed tooth aligners (Invisalign) have gained a great deal of attention from patients who desire invisible braces. The principles of removable appliances apply to these appliances as well. With the introduction of three-dimensional computer technology, Invisalign appliances have gained ground in the precision of treatment that can be provided using them, when compared to traditional removable orthodontic appliances. Even with the advent of this new technology, the responsibility for diagnosis and treatment planning orthodontic care remains the dentist's. When developing a treatment plan for patients using clear aligners, their indications and limitations should be considered. These limitations must be communicated to other doctors who may be involved in the patient's care as well as to the patient. For example, Invisalign is indicated only for the treatment of patients with no skeletal discrepancies with mild to moderate crowding (1–6 mm), and mild to moderate spacing (1–6 mm). Another indication is in the treatment of patients who have had a relapse of fixed orthodontic treatment. Treatment outcomes using clear aligners, compared to those of fixed appliances, are still unclear. Further research is necessary to explore the potential of these appliances.

Fixed appliances

▶ Fixed appliances (FA) should only be used in cooperative patients with good oral hygiene, to minimize damage.

As the name implies, fixed appliances are attached to the teeth. They vary in complexity, from a single bracket used in conjunction with a removable appliance, to attachments on all teeth. Removable appliances are limited to tilting movements, but fixed appliances can tilt, rotate, intrude, extrude, and move teeth bodily. Not surprisingly, fixed appliances have a greater propensity for things to go awry. Therefore, only those with the skills and training for their use should use them.

Principles

- Rx planning (p. 134) is important, but with increased attention to anchorage requirements, especially if apical movement is planned.
- As fixed appliances are able to achieve bodily movement, it is possible (within limits) to move teeth to compensate for a skeletal discrepancy.
- Fixed appliances can be used in conjunction with other appliances and/or headgear.
- For initial alignment flexible archwires are used, but to minimize unwanted movements, progressively more rigid archwires are necessary.
- Archwires should be based on the pre-Rx lower-arch form for stability.
- Mesiodistal movement is achieved by either 1 sliding the teeth along the archwire with elastic force (sliding mechanics) or 2 moving the teeth with the archwire.
- Intermaxillary traction is often used to aid AP correction and increase anchorage.

Components of fixed appliances

Bands These are usually used on molar teeth so that the end of the arch wire is retained even if the band becomes loose. They are indicated for other teeth if bonds fail or lingual attachment is required for de-rotation. If tooth contacts are tight these will need to be separated prior to band placement using an elastic doughnut stretched around the contact point for 1–7 days. Use of GI cements helps to reduce decalcification.

Bonds are attached to enamel with (acid-etch) composite. There are three types: 1 metal (poor aesthetics), 2 plastic (become stained), and 3 ceramic (prone to # and can cause enamel wear).

Archwires Flexible nickel titanium (NiTi) archwires are used in the initial stages of Rx and more rigid stainless steel wires for the planned tooth movements. Tungsten molybdenum, and cobalt chromium alloys are also popular.

Auxiliaries Elastic rings or wire ligatures are used to tie the archwire to the brackets. Forces can be applied to the teeth by auxiliary springs or elastics.

Types of fixed appliance

There is an almost infinite variety, but most are based on the following:

Begg uses round wires that fit loosely into a vertical slot in the bracket, thus allowing the teeth to tip freely. Auxiliaries are required to achieve apical and rotational movements. This type is now superseded by tip-edge.

Edgewise uses rectangular brackets that are wide mesiodistally for rotational control. Round wires are used initially for alignment, but rectangular wires are necessary for apical control. This is largely a historical type.

Preadjusted systems These "prescribed" brackets allow increased use of preformed archwires. As each tooth has its own individual bracket with a built-in prescription for that tooth, these systems are more expensive, but that is offset by savings in operator time.

Tip edge is based on the Begg philosophy but the brackets also have preadjusted values incorporated to give the "finish" produced by using a straight wire appliance.

Lingual appliances These are popular with patients, but not with orthodontists, as they are difficult to adjust!

Damon brackets have a clip mechanism to hold the archwire in place, which reduces friction, making space closure quicker.

More details can be found in specialist texts.

Functional appliances—rationale and mode of action

Definition Functional appliances use, eliminate, or guide the forces of muscle function, tooth eruption, and growth to correct a malocclusion.

Philosophy The term *functional appliance* dates back to a belief that by eliminating abnormal muscle function normal growth and development would follow. Today, the importance of both genetic and environmental factors in the etiology of malocclusion is acknowledged, but functional appliances are still successfully used to correct Class II malocclusions by dental and limited skeletal effects. Functional appliances can also be used in the Rx of anterior open bite and Class III, but generally alternative approaches are more successful; thus, we shall only consider Class II malocclusions.

Mode of action In the average child, the maxilla and mandible grow downward and forward relative to the cranial base. Functional appliances are intended to help harness this change to correct Class II malocclusions through a combination of force application and force elimination. The relative contributions of each depend on the design of appliance. Force application usually takes the form of intermaxillary traction, i.e., a restraining effect on the maxilla and maxillary teeth and a forward pressure on the mandible and mandibular teeth. A similar effect is produced with Class II elastics (p. 156). Functional appliances are ineffective for individual tooth movement.

Application
1 To achieve some AP correction for a Class II malocclusion prior to fixed appliances with extractions. Ideally, for Class II/1 with mandibular retrusion, average or reduced LFH, or upright or retroclined lower anterior teeth. A useful test is to examine the profile with patient postured forward to a Class I incisor relationship, and if not improved, consider another appliance.
2 Can be used as sole appliance in milder cases with well-aligned arches.

Changes produced by functional appliances
Skeletal
• Some proponents of functional appliances have claimed increased mandibular growth. Research supports the idea that changes seen are small and unsubstantiated over the long term. The debate continues! It is better to consider functional appliances as providing an environment for achieving an individual's best mandibular growth potential.
• Forward remodeling of the glenoid fossa
• Increase in LFH

Dental
- Palatal tipping of the upper incisors
- Labial tipping of the lower incisors
- Inhibition of forward movement of the maxillary molars
- Mesial and vertical eruption of the mandibular molars

Keys to success with functional appliances
- Cooperative and keen patient. Remember that cooperation is finite.
- Favorable growth

Types of functional appliance and practical tips

Choice of appliance

Except for those designed for cases with increased LFH, the effects produced by the different types of appliance are similar. It is wiser to become familiar with one particular design. For each appliance well-extended upper and lower impressions are required. A wax bite should be recorded with the mandible postured forward 7–10 mm.

Some of the more popular types are the following:

Twin block comprises a separate upper removable appliance and lower removable appliance that, through sloping buccal blocks, help to posture the mandible forward. They are well tolerated by patients and can be worn for meals. In addition, a screw can be incorporated in the upper twin block if expansion is required, as well as springs (e.g., to align 2̲).

Frankel is advocated for cases with abnormal soft-tissue pattern, e.g., lower lip trap. There are several subtypes, of which FRII is the most popular. Buccal shields allow expansion of the arches, but the long-term stability of this is unsubstantiated. Construction bite is forward 6 mm and open 3–4 mm in premolar region. It is worn full-time. This type is difficult to repair or adjust, but can be reactivated by dividing buccal shields and advancing.

Medium opening activator A preliminary phase of upper arch expansion is required in most patients to coordinate arch widths. Construction bite is as for Frankel. It is worn full-time. This type must be made in heat-cure acrylic as lower arch extensions are prone to fracture.

Functionals in Class II/1 with increased LFH

An appliance with molar capping is needed to try and prevent molar eruption, encourage autorotation of the mandible, and thus reduce LFH. Increasing the bite opening of an appliance is thought to result in a more forward direction of mandibular growth.[1] Some designs include high-pull headgear to restrain vertical maxillary growth.

Practical tips

- Advise patient to wear appliance full-time. Only the twin block appliance can be worn for eating. See patient every 2 months.
- Increasing daytime wear often cures problems with appliances that fall out in bed at night.
- Expect at least 1 mm o/j reduction per month.
- It is wise to continue until o/j is almost edge to edge.
- Retain by wearing nights only, for about 3 months before progressing on to fixed appliance.

---

1 S. E. Bishara 1989 *Am J Orthod Dentofac Orthop* **95** 250.

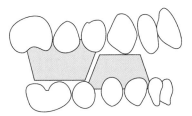

Diagram showing how the inclined bite blocks of the twin block appliance hold the mandible forward in a postured position.

Orthodontics and orthognathic surgery

Orthognathic surgery is the correction of skeletal discrepancies beyond the limits of orthodontic Rx alone, because of either their severity or a lack of growth. Surgery is usually deferred until growth is complete.

Diagnosis and treatment planning

This is best undertaken jointly by an orthodontist and maxillofacial surgeon. The following information is required:

Patient's perception of problem Clinical observations of appearance of jaws or teeth; speech; are there problems with eating? Are patient's expectations realistic?

Clinical examination Assessment of the balance and proportions of full face and profile.

Study models For bimaxillary procedure mount on semi- or fully adjustable articulator.

Radiographs require panoramic radiograph and lateral skull, plus PA skull for asymmetries. It is helpful to compare patient's cephalometric tracing with the ideal to visually assess areas of discrepancy. A number of computer programs are available to aid in diagnosis and planning, of varying complexity and cost. However, these should not supersede clinical assessment in planning.

Photographs are required, as pre-Rx record and can also be manipulated with lateral skull for visual predictions.

It is important to correlate desired facial changes with patient's occlusion. Presurgical orthodontics will be required to decompensate teeth so that a full surgical correction is possible.

Include the patient in Rx planning so they understand what is involved.

Sequence of treatment

Presurgical orthodontics The aim of orthodontic Rx is to align and coordinate the arches so that the teeth will not interfere when the jaws are placed in their correct position. This usually involves decompensation, i.e., removal of any dentoalveolar compensation for the skeletal discrepancy so that the teeth are at their correct axial inclinations and a full surgical correction can be achieved. If a segmental procedure is planned, space will be needed interdentally for surgical cuts. It is inefficient to carry out movements that can be accomplished more readily at surgery (e.g., expansion of upper arch if Le Fort 1 planned), or following surgery (e.g., leveling of lower arch in Class II/2). In addition, the fixed appliance provides a means of fixation at surgery.

Surgery See p. 416.

Postsurgical orthodontics Lighter round wires and intermaxillary traction are used to detail occlusion. Then patients are placed in retention, usually with removable retainers.

Relapse can be surgical or orthodontic or both. Relapse is more likely in Rx of deficiencies, as soft tissues are under greater tension postoperatively.

Cleft lip and palate (CLP)

Prevalence CLP varies with racial group and geographically. It occurs in 1:750 Caucasian births, but prevalence is increased in M > F. If unilateral, L > R. There is a family history in 40% of cases.

Isolated cleft palate occurs in 1:2000 births, F > M. A family history is in 20% of cases.

Etiology Polygenic inheritance with a threshold. Environmental factors may precipitate susceptible individuals toward threshold.

Classification Many exist, but the best approach is to describe cleft: primary and/or secondary palate; complete or incomplete; unilateral or bilateral. Submucous cleft is often missed until poor speech is noticed, as overlying mucosa is intact.

Problems

Embryological anomalies Tissue deficit, displacement of segments, abnormal muscle attachments.

Postsurgical distortions Unrepaired clefts show normal growth. In repaired clefts maxillary growth is impaired anteroposteriorly, transversely, and vertically. Mandibular growth is also impaired.

Hearing and speech are impaired.

Other congenital anomalies occur in up to 20% of cases with CLP and are more likely in association with isolated clefts of palate than of lip.

Dental anomalies In CLP, prevalence of hypodontia and supernumerary teeth (especially in region of cleft) is increased. Incidence of hypoplasia and delayed eruption are also increased.

Management (of unilateral complete CLP)

The treatment team usually includes a cleft surgeon, secondary surgeon, ENT surgeon, health visitors, orthodontist, speech therapist, clinical psychologist, and central coordinator. Centralization of care and audit of outcome gives better results.

Birth Parents need explanation, reassurance, and help with feeding. Presurgical orthopedics is now out of vogue, as benefits are not proven.

Lip closure Most centers do lip repair at about 3 months, but some surgeons carry out neonatal repair. Delaire or Millard and/or modifications are the most popular. Some surgeons do Vomer flap at the same time. Bilateral lips are closed in either one or two operations.

Palatal closure is usually between 9 and 18 months. Deferring repair until the patient is older reduces growth disturbance, but resultant poor speech has a greater psychological impact.

Primary dentition Lip revision may be carried out before the patient starts school. Speech and hearing assessments are required.

Mixed dentition may be necessary to procline upper incisors if they erupt into linguo-occlusion, otherwise orthodontic Rx is better deferred until just prior to secondary bone grafting at 8–10 yr.

Secondary bone grafting involves grafting cancellous bone from the iliac crest into the cleft alveolus. Advantages include the following:

1 Provides bone for 3 to erupt through (ideally before eruption of 3)
2 Allows tooth movement into cleft site
3 Increases bony support for alar base
4 Aids closure of oronasal fistulae

Orthodontic expansion of collapsed arches and alignment of the upper incisors is required prior to grafting to improve access. Closure is with local keratinized flaps; thus, if any extraction is planned, these should be carried out in advance.

Permanent dentition Once permanent teeth have erupted, fixed appliances are usually required for alignment and space closure. Ideally, if 2 is missing, Rx should aim to bring 3 forward to replace it, thus avoiding a prosthesis.

Growth complete A final nose revision is often performed at this stage. Orthognathic surgery to improve facial esthetics (p. 416) may also be considered, in which case it is preferable to postpone the nose revision until bony surgery complete.

Periodontology

Principal sources: F. A. Carranza 2002 Carranza's Clinical Periodontology 9th ed., Saunders. L. F. Rose 2003 Periodontics: Medicine, Surgery, and Implants, 1st ed., Elsevier Mosby.

Oral microbiology

Microorganisms colonize the mouth a few hours after birth, mainly by aerobic and facultative anaerobic organisms. The eruption of teeth allows the development of a complex ecosystem of microorganisms, and the healthy mouth depends on maintaining an environment in which these organisms coexist without damaging oral structures.[1]

About 500–600 bacterial taxa have been detected in samples from the oral cavity.[2] Most putative periodontal pathogens are Gram-negative anaerobic rods. Other pathogens include Gram-positive facultative and anaerobic cocci and rods and Gram-negative facultative rods.[3]

Association between putative periodontal pathogens and periodontitis[3]

Very strong
- *Porphyromonas gingivalis*
- *Actinobacillus actinomycetemcomitans*
- *Tannerella forsythensis*
- Spirochtes of acute necrotizing gingivitis

Strong
- *Preveotella intermedia*
- *Dialister pneumosintes/Dialister invisus*
- *Eubacterium nodatum*
- *Treponema denticola*

Moderate
- *Campylobacter rectus*
- *Peptostreptococcus micros*
- *Fusobacterium nucleatum*
- *Selenomonas noxia*
- Beta-hemolytic streptococci
- Eikenella corrodens

Early stage of investigation
- Gram-negative enteric rods
- *Pseudomonas* species
- *Staphylococcus* species
- *Enterococcus faecalis*
- *Candida albicans*

1 J. M. Hardie 1992 *BDJ* **172** 271.
2 S. S. Socransky 2002 *Periodontology 2000* **28** 12.
3 AAP Position Paper 2004 *J Periodontol* **75** 1553.

Plaque

Dental plaque, which is a biofilm, is composed of a myriad of microbial clusters surrounded by an adherent matrix of polysaccharides and glyco-proteins produced by bacteria within the plaque.[1] Plaque is not easily removed with a water spray or vigorous rinsing, but it can be mechanically removed by effective brushing and flossing.

Attachment To colonize smooth tooth surfaces plaque needs the presence of an *acquired pellicle*, a thin layer of salivary glycoproteins that formed on the tooth surface within minutes of polishing. The pellicle has an ion-regulating function between tooth and saliva and contains immunoglobulins, complement and lysozyme.

Development The development of dental plaque has been studied in humans as well as nonhuman animal model systems. One of the most commonly used models of plaque development is referred to as the "experimental gingivitis" model.[2] Three phases of plaque morphogenesis have been described based on time (days). Phase 1 (days 1–2) is characterized by a sparse flora to a dense mat of gram-positive cocci and short rods. During phase 2 (days 2–4), filamentous forms and rods increase. Phase 3 (days 6–10) is associated with a gradual shift to vibrios and spirochetes. This overall pattern observed in dental plaque development is a very characteristic shift from the early predominance of gram-positive facultative microorganisms to the later predominance of gram-negative anaerobic microorganisms, as the plaque mass accumulates and matures. This developmental progression is also reflected in the shifts in predominant microorganisms observed in the transition from health to disease.

Plaque in periodontal disease There is a direct correlation between the amount of plaque at the cervical margin of teeth and the severity of gingivitis,[3] and experimental gingivitis can be produced and abolished by suspending and reintroducing oral hygiene.[2] It is commonly accepted that plaque accumulation causes gingivitis, the major variable being host susceptibility. While there are numerous interacting components that determine the progression of gingivitis to periodontitis, particularly host susceptibility, the presence of plaque, particularly "'old" plaque with its high anaerobe content, is widely held to be crucial, and most treatment is based on the meticulous, regular removal of plaque.

1 L. F. Rose 2004 *Periodontics: Medicine, Surgery, and Implants*, p. 505, Elsevier Mosby.

2 H. Löe 1965 *J Periodontol* **36** 177.

3 M. Ash 1964 *J Periodontol* **35** 424.

Calculus

Calculus (tartar) is a calcified deposit found on teeth and/or restorations and is formed by mineralization of plaque deposits. It can be subdivided into the following categories:

- *Supragingival calculus* is most often on the lingual of the lower anterior teeth and on the facial surfaces of upper molars, near the openings of submandibular and parotid salivary glands. It is usually yellow, but can become stained a variety of colors.
- *Subgingival calculus* is found underneath the gingival margin and is firmly attached to tooth roots. It tends to be brown or black, is extremely tenacious, and is most often found on interproximal and lingual surfaces. It may be identified visually, by exploration, or on radiographs. With gingival recession it can become supragingival.

Composition Calculus consists of up to 80% inorganic salts, mostly crystal-line, the major components being calcium and phosphorus. The microscopic structure is basically that of a randomly orientated crystal formation.

Formation is always preceded by plaque deposition, the plaque serving as an organic matrix for subsequent mineralization. Calculus formation may begin in as little as 4 to 8 h and calcifying plaques may become 50% mineralized in 48 h. The principal mineral source for supragingival and subgingival calculus is saliva and gingival crevicular fluid (GCF).

Pathological effect Calculus (particularly subgingival calculus) is associated with periodontal disease, likely because a layer of plaque covers it. Its principal detrimental effect is probably that it acts as a retention site for plaque and bacterial toxins. The presence of calculus makes it difficult to implement adequate oral hygiene.

Etiology of periodontal disease

Plaque is the principal etiological factor in most all forms of periodontal disease. Periodontal damage is almost certainly the direct consequence of colonization in the gingival sulcus by organisms within dental plaque. However, the progression from gingivitis to periodontitis is far more complex than this statement suggests, as it involves host defense, the oral environment, the pathogenicity of organisms, and plaque maturity. It is probably easiest to regard periodontal disease as a complex multi-factorial infection complicated by the inflammatory response of the host. Various elements of this process are worthy of special note.

Microbiology

As was reviewed previously, specific bacteria or the interaction of a number of different bacterial species may cause destruction of the perio-dontal attachment apparatus. The inflammatory response of gingiva to the presence of initial young plaque creates a minute gingival pocket, which serves as an ideal environment for further bacterial colonization, providing all the nutrients required for the growth of numerous fastidious organisms. In addition, there is an extremely low oxygen level within gingival pockets, which favors the development of obligate anaerobes, several of which are closely associated with the progression of periodontal disease. High levels of carbon dioxide favor the establishment of the capnophilic organisms, some of whom are associated with localized aggres-sive periodontitis. However, to date it has not been possible to identify one particular organism or group of microorganisms solely responsible for the initiation and progression of periodontal disease, although the general concepts outlined reflect current working data.

Immunopathology

The inflammatory response to the presence of dental plaque is detectable both clinically and histologically and is responsible for at least some of the periodontal destruction that occurs. Both inflammatory and immunologi-cally mediated pathways contribute to periodontal damage. Antigenic substances released by plaque organisms elicit both cell-mediated and humoral responses, which, while designed to be protective, also cause local tissue damage, usually by complement activation (bystander damage). Non-immune-mediated damage is caused by one or all of the major endo-genous mediators of inflammation: vasoactive amines (histamine), plasma proteases (complement), prostaglandins and leukotrienes, lysosomal acid hydrolases, proteases, free radicals, and cytokines.

Host

Local and systemic modifying factors influence progress of the disease.

Local factors are tooth position and morphology, calculus, overhangs and appliances, occlusal trauma, and mucogingival state.

Systemic factors include immune status, stress, endocrine function (e.g., diabetes), smoking, drugs, age, and nutrition. There has been evidence reported suggesting a link between periodontitis, ischemic heart disease, cerebrovascular disease, and preterm low birth weight. It is unclear if this is a cause-and-effect relationship.

Epidemiology of periodontal disease

Epidemiology is the study of the health and disease in populations and of how these states are influenced by heredity, biology, physical environment, social environment, and personal behavior.[1]

Incidence is the number of new cases in a population over a given time period.

Prevalence is the number of cases of a disease in a designated population at a given point.

Prevalence of gingivitis

National survey data show that gingivitis is found in early childhood, is more prevalent and severe in adolescence, and then tends to level off in older age groups.[2] The prevalence of gingivitis among schoolchildren in the United States has ranged from 40% to 60% in national surveys.[3] In the third National Health and Nutrition Examination Survey (NHANES III), 50% of adults were found to have gingivitis on at least three or four teeth.[4] Plaque deposits are closely correlated with gingivitis, a relationship long considered one of cause and effect.[1]

Prevalence of periodontitis

Periodontitis, viewed for years as primarily the outcome from infection, is now seen as resulting from a complex interplay between bacterial infection and host response, often modified by behavioral factors.[5] Today it is well documented that only some 5% to 15% of any population suffers from severe generalized periodontitis, even though moderate disease affects a majority of adults.[6] What epidemiology has demonstrated is that the majority of adult populations have chronic periodontis to some degree, and the mild attachment loss (clinical attachment loss of 2 mm or so) is common and may be seen in clinically healthy gingiva.[1]

Risk determinant: Risk factors that cannot be modified.

Risk factor An environmental exposure, aspect of behavior, or inherent characteristic that is associated with a disease. Confirmed in longitudinal studies.

Risk indicator Plausible correlates of disease identified in cross-sectional studies.

Risk marker A factor associated with increased probability of future disease but where causality is not usually implied.

Determinants of periodontitis[1]
- *Age* Prevalence and severity of clinical attachment loss (CAL) increases with age.
- *Gender* CAL of all levels of severity is generally more prevalent in males than in females.
- *Socioeconomic status* Those who are better educated, wealthier, and live in more desirable circumstances enjoy better health status.
- *Genetics* A specific genotype of the polymorphic IL-1 gene cluster is associated with severe periodontitis.

Risk factors for periodontitis[1]
- Plaque, microbiota, and lack of oral hygiene
- Tobacco

Periodontal indices

The original purpose of periodontal indices was to study the extent of disease within population groups; however, indices in the screening and management of individual patients are valuable. Examples of indices are shown below.

Plaque Index[7]

Score	Criteria
0	No plaque
1	No plaque visible by the unaided eye, but plaque is visible on the point of the probe after it has been moved across
2	Gingival area is covered with a thin to moderately thick layer of plaque
3	Heavy accumulation of soft matter

Gingival Index[8]

Score	Criteria
0	Normal gingiva
1	Mild inflammation
2	Moderate inflammation
3	Severe inflammation

Periodontal Index[9]

Score	Criteria
0	Normal gingiva
1	Mild gingivitis
2	Gingivitis
3	Gingivitis with pocket formation
4	Advanced destruction with loss of masticatory function

1 AAP Position Paper 2005 *J Periodontol* **76** 1406.

2 J. W. Stamm 1986 *J Clin Periodontol* **13** 360.

3 M. Bhat 1991 *J Public Health Dent* **51** 5.

4 R. C. Oliver 1998 *J Periodontol* **69** 269.

5 R. C. Page 1997 *Periodontology 2000* **14** 216.

6 R. C. Oliver 1998 *J Periodontol* **69** 269.

7 P. Silness 1964 *Acta Odontol Scand* **22** 123.

8 H. Löe 1963 *Acta Odontol Scand* **21** 533.

9 A. L. Russell 1956 *J Dent Res* **35** 350.

Chronic gingivitis

Chronic gingivitis is, as the name suggests, inflammation of the gingival tissues. It is **not** associated with alveolar bone resorption or apical migration of the junctional epithelium. Pockets >2 mm can occur in chronic gingivitis due to an increase in gingival size because of edema or hyperplasia (false pockets). Four different types of gingivitis are described; the most common type is plaque induced.

Plaque-induced gingivitis This is present in virtually all mouths to some extent. The classic triad of redness, swelling and bleeding on gentle probing are diagnostic and are usually associated with a complaint by the patient that their "gums bleed when they brush." False pocketing may also be present. This gingivitis occurs as a result of low-grade infection caused by the presence of undisturbed dental plaque, which is associated with a change in the flora from gram-positive aerobes to gram-negative anaerobes. This gives rise to inflammatory changes in the associated gingiva; these are detectable histologically prior to the appearance of overt clinical gingivitis, which is observed after about 7 days of undisturbed plaque accumulation. The inflammatory response seen comprises an alteration in the integrity of the gingival microcirculation, an increase in the numbers of inflammatory cells in the gingival connective tissue (i.e., plasma cells, lymphocytes, macrophages, and neutrophils), a decrease in the number of fibroblasts, and a decrease in collagen density. These inflammatory changes are easily reversible after institution of effective plaque control. While gingivitis is reversible, it should be remembered that calculus and other factors that promote plaque retention (e.g., overhanging restorations) will make adequate oral hygiene difficult. These factors should be corrected by scaling and appropriate restorative treatment in addition to OHI. Gingivitis may be a precursor to, or marker of, chronic periodontitis, and must be differentiated from periodontitis by measuring attachment levels and by visualizing alveolar bone levels radiographically.

Gingivitis modified by systemic factors These would include puberty-associated gingivitis, menstrual cycle–associated gingivitis, pregnancy-associated gingivitis, pyogenic granuloma, diabetes mellitus–associated gingivitis, and gingivitis associated with blood dyscrasias (e.g., leukemia-associated gingivitis).

Gingivitis modified by medications These would include drug-influenced gingival enlargement and drug-induced gingivitis (e.g., oral contraceptive–associated gingivitis and drug-induced gingival overgrowth due to phenytoin or cyclosporine).

Gingival disease modified by malnutrition These would include ascorbic acid-deficiency gingivitis (scurvy) and gingivitis due to protein deficiency.

Classification of periodontal disease[1]

Classification systems are necessary to provide a framework in which to scientifically study the etiology, pathogenesis and treatment of diseases in an orderly fasion.[1] A new periodontal disease classification system was recommended by the 1999 International Workshop for a Classification of Periodontal Disease and Conditions and has been accepted by the American Academy of Periodontology (AAP).

One of the most significant changes included the addition of a detailed section on gingival diseases and lesions. Another important change was the discontinuation of terms related to age of presentation and rate of progression of the diseases. This new classification has numerous subcategories; only the major categories will be discussed here.

I	Gingival diseases
II	Chronic periodontitis
III	Aggressive periodontitis
IV	Periodontitis as a manifestation of systemic diseases
V	Necrotizing periodontal diseases
VI	Abscesses of the periodontium
VII	Periodontitis associated with endodontic lesions
VIII	Development or acquired deformities and conditions

Changes to the periodontal classification system

- Addition of a gingival disease component
- Replacement of "adult periodontitis" with "chronic periodontitis"
- Replacement of "early-onset periodontitis" with "aggressive periodontitis"
- Elimination of "refractory periodontitis" as a separate entity
- Further subclassification of "periodontitis as a manifestation of systemic diseases"
- Replacement of "necrotizing ulcerative periodontitis" with "necrotizing periodontal diseases"
- Addition of a category on "periodontal abscess," "periodontic-endodontic lesions," and "developmental or acquired deformities and conditions"

1 G. C. Armitage 1999 *Ann Periodontol* **4** 1.

Chronic periodontitis[1]

Chronic periodontitis is an infectious disease resulting in inflammation within the supporting tissues of the teeth, with progressive attachment and bone loss. It is characterized by pocket formation and/or gingival recession. It is recognized as the most frequently occurring form of periodontitis. Its onset may be at any age, but is most commonly detected in adults. The prevalence and severity of the disease increase with age. It may affect a variable number of teeth, and it has variable rates of progression.

Chronic periodontitis is initiated and sustained by bacterial plaque, but host defense mechanisms play an integral role in its pathogenesis. It is reasonable to assume that the disease will progress further if treatment is not provided.

Risk factors and determinants associated with chronic periodontitis
- Plaque, poor oral hygiene
- Tobacco
- Genetic predisposition
- Psychosocial stress
- Diabetes
- Systemic disease

Microbiology Several bacterial species residing in a biofilm on tooth surfaces referred to as dental plaque have been closely associated with periodontitis.[2] These include *Prophyromonas gingivalis, Actinobacillus actinomycetemcomitans, Bacteroides forsythus,* non-classified spirochetes, *Prevotella intermedia, Campylobacter rectus, Eubacterium nodatum, Treponema denticola, Streptococcus intermedia, Preveotella nigrescens, Peptostreptococcus micros, Fusobacterium nucleatum,* and *Eikenella corrodens.* Thus, it appears that various complexes of putative periodontal pathogens can initiate and perpetuate the disease in a susceptible host.[3,4]

Diagnosis is based on the following:
- Bleeding on probing, probing depth, and clinical attachment loss
- Testing teeth for mobility
- Radiographic examination (vertical bitewings and periapical views)

Treatment includes the following:
- Scaling and root planning
- Pharmacological therapy
- Surgical therapy
- Occlusal adjustment

1 AAP Consensus Report 1999 *Ann Periodontol* **4** 38.

2 T. F. Flemming 1999 *Ann Periodontol* **4** 32.

3 A. D. Haffajee 1994 *Periodontol 2000* **5** 78.

4 R. P. Darveau 1997 *Periodontol 2000* **14** 12.

Pocketing

The periodontal *pocket*, defined as a pathologically deepened gingival sulcus, is one of the most important clinical features of periodontal disease.[1]

Gingival (pseudo) pockets are due to gingival enlargement with the pocket epithelium at or above the cementoenamel junction.

Periodontal pockets imply apical migration of the junctional epithelium beyond the cementoenamel junction and can be divided into suprabony and intrabony pockets. In a suprabony pocket, the bottom of the pocket is coronal to the underlying alveolar bone.[1] In the case of an intrabony pocket, the bottom of the pocket is apical to the level of the adjacent alveolar bone. In this second type, the lateral pocket wall lies between the tooth surface and the alveolar bone.[1]

Pocket contents Periodontal pockets contain debris consisting principally of microorganisms and their products (enzymes, endotoxins, and etc.), gingival crevicular fluid, food remnants, salivary mucin, desquamated epithelial cells, and leukocytes.[1]

Pocket depths are measured from the gingival margin to the estimated base of the pocket. Because a pocket can develop at any point around a tooth, its entire circumference must be probed. Clinical attachment levels are measured from a fixed reference point: the cementoenamel junction to the base of the pocket.

Periodontal probes are the key instruments in detecting pockets. Numerous designs exist, and while individual preference will influence choice, it is sensible to reduce variability by selecting a single type of probe and using that type of probe throughout any one individual's treatment. An attempt should be made to probe parallel to the long axis of the tooth each time. The exception to this rule is when probing interproximal areas where it is necessary to angle the probe slightly so that the site directly under the contact point can be reached. The other crucial indicator of periodontal disease, bleeding, is also detected using a probe (gently); again, consistency with a single type of probe is necessary.

Probing variables The depth of penetration depends on the following:
• Type of probe and its position
• Amount of pressure used
• Degree of inflammation[2]

In the presence of inflammation, a probe tip can pass through the inflamed tissues until it reaches the most coronal dentogingival fibers, about 0.5 mm apical to the apical extent of the junctional epithelium. The amount of penetration into the tissues varies directly with the degree of inflammation, so that, following resolution of inflammation, an underestimate of attachment levels may be given. Formation of a tight, long junctional epithelium following treatment may also give a false sense of security if probing measurements are not interpreted with a degree of caution.

In an attempt to overcome some of the technical problems associated with conventional manual periodontal probes, numerous electronic periodontal probes have been developed that permit probe insertion with a controlled force.[3] However, comparative reproducibility data from multiple studies do not show any major differences between conventional and various types of controlled-force probes.[4]

1 F. A. Carranza 2002 *Carranza's Clinical Periodontology*, **9** 336, Saunders.

2 M. A. Listgarten 1980 *J Clin Periodontol* **7** 165.

3 G. C. Armitage 1996 *J Periodontol* **1** 37.

4 L. F. Rose 2004 *Periodontics: Medicine, Surgery, and Implants*, p. 140, Elsevier Mosby.

Diagnostic tests and monitoring

Despite our increased understanding of the etiology and pathogenesis of periodontal infections, the diagnosis and classification of these diseases is still based almost entirely on traditional clinical assessments.[1] Even though bleeding on probing has traditionally been the most useful indicator of disease activity, only 30% of sites that bleed will lose attachment.[2]

Traditional approach to diagnosis[1]

- Presence or absence of clinical signs of inflammation
- Probing depths
- Extent and pattern of loss of clinical attachment and bone
- Patient's medical and dental histories
- Presence or absence of miscellaneous signs and symptoms

In some situations, supplemental qualitative or quantitative assessments of the GCF and subgingival microflora are performed.[1] In addition, a genetic test for susceptibility to chronic periodontitis has become commercially available.[3] However, it should be emphasized that the supplemental information on GCF components, the subgingival microflora, and genetic susceptibility are not commonly used by practitioner in arriving at a diagnosis since the diagnostic utility of this information has not been validated.[1]

Advances in traditional diagnostics methods

- Instruments have been developed that measure the temperature in the gingival tissue.
- Comparable repeatability values have been obtained with computer-linked, controlled-force electronic periodontal probes.[4] Electronic probes have the advantages of controlling insertion forces and automatically recording clinical information into a computer.[4]
- Advanced direct digital radiographic and computed tomographic techniques have been developed to the stage where they are already being used on a daily basis in practice.[5]
- Intraoral radiographs (long cone technique) supplemented with vertical or horizontal bitewings provide a considerable amount of information about the periodontium that cannot be obtained by other noninvasive means.[1]

Many of the criteria used in the diagnosis and classification of the different forms of periodontal disease are also used in the development of a prognosis. Examples of typical periodontal prognostic criteria follow.

Prognostic Categories[6]

- *Good prognosis:* adequate remaining periodontal support and ease of maintenance.
- *Fair prognosis:* attachment loss to the point that the tooth cannot have a good prognosis; Class I furcation (maintainable).
- *Poor prognosis:* moderate attachment loss with Class I or Class II furcation lesions (can be maintained with difficulty).
- *Questionable prognosis:* poor crown-to-root ratio; poor root form; root proximity; Class II or III furcation lesions; mobility of 2+ or greater.

- *Hopeless prognosis:* inadequate attachment to maintain the tooth in health, comfort, and function. In such cases, extraction is recommended.

In summary, the evaluation of a patient's periodontal status requires a relevant medical and dental history as well as a thorough clinical and radiographic examination including an evaluation of extraoral and intraoral structures.[7]

1 AAP Position Paper 2003 *J Periodontol* **74** 1237.

2 N. Lang 1986 *J Clin Periodontol* **13** 590.

3 G. C. Armitage 1995 *Periodontology 2000* **7** 39.

4 G. C. Armitage 1996 *Periodontology 2000* **12** 40.

5 M. K. Jeffcoat 1995 *Periodontology 2000* **7** 54.

6 M. K. McGuire 1991 *J Periodontol* **62** 51.

7 AAP Parameters of Care Supplement 2000 *J Periodontol* **71** 847.

Acute periodontal disease[1]

Acute periodontal diseases are clinical conditions of rapid onset that involve the periodontium or associated structures, and may be characterized by pain or discomfort and infection.

Clinical features

Acute periodontal infections include the following:
1 Gingival abscess
2 Periodontal abscess
3 Necrotizing periodontal disease
4 Herpetic gingivostomatitis
5 Pericoronal abscess (pericoronitis)
6 Combined periodontal–endodontic lesions

Gingival abscess

Definition A localized purulent infection that involves the marginal gingiva or interdental papilla.

Clinical features A localized area of swelling in the marginal gingiva or interdental papilla, with a red, smooth, shiny surface. The lesion may be painful and appear pointed. Purulent exudates may be present.

Treatment Drainage to relieve the acute symptoms and mitigation of the etiology.

Periodontal abscess

Definition A localized purulent infection within the tissue adjacent to the periodontal pocket that may lead to the destruction of periodontal ligament and alveolar bone.

Clinical features A smooth, shiny swelling of the gingiva; pain associated with the area of swelling with tender to touch; a purulent exudate. The tooth may be sensitive to percussion and mobile. Rapid loss of periodontal attachment may occur.

Treatment Establish drainage by debriding the pocket and remove plaque, calculus and other irritants. Other treatments may include irrigation of the pocket, limited occlusal adjustment, and administration of antimicrobials and management of patient comfort. In some circumstances, extraction of the tooth may be necessary.

Necrotizing Periodontal Disease

Definition Necrotizing ulcerative periodontal disease (NUP) is an acute infection of the gingiva.

Clinical features Necrosis and ulceration of the tips of the interdental papilla or gingival margin, and painful, bright red marginal gingiva that bleed on slight manipulation. The mouth may have a malodor and systemic manifestations may be present. NUP may be associated with HIV/AIDS and other diseases where the immune system is compromised.

1 AAP 2000 *J Periodontol* **71** 863.

Treatment Irrigation and debridement of the necrotic areas and tooth surfaces; oral hygiene instructions and the use of oral rinses, pain control, and management of systemic manifestations, including appropriate antibiotic therapy as necessary.

Herpetic gingivostomatitis See p. 430

Pericoronal abscess (pericoronitis) See p. 372

Combined periodontal/endodontic lesions (abscesses) See p. 218

Periodontitis in children and adolescents

Children and adolescents can have any of the several forms of periodontitis as described in the proceedings of the 1999 International Workshop for a Classification of Periodontal Diseases and Conditions (*aggressive periodontitis, chronic periodontitis* and *periodontitis as a manifestation of systemic diseases*).[1] However, chronic periodontitis is more common in adults, while aggressive periodontitis may be more common in children and adolescents.[2]

Localized aggressive periodontitis (LAgP)

Patients with LagP have interproximal attachment loss on at least two permanent first molars and incisors, with attachment loss on no more than two teeth other than first molars and incisors.[1] LAgP occurs in children and adolescents without clinical evidence of systemic disease and is characterized by the severe loss of alveolar bone around permanent teeth.[3] Retrospective studies have suggested it may affect primary dentition.[4] The gingiva around affected teeth may appear entirely normal despite deep periodontal pockets. The degree of periodontal destruction seems out of proportion to the deposits of plaque and calculus.

Prevalence Reported estimates of the prevalence of LAgP in geographically diverse adolescent populations range from 0.1% to 15%.[1] Most reports suggest a low prevalence (0.2%), which is markedly greater in African-American populations.[1]

Microbiology Bacteria of probable etiologic importance include highly virulent strains of *Actinobacillus actinomycetemcomitans* in combination with *Bacteriodes*-like species.[5,6] In some populations, *Eubacterium* species have been associated with the presence of LAgP.[7] To date, no single species is found in all cases of LAgP. A variety of functional defects have been reported in neutrophils from patients with LAgP. These include anomalies of chemotaxis, phagocytosis, bactericidal activity, superoxide production, FcγRIIIB (CD16) expression, leukotriene B4 generation, and Ca^{2+} channel and second messenger activation.[1] The influence of these functional defects on the susceptibility of individuals to LAgP is unknown, but it is possible that they play a role in the clinical course of disease in some patients.[1]

Treatment Meticulous oral hygiene, surgical and nonsurgical root debridement in conjunction with antimicrobial (antibiotic) therapy. The most successful antibiotics reported are the tetracyclines, metronidazole, and metronidazole in combination with amoxicillin.

Generalized aggressive periodontitis (GAgP)

Patients with GAgP exhibit generalized interproximal attachment loss including at least three teeth that are not first molars and incisors.[1] GAgP can begin at any age and often affects the entire dentition. Individuals with GAgP exhibit marked periodontal inflammation and have heavy accumulations of plaque and calculus.[8]

Prevalence In the United States, the reported prevalence in adolescents (14–17 years of age) is 0.13%.[9]

Microbiology High percentages of nonmotile, facultatively anaerobic, gram-negative rods including *Porphyromonas gingivalis*.[10] In common with LAgP, these patients have neutrophils with suppressed chemotaxis.[10]

Treatment Meticulous oral hygiene, surgical and nonsurgical root debridement in conjunction with antimicrobial (antibiotic) therapy. The most successful antibiotics reported are the tetracyclines, metronidazole, and metronidazole in combination with amoxicillin.

Periodontitis as a manifestation of systemic diseases

In patients with one of several systemic diseases that predispose to highly destructive disease of the primary teeth (up to the age of 4 or 5 years), the diagnosis is periodontitis as a manifestation of systemic disease. Such systemic diseases include Papillon-Lefèvre syndrome, cyclic neutropenia, agranulocytosis, Down syndrome, hypophosphatasia, and leukocyte adherence deficiency.[1] The disease occurs in localized and generalized forms.[1] In the localized form, affected sites exhibit rapid bone loss and minimal gingival inflammation. In the generalized form, there is rapid bone loss around nearly all teeth and marked gingival inflammation.

Microbiology High percentages of *A. actinomycetemcomitans*, *Prevotella intermedia*, *Eikenella corrodens*, and *Capnocytophaga sputigena*.

Pathology It is probable that defects in neutrophil and immune cell function associated with these diseases play an important role in increased susceptibility to periodontitis and other infections.

Treatment Similar to treatment of LAgP and GAgP in the permanent dentition and has been reported to include surgical and nonsurgical mechanical debridement and antimicrobial therapy.[1]

1 AAP 2003 *J Periodontol* **74** 1696.

2 G. Armitage 1999 *Ann Periodontol* **4** 1.

3 P. N. Baer 1971 *J Periodontol* **42** 516.

4 B. Sjödin 1993 *J Clin Periodontol* **20** 32.

5 V. Haraszthy 2000 *J Periodontol* **71** 912.

6 K. S. Kornman 1985 *J Periodontol* **56** 443.

7 W. E. C. Moore 1985 *Infect Immun* **48** 507.

8 R. C. Page 1983 *J Periodontol* **54** 197.

9 H Löe 1991 *J Periodontol* **62** 608.

10 M. E. Wilson 1985 *J Periodontol* **56** 457.

Prevention of periodontal disease

Periodontal diseases are typically characterized by asymptomatic clinical signs such as bleeding on probing and loss of clinical attachment.[1] This means patients often are unaware of their periodontal status. Thus, patients must be educated to understand that unchecked periodontal diseases may eventually lead to tooth loss.[1] Following the comments on the pages covering the etiology and epidemiology of periodontal disease, it is quite clear that dental plaque is the main cause of the problem and its elimination will prevent periodontal disease. This is easier said than done—remember, most of the world's population has gingivitis and/or periodontitis. The key to prevention is regular and thorough plaque removal.

Oral hygiene instruction is probably the most useful advice you can give to your patients. OHI should include an explanation of the nature of the patient's disease and hence the reasons for good oral hygiene. Identify and demonstrate to the patient the disease (such as swollen gingiva and bleeding on probing) using a hand mirror, then demonstrate the cause (plaque), either directly by scraping off a deposit or by disclosing solution. Explain how plaque starts to grow immediately after tooth brushing, so that regular removal is necessary, and that it cannot be rinsed away. Then demonstrate how to remove it, avoiding overt criticism of the patient's present efforts, as this is often counterproductive. Since smoking exacerbates periodontal disease and adversely affects treatment outcome, patients should be advised of this link.

Tooth brushing requires a brush, ideally with a small head and even nylon bristles (3–4 tufts across by 10–12 lengthways), which should be renewed at least monthly. Currently, it is safe to assume that the differences among manual brushes are likely to be insignificant compared with the frequency of use and operator dexterity.[1] Toothpaste makes the process more pleasant and is a useful medium for topical fluoride and other agents. Numerous brushing methods can be described, based on the movement of the brush stroke: rolling, vibratory, circular, vertical or horizontal. The best is the one that works for the individual patient and does no harm to tooth or gingiva. The horizontal scrub is notorious for exacerbating gingival recession. Modifications to toothbrushes and brushing technique are often required in children, the elderly, and those with disabling diseases.

Interdental cleaning Brushing alone is unlikely to clean the interdental spaces. Dental floss, floss holders, mini-interdental brushes (particularly good for concave root surfaces), automated interdental cleaners, and toothpicks are available for interdental cleaning. The use of dental floss must be learned by demonstration and observation of the patient's techniques.

Professional preventive techniques

Regular periodic examination for periodontal disease, which is largely a-symptomatic, is essential. This requires a complete oral examination, including probing for pockets as part of a routine examination. In patients who have been demonstrated to have periodontal disease, 3-month follow-ups are advisable. Routine scaling and polishing is of little value unless accompanied by intensive education and motivation of the patient, as it is the patient's efforts that will prevent the re-formation of plaque and initiation of periodontal disease. Elimination, avoidance and prevention of iatrogenic problems, such as overhanging margins on restorations, ill-fitting crown margins, poorly designed appliances, etc., are mandatory.

1 L. F. Rose 2004 *Periodontics: Medicine, Surgery, and Implants*, pp. 217, 298, Elsevier Mosby.

Principles of treatment

1 Establish a diagnosis.
2 Periodontal disease is an infection due to the presence of plaque. Daily plaque control is the key to success. More complex treatments will always fail in the absence of effective plaque control.
3 The aims of corrective techniques such as scaling, root planing, periodontal surgery, restorative work, endodontics, occlusal adjustment, etc., focus on
   • eliminating pathological periodontal pockets, and creating a tight epithelial attachment where the pocket once existed;
   • arresting loss of and, in some cases, improving the alveolar bone support; and
   • creating an oral environment that is relatively simple for the patient to maintain plaque-free.

The overall aim could be summarized as the creation of a healthy mouth that the patient is both able and willing to maintain.

It is often convenient to divide the principles of periodontal therapy into three phases:
1 The *initial* (cause-related) phase, where the aim is to control or eliminate gingivitis and arrest any further progression of periodontal disease by the removal of plaque and other contributory factors.
2 The *corrective* phase is designed principally to restore function and, where relevant, aesthetics.
3 The *maintenance* (supportive) phase aims to reinforce patient motivation so that their OH is adequate to prevent recurrence of disease. Keep in mind that the patient cannot easily detect subgingival plaque buildup.

Nonsurgical therapy—1

Nonsurgical therapy in periodontal disease consists of oral physiotherapy, scaling and root planing, and chemotherapeutic agents to prevent, arrest, or eliminate periodontal disease.[1]

Oral physiotherapy[1] The goal of oral hygiene is the physical and chemical disruption of the biofilm on a frequent basis. A variety of devices and techniques, such as manual toothbrushes, electromechanical toothbrushes, dental floss, floss holders, toothpicks, interdental brushes, proxabrushes, and rubber tips have been used in this pursuit.

Scaling is the process by which plaque and calculus are removed from both supragingival and subgingival tooth surfaces, either with hand instruments (curettes and scalers) or with mechanical instruments (sonic and ultrasonic scalers).[2]

Root planing is the process by which residual embedded calculus and portions of cementum are removed from the roots to produce a smooth, hard and clean surface. It is customary to make use of an ultrasonic scaler for the bulk of the work and finish off, particularly subgingivally, with hand instruments. The precise use of hand instruments is largely a matter of personal preference; however, it is essential to use controlled force and a secure finger-rest. Ultrasonic instruments are quicker, but they can be uncomfortable and leave an uneven root surface (though the significance of the latter is controversial). Ultrasonic scaling employs a frequency of 18,000 to 42,000 cycles/sec. Another instrument, known as a sonic scaler and vibrating at 3000–8000 cycles/sec, has been shown to be equally effective at removing calculus.

The teeth are usually polished after scaling, preferably using a rubber cup and a fluoride-containing paste. Patients can then appreciate the feeling of a clean mouth that they must then maintain; however, this may result in increased sensitivity to cold due to the exposed root surfaces.

Local delivery of medicaments

Due to controversy over the efficacy and unwanted effects of systemic antibiotics, methods of direct delivery into the pocket have been explored. These have included using injected pastes or gels, or by impregnated fibers. This gives a high local dose, low systemic uptake, and prolonged exposure of the pathogens to the drug. The rate of crevicular fluid turnover is such that the substantivity of these agents is low.

Examples Tetracycline fibers (Actisite), chlorhexidine chips (PerioChip), doxycycline gels (Atridox), minocycline microspheres (Arestin), metronidazole gel, and minocycline ointment and gel.

However, only small increases in attachment levels have been reported, and currently local adjunctive antibiotics are only indicated as adjuncts to conventional mechanical therapy.

---

1 L. F. Rose 2004 *Periodontics: Medicine, Surgery, and Implants*, p. 238, Elsevier Mosby.

2 F. A. Carranza 2002 *Carranza's Clinical Periodontology*, **9** 631, Saunders.

Nonsurgical therapy—2

Antiseptics and antibiotics

The microbial etiology of inflammatory periodontal diseases provides the rationale for the use of antimicrobial medication in periodontal therapy.[1] This concept is based on the premise that specific microorganisms cause destructive periodontal disease, and that the antibiotic agent in vivo can exceed concentrations necessary to kill or inhibit the pathogens.[1]

Antiseptics The antiseptic of greatest proven value is chlorhexidine gluconat (0.12% mouthwash), which provides antimicrobicidal activity during oral rinsing. Microbiologic sampling of plaque has shown a general reduction of both aerobic and anaerobic bacterial counts ranging from 54% to 97% through 6 months' clinical use. Rinsing with chlorhexidine inhibits the buildup and maturation of plaque by reducing certain microbes regarded as gingival pathogens, thereby reducing gingivitis. A standard regimen is 15 ml of solution rinsed for 30 sec twice a day. Side effects from this medication include staining of oral surfaces, such as tooth surfaces, restorations, and the dorsum of the tongue. Some patients may experience an alteration in taste perception and increase in the formation of calculus.

Antibiotics Patients with gingivitis or chronic periodontitis usually respond well to mechanical debridement and topical antiseptics and may not derive clinically significant additional benefit from antibiotic therapy.[2] Nevertheless, there is a clear place for antibiotics/antiseptics as adjuncts in selected types of periodontal disease, e.g., aggressive periodontitis and acute or severe periodontal infections.

Antibiotic prescription is suitable for the following:[1]

- Periodontal patients who do not respond to conventional mechanical therapy
- Patients with acute periodontal infections associated with systemic manifestations
- Prophylaxis in medically compromised patients
- Adjunct to surgical and nonsurgical periodontal therapy

Selection of antibiotics[1]

Tetracycline (tetracycline-HCl, doxycycline and minocycline) may be indicated in periodontal infections in which *Actinobacillus actinomycetemcomitas* is the prominent pathogen. It can be administered either systemically or directly into the pocket via a slow-release mechanism. It is most useful in the treatment of LAgP. Minocycline and doxycycline are currently popular. In addition to being antibacterial, tetracyclines decrease host neutrophil collagenases and bone loss.

Metronidazole may arrest disease progression in recurrent periodontitis patients with *Porphyromonas gingivalis* and/or *Prevotella intermedia* infections with few or no other potential pathogens. It is effective against protozoa and strict anaerobes and capable of eliminating all the strict anaerobes found in periodontal pockets. As it does not interfere with aerobes or facultative anaerobes, it is highly unlikely to allow the development of opportunist pathogens. There is frequent mention of the mutagenicity and teratogenicity of this drug in animal studies, but despite widespread use in medicine, no clinical evidence has emerged to support this. It is, in fact, an extremely safe and useful drug. When combined with mechanical pocket therapy, significant improvements in terms of probing depth have been demonstrated.[2] Although adverse effects are relatively minor, there is an important interaction of metronidazole with warfarin and alcohol.

Clindamycin has demonstrated efficacy in recurrent periodontitis and may be considered with periodontal infection of *Peptostreptococcus*, β-hemolytic streptococci, and various oral gram-negative anaerobic rods. Clindamycin should be prescribed with caution because of the potential for psedomembranous colitis as a result of intestinal overgrowth with *Clostridium difficile*.

Fluoroquinolones (ciprofloxacin) are effective against enteric rods, pseudomonads, staphylococci, *Actinobacillus actinomycetemcomitans*, and other periodontal microorganisms. Fluoroquinolones may induce tendinopathy and strenuous exercise should be avoided during therapy.

Azithromycin exhibits an excellent ability to penetrate into both normal and pathological periodontal tissues, and is highly active against many periodontal pathogens.

Metronidazole plus amoxicillin provides a relatively predictable eradication and suppression of Actinobacillus actinomycetemcomitans and Porphyromonas gingivalis.

Metronidazole plus ciprofloxacin may substitute for metronidazole plus amoxicillin in individuals who are allergic to β-lactam drugs and are at least 18 years of age.

Even though antibiotics are beneficial in some patients, problems with their use include the unwanted side effects of such chemicals, development of resistance, mode of delivery, and, most importantly, the fact that no single organism has been identified as the main pathogen in periodontal disease.

Common antibiotic therapies in the treatment of periodontitis[1]

Antibiotic	Adult dosage
Metronidazole	500 mg/tid/8 days
Clindamycin	300 mg/tid/8 days
Doxycycline or minocycline	100–200 mg/qd/21 days
Ciprofloxacin	500 mg/bid/8 days
Azithromycin	500 mg/qd/4–7 days
Metronidazole + amoxicillin	250 mg/tid/8 days of each drug
Metronidazole + ciprofloxacin	500 mg/bid/8 days of each drug

1 AAP Position Paper 2004 *J Periodontol* **75** 1553.

Minimally invasive therapy—1

There has been a progressive move away from pocket elimination surgery and toward the creation of a healthy periodontium, which gives access for both professional and home cleaning. Recognition that periodontal disease is a localized infection due to the presence of dental plaque, and that its arrest and prevention depend on the removal of plaque and plaque-retaining factors, has allowed a far more rational and conservative approach to therapy to develop.

The primary aims of periodontal surgery are to

- remove deposits from root surfaces;
- create subgingival root surfaces that are accessible for cleaning, either by professionals or by the patient; and
- maximize the potential for healing of damaged periodontal tissues.

Minimally invasive techniques include deep subgingival scaling/root planing and the modified Widman flap (open flap debridement). These are suitable for those patients who, despite good supragingival plaque control, still have true pockets but do not need recontouring of the gingival margins.

Scaling and root planing Deep subgingival scaling and root planing are best carried out under LA. Root planing is a procedure through which plaque and calculus are removed from the root surface; it differs from supragingival scaling simply in its thoroughness and the discomfort it causes. Root planing is a technique whereby endotoxin-damaged cementum is removed from the root surface by scraping the root. The same instruments are used for both procedures (p. 197), and in practice it is probably impossible to differentiate between subgingival scaling and root planing, as in both techniques plaque, calculus, root cementum, and small amounts of dentine will be removed. These are the core procedures for all periodontal techniques; the only real difference with formal surgery is that it allows treatment under direct vision, osseous recontouring and sculpting if desired, and repositioning of the gingiva. It is often most effective to treat one quadrant at a time under LA. The choice of instruments is less important than the end result, as effective debridement of the root surface is essential. Maintaining sharp instruments is essential and having a sterile sharpening stone allows the operator to maintain instrument sharpness during the procedure. Success therapy will allow tight adaptation of the pocket epithelium to the root, creating a *long junctional epithelium*. Because smoking decreases outcome of treatment, some periodontists offer limited treatment options in those patients who continue to smoke. While periodontal surgery hardly has the public impact of cardiac surgery, the ethical problem is the same.

Practical tips for periodontal surgery

Local anesthesia The infiltration, block, and/or lingual/palatal injections required will be determined by the site of surgery. Both LA and hemostasis are improved by injecting directly into the gingival margin and interdental papilla until blanching is seen.

Suturing techniques Interrupted interproximal sutures are used when buccal and lingual flaps are being reapposed at the same level. When flaps are repositioned at different levels, a suspensory suture is used, where the suture only passes through the buccal flap and is suspended around the cervical margins of the teeth.

Periodontal dressing These are essential after gingivectomy to decrease postoperative discomfort. Many practioners favor them after all periodontal surgery to help reappose the flap to bone. Eugenol dressings (e.g., ZOE) have the advantage of being mildly analgesic but can cause sensitivity reactions. Eugenol-free dressings (e.g., Coe-pak) are more popular.

Minimally invasive therapy—2

The modified Widman flap[1]

This is a technique that enables open debridement of the root surface, with a minimal amount of trauma. There is no attempt to excise the pocket, although a superficial collar of tissue is removed. This has the advantage of allowing close adaptation of the soft tissues to the root surface with minimal trauma to and exposure of underlying bone and connective tissue, thus causing fewer problems with postoperative sensitivity and aesthetics.

Technique

A scalloped incision is made parallel to the long axis of the teeth involved 1 mm from the crevicular margin, except when pockets are <2 mm deep, when an intracrevicular incision is made. This incision is extended interproximally as far as possible, separating the pocket epithelium from the flap to be raised, and then extended mesially and distally, allowing the flap to be raised as an envelope without relieving incisions. The flap should be as conservative as possible and only a few millimeters of alveolar bone exposed by a second incision intercrevicularly to release the collar of pocket epithelium and granulation tissue. A third incision at 90° to the tooth separates the pocket epithelium, and this is removed along with accompanying granulation tissue with curettes and hoes. The root surface is then thoroughly scaled and root planed. Although bony defects can be curetted, **no** osseous surgery is carried out. The flaps are then repositioned to cover all exposed alveolar bone and sutured into position. Postoperatively 0.12% chlorhexidine rinse is prescribed for 30 sec two times a day, and most periodontists prefer to use a periodontal dressing to improve patient comfort postoperatively.

Notes

There continues to be considerable confusion about nomenclature with this type of flap. The original Widman flap, described in 1918 by Leonard Widman, used relieving incisions and osseous surgery, and attempted to eliminate the pocket. The Neumann flap used an intracrevicular incision, again attempting to excise the pocket, but the "modified flap operation," described by Kirkland in 1931, did not require removal of inflamed tissues or apical displacement of the gingival margin. The latter was, of course, the precursor of the modified Widman flap.

---

1 S. Ramfjord 1974 *J Periodont* **45** 601.

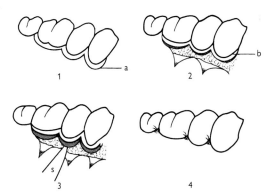

Modified Widman flap.
1 Design of flap
  a. Incision
2 Flap elevated
  b. Gingival cuff to be discarded
3 Excision of supra-alveolar pocket
  s. Scalpel blade
4 Flap repositioned and sutured in place

Periodontal surgery

Gingivectomy

Gingivectomy is the term used to describe the surgical excision of the gingiva performed to treat the pathologic effects of gingivitis, periodontitis and other conditions that result in alterations in normal gingival form.[1] Although gingivectomy was once a commonly performed surgical procedure, it has been supplanted by a variety of other surgical procedures.[2]

Indication[2]

1 To eliminate gingival pockets (suprabony pockets) and soft tissue craters
2 To create an aesthetic gingival form in case of delayed passive eruption
3 To reduce gingival enlargements resulting from medications or genetic factors

Contraindication[2]

1 Inadequate oral hygiene
2 Acutely inflamed gingiva
3 Inadequate keratinized gingiva
4 Presence of interdental osseous craters and infrabony defects

Technique Identification of the base of the pocket is usually accomplished by use of the periodontal probe or a mechanical device such as the Crane-Kaplan or Goldman-Fox pocket marker.[2] After establishment of the bleeding points, a coronally directed external bevel incision (45° angle) is made, using an appropriate surgical knife.[2] This bevelled incision excises supragingival pockets and allows for gingival recontouring. After completion of the primary incisions, the interdental incisions are made to sever the interproximal portion of the soft tissue pockets with the same interproximal angle used in the primary incision.[2] The exposed root surfaces are then curetted, and the margins of the gingiva may be refined by gingivoplasty.[2] Surgical periodontal dressing may be applied and oral hygiene procedures can be supplemented with oral saline rinses or with antibacterial mouthwashes such as 0.12% chlorhexidine.[3]

Disadvantages Loss of attached gingival and exposed root surface (which increases the likelihood of sensitivity and caries). Some remodeling of alveolar bone occurs, despite there being no operative interference.

Apically repositioned flap

This procedure is used to expose alveolar bone and includes the option for osseous surgery to correct infrabony defects. It allows excellent access to the root surface for debridement. The principal difference between this procedure and the modified Widman flap is the deliberate exposure of alveolar bone and the apical repositioning of the flap with postoperative exposure of the root surfaces. This is primarily a buccal procedure for the maxilla. The palatal procedure includes a conventional or reverse-bevel gingivectomy approach.

Technique A reverse bevel incision is made in the attached gingiva angled to excise the periodontal pocket in a scalloped outline with vertical relieving incisions at either end. A split-thickness flap is made down to bone and then converted to full thickness, leaving a residual collar of tissue around the root surfaces. This combination of pocket epithelium and granulation tissue is removed with a curette. If indicated, the alveolar crest can be reshaped.

Advantages include exposure of alveolar bone with controlled bone loss, exposure of furcation area, minimal postoperative pocket depth, ability to reposition the flap, and primary closure of the wound. In addition, keratinized gingiva is preserved.

Disadvantages include exposure of root surface (leading to increased susceptibility to caries and sensitivity) and increased loss of alveolar bone height, which accompanies full exposure of the bone at operation.

Osseous surgery

Bone recontouring has become less popular, as it is always accompanied by some degree of alveolar resorption and decreased support for the tooth. The basis for performing resective osseous surgery lay in the fact that periodontal disease attacks the underlying or supportive bony architecture.

Osteoplasty is conservative recontouring of the bone margin (i.e., non-supporting bone).

Ostectomy is excision of tooth-supporting bone, aimed at eliminating infra-alveolar pocketing, but unfortunately it also decreases alveolar support. The aim of osseous surgery should be establishing a more anatomically correct relationship between bone and tooth while maintaining as much alveolar support as possible.

Indication[4]
1 Sufficient bone remaining without attachment compromise
2 Elimination of interdental craters
3 Intrabony defects not amenable to regeneration
4 Horizontal bone loss with irregular marginal bone height
5 No aesthetic or anatomic limitations

Contraindication[4]
1 Anatomic and aesthetic limitations
2 Areas of insufficient remaining attachment

Advantages[4]
1 Predictable pocket elimination
2 Establishment of physiologic gingival and osseous architecture
3 Establishment of a favorable prosthetic environment

Disadvantages[4]
1 Loss of attachment
2 Aesthetic compromise
3 Increased root sensitivity

Technique With the flaps reflected, vertical interradicular grooving is done using a round no. 6, 8, or 10 bur with a high-speed handpiece with copious amounts of water to establish width and thin bone interdentally. Once the vertical grooves are completed, radicular blending is done to reduce thick bony margins and establish physiologic form. The final bony contours should mirror or approximate the healthy preoperative gingival form.

Other flap procedures

These include simple replaced flaps that give increased bony access compared to that with the modified Widman flap. There are also crown-lengthening procedures, which can range from a simple gingivectomy to an apically repositioned flap with or without bone removal. In addition, many periodontists have their own modification of these techniques.

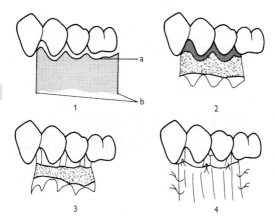

Apically repositioned flap.
1 Design of flap
   a Reverse bevel incision
   b Relieving incisions
2 Elevating the flap. Tissue enclosing pocketing to be discarded is hatched.
3 Flap is elevated, pockets excised. Osseous surgery can be performed at this stage.
4 Flap is apically repositioned and sutured in position.

1 H. Goldman 1946 *Am J Orthod* **32** 323.

2 L. F. Rose 2004 *Periodontics: Medicine, Surgery, and Implants*, p. 505, Elsevier Mosby.

3 P. N. Baer 1960 *Oral Surg* **13** 494.

4 E. S. Cohen 1989 *Atlas of Cosmetic and Reconstructive Periodontal Surgery*, **2** 84, Williams & Wilkins.

Regenerative techniques

Periodontal regeneration and repair

- *Periodontal repair* Healing by replacement with epithelium or connective tissue, or both.
- *Periodontal regeneration* Restoration of lost periodontium that involves the formation of alveolar bone, functionally aligned periodontal ligament (PDL), and new cementum.
- *New attachment* The union of connective tissue or epithelium with root surface that has been deprived of its original attachment apparatus. It is the ideal aim of periodontal therapy.
- *Reattachment* The reunion of epithelial and connective tissues with root surfaces and bone such as occurs after an incision or injury.

When the periodontium is damaged by inflammation or as a result of surgical treatment, the defect heals either through one of the above means. Histologic analysis is the only definitive method for determining the type of healing. Currently, the most widely used methods of evaluating whether a treatment modality can potentially result in periodontal regeneration are to provide histologic evaluation of periodontal regeneration in animal models when human biopsy materials are not available and to provide supportive clinical and radiographic data.[1]

A number of periodontal regenerative approaches have been attempted with varying degrees of success, described below.[1]

Root conditioning procedures

One approach toward improving periodontal healing is to clean and enhance the root surface so that it is biologically compatible. This strategy focuses on treatment with citric acid, tetracycline, or edetate disodium (EDTA) to demineralize the root surface. The conditioned root surface may enhance the formation of new connective tissue attachment.

Bone grafts and grafting materials

Bone grafts such as autografts (intraoral or extraoral bone sites), allografts (demineralized freeze-dried bone allografts and freeze-dried bone allografts), xenografts (anorganic bovine bone), and alloplasts (β-tricalcium phosphate-hydroxyapatite, bioactive glass polymers) may be used in repairing periodontal defects. Correction of osseous aspects of the periodontal defect occurs by osteoinduction (graft material induces bone formation) or osteoconduction (graft material acts as scaffold).

Guided-tissue regeneration

The recognition that epithelium migrates along the root surface before any other cell type after periodontal surgery and creates the *long junctional epithelium* that prevents new attachment raised the possibility that prevention of epithelium migration would allow new connective tissue attachment.[2]

The use of an occlusive membrane barrier to promote the formation of new periodontium and prevention of epithelial migration is called guided-tissue regeneration (GTR). This enables stem cells from the PDL and perivascular tissue to repopulate the root area and differentiate into a new periodontal supporting apparatus. Membranes may be used either alone or in combination with a bone graft or alloplastic material. Original barriers were either Millipore filters or ePTFE (expanded polytetrafluoroethylene membranes). Currently, both resorbable (polyglycoside synthetic polymers, collagen, and calcium sulfate) and nonresorbable membranes (ePTFE) in a variety of shapes are widely used. A nonresorbable membrane has to be removed at 4–6 weeks while resorbable membranes do not require a second surgical procedure for retrieval.

Bony infill in osseous defect There are a number of studies suggesting that complete regeneration may occur in up to 70% of three-walled infrabony defects. This success rate, however, is not consistent, especially in combined and two-walled defects.

Biologic and biomimicry mediators

Research has focused on the use of biologic mediators to selectively enhance cellular repopulation of the periodontal wound. Purified biologic (enamel matrix derivative) or synthetic biomimicry agents (platelet-derived growth factors and bone morphogenetic proteins) have emerged as potential agents to enhance periodontal regeneration.

Emdogain is a product containing enamel matrix derivative (EMD) proteins. These substances (e.g., amelogenin) are found in Hertwig's sheath and induce root formation in the developing tooth. Locally applied enamel matrix proteins might help form acellular cementum, the key tissue in the development of a functional periodontium.

Technique Access to the root surface is gained surgically, the cementum is mechanically cleaned, and EMD solution is applied to the root surfaces. The access flaps are then repositioned and sutured.

Outcome Regeneration of cementum, periodontal ligament, and alveolar bone appears to be possible experimentally; long-term clinical outcome awaits prospective randomized controlled clinical trials (RCCTs).

Even though periodontal regeneration continues to be one of the primary therapeutic approaches toward the management of periodontal defects, it is difficult to achieve. Some of the factors that influence therapeutic success are:[3]

- Poor plaque control and OH compliance
- Smoking
- Tooth and defect factors
- Poor surgical management

The crucial challenge for the clinician is to critically assess whether a periodontal defect can be corrected with a regenerative approach or whether it would be better managed with other treatment options.[1]

1 L. F. Rose 2004 *Periodontics: Medicine, Surgery and Implants*, p. 578, Elsevier Mosby .

2 A. H. Melcher 1976 *J Periodontal* **47** 256.

3 M. A. Reynolds 2003 *Ann Periodontol* **8** 227.

Peri-implantitis

The long-term predictability of osseointegrated implants has been documented.[1] Nevertheless, a significant number of early and late complications have also been reported.[2] The current hypothesis postulates bacterial infection and/or biomechanical overload as etiologic factors of late implant failure.[3] For example, infected sites around failed implants may harbor a complex microbiota with a large proportion of *Porphyromonas gingivalis*, *Prevotella intermedia,* and *Fusobacterium nucleatum.*[4]

The term *peri-implantitis* was introduced in the 1980s to describe the destructive inflammatory process affecting the soft and hard tissues around osseointegrated implants, leading to the formation of a peri-implant pocket and loss of supporting bone.[5] A peri-implantitis defect usually assumes the shape of a saucer around the implant and is well demarcated. In general, peri-implantitis begins at the coronal portion of the implant, while the more apical portion of the implant maintains an osseointegrated status. Signs of peri-implantitis include redness, increased probing depth, bleeding on probing, swelling, suppuration, and radiographic bone loss. Thus, peri-implantitis, like periodontitis, if left untreated may result in bone loss and ultimately implant loss. Patients with a history of periodontitis may represent a group of individuals with an elevated risk of developing peri-implantitis.[6]

Therefore, the current recommendation is that patients with implants be evaluated at regular visits for periodontal maintenance procedures, and any clinical signs and symptoms of peri-implant disease should be recorded and treated.[7] Reports indicate that steel curettes should not be used to remove calculus as they may scratch abutments, leading to further plaque accumulation.[8,9]

Several procedures have been described for the treatment of the inflammatory component and the resulting bony defect associated with infection of the peri-implant mucosa, including antimicrobial therapy, and resective or regenerative procedures.[10–13] Additional data indicate that a lack of keratinized tissue attached to an abutment or machined surface implant may have no adverse effect on implant survival.[14,15]

1 T. Albrektsson 1986 *Int J Oral Maxillofac Implants* **1** 11.
2 P. Worthington 1987 *Int J Oral Maxillofac Implants* **2** 77.
3 A. Mombelli 1987 *Oral Microbiol Immunol* **2** 145.
4 V. J. Iacono 1991 *Recent Adv Periodontol* **2** 85.
5 A. Mombelli 2002 *Periodontol 2000* **28** 177.
6 F. A. Carranza 2002 *Carranza's Clinical Periodontology,* **9,** p. 933, Saunders.
7 L. Sbordone 1999 *J Periodontol* **70** 1322.
8 AAP 1998 *J Periodontol* **69** 405.
9 AAP 1998 *J Periodontol* **69** 502.
10 U. Grunder 1993 *Int J Oral Maxillofac Implants* **8** 282.
11 M. B. Hürzeler 1995 *Int J Oral Maxillofac Implants* **10** 474.
12 L. B. Persson 1996 *Clin Oral Implants Res* **7** 366.
13 A. C. Wetzel 1999 *Clin Oral Implants Res* **10** 111.
14 J. L. Wennström 1994 *Clin Oral Implants Res* **5** 1.
15 R. Mericske-Stern 1994 *Clin Oral Implants Res* **5** 9.

Mucogingival surgery

Mucogingival surgery encompasses those techniques aimed at the correction of local gingival defects and provides a functionally adequate zone of keratinized attached gingiva. The rationale for this type of surgery has been hotly debated over many years, and no standard width of keratinized attached gingiva has been established. Initially it was felt that a margin of attached gingiva of approximately 3 mm was required to protect the periodontium during mastication and to dissipate the pull to the gingival margin from frenal attachments. In fact, data from properly conducted experimental work have demonstrated that the width of attached gingiva and the presence or absence of an attached portion are **not** of decisive importance for the maintenance of gingival health.[1] As a result of this finding, the indications for mucogingival surgery have been rationalized:

• Where change in the morphology of the gingival margin would improve plaque control, e.g., presence of high frenal attachments or deep areas of recession
• Areas where recession creates root sensitivity that cannot be controlled with fluoride or desensitizing toothpaste
• Esthetic problems
• A very thin layer of attached gingiva overlying a tooth to be moved orthodontically or to receive prosthetic or restorative dentistry

Gingival recession

Gingival recession is one of the most common reasons for carrying out mucogingival surgery. The two most common causes are plaque-induced gingival inflammation and toothbrush trauma, revealing dehiscences in alveolar bone. Basic periodontal care and correction of faulty toothbrushing technique are the first lines of treatment. Other factors that can predispose to gingival recession include tooth malposition, prominent roots, bone dehiscence, thin marginal soft tissue, high frenal attachment, inflammation, inflammatory viral eruption, and dental procedures such as orthodontic, restorative, and periodontal treatments.[2]

Classification of gingival recession (Miller Classification)[3]

• Class I: marginal recession coronal to the mucogingival junction with no periodontal loss in the interdental areas
• Class II: also shows no interdental periodontal loss but recession extends beyond the mucogingival junction
• Class III: recession extending to or beyond the mucogingival junction, but with some soft tissue or bone loss in the interdental areas
• Class IV: similar to class III defects except there is severe bone or soft tissue loss interdentally

Mucogingival techniques

The surgical methods available for correction of mucogingival problems are as follows:

Free gingival grafts are the most widely used, most predictable technique for increasing the zone of attached gingiva. Thin or intermediate-thickness grafts of approximately 0.5 to 0.75 mm are ideal thickness for increasing the zone of keratinized attached gingival.[4] Thick or full-thickness grafts of 1.25 to 2 mm or greater are indicated for root coverage and ridge augmentation procedures.

Advantages[5]
- High degree of predictability
- Simplicity
- Ability to treat multiple teeth at the same time
- Can be performed when keratinized gingiva adjacent to the involved area is insufficient

Disadvantages[5]
- Two operative sites
- Compromised blood supply
- Lack of predictability in attempting root coverage
- Greater palatal discomfort due to secondary intention healing

Pedicle grafts are not separated from their blood supply. Commonly used pedicle grafts are the laterally positioned pedicle flap and the double papilla laterally positioned flap. These techniques may be of some value in very narrow areas of isolated gingival recession. Technically, of course, these are flaps, **not** grafts.

Advantages[5]
- One surgical site
- Good vascularity of the flap
- Ability to cover a denuded root surface

Disadvantages[5]
- Limited by the amount of adjacent keratinized attached gingiva
- Possibility of recession at the donor site
- Dehiscence or fenestration at the donor site
- Limited to one or two teeth with recession

Connective tissue grafts are an effective way to achieve predictable root coverage with a high degree of cosmetic enhancement. The procedure is basically a combination of a partial-thickness coronally or laterally reposi-tioned flap and a free connective tissue graft.

Advantages[5]
- Aesthetics
- Predictability
- Minimum palatal trauma
- Treat multiple teeth
- Increased graft vascularity

Disadvantages[5]
- High degree of technical skill required
- Complicated suturing

Guided tissue regeneration a technique employing either a bioabsorbable or nonresorbable membrane used for recession defect coverage. The membrane is sutured into place and covered with a coronally positioned flap. An advantage of this technique is that it is theoretically possible to regenerate bone and periodontal ligament rather than just gain soft tissue coverage alone. Another advantage is that a secondary surgical site to obtain donor tissue is not necessary.

Acellular dermal matrix (ADM) is used as a substitute for connective tissue when covered by a coronally positioned flap. ADM is obtained from human dermis harvested and treated to remove all cells while preserving the intact structure of the extracellular matrix, including an intact vascular network.[2] The ability to cover an unlimited number of sites without the need for a second surgical site to obtain donor tissue is a significant advantage of this material.

Enamel matrix derivative (Emdogain) applied to a coronally positioned flap may enhance root coverage, although some studies show no advantage to its use.

1 J. Wenstrom 1987 *J Clin Periodont* **14** 181.

2 Academy Report *J Periodontol* 2005 **76** 1588.

3 P. D. Miller 1985 *Int J Periodontics Restorative Dent* **2** 15.

4 E. E. Soehren 1973 *J Periodontol* **44** 727.

5 E. S. Cohen 1989 *Atlas of Cosmetic & Reconstructive Periodontal Surgery*, **2** 84, Williams & Wilkins.

Role of occlusion

The relation between occlusion and periodontal therapy is not clear. Current evidence-based research is inconclusive.

Forces that exceed the adaptive capacity of the periodontium produce injury called "trauma from occlusion." In the past it was thought that angular bony defects and ↑ mobility were directly attributable to trauma from the occlusion. This belief is currently less common as angular defects can be found around teeth in traumatic and in atraumatic occlusion.[1] In the absence of inflammation, the changes caused by traumatic occlusion are reversible in that they can be repaired if the offending forces are removed. However, when combined with inflammation, traumatic occlusion might enhance the bone destruction caused by the inflammation.[2]

Occlusal trauma[3]

- *Primary:* injury resulting in tissue changes from excessive occlusal forces applied to a tooth or teeth with normal support. It occurs in the presence of (1) normal bone levels, (2) normal attachment levels, and (3) excessive occlusal force(s).
- *Secondary:* injury resulting in tissue changes from normal or excessive occlusal forces applied to a tooth or teeth with reduced support. It occurs in the presence of (1) bone loss, (2) attachment loss, and (3) normal and/or excessive occlusal force(s).

Clinical and Radiographic Signs
Excessive tooth mobility
Radiographic evidence of widened PDL space
Vertical or angular bone destruction
Infrabony pockets
Pathologic migration
Loss of lamina dura
Root resorption

Tooth mobility

Tooth mobility may simply be a result of loss of periodontal attachment and bony support. It may also result purely as a localized effect due to a heavy occlusal loading, causing a widening of the periodontal membrane space, though this is usually iatrogenic in origin. Transient tooth mobility can also be a result of orthodontic treatment or periodontal surgery.

Miller's Mobility Index[4]
Grade 1 First distinguishable sign of movement greater than "normal"
Grade 2 Movement of the crown up to 1 mm in any buccal-lingual direction
Grade 3 Movement of the crown more than 1 mm in any direction and/or vertical depression or rotation of the crown in its socket

Fremitus A palpable or visible movement of a tooth when subjected to occlusal forces.

Treatment The first priority should be to diagnose and treat any existing periodontal disease and correct any preexisting iatrogenic causes, e.g., poor crowns or bridges, high restorations, etc. If tooth mobility persists as a direct result of diagnosable occlusal trauma, occlusal adjustment should be implemented. If the tooth is mobile as a result of lack of alveolar bone support, this is not automatically an indication for splinting.

Splinting is indicated in the following situations:
- Tooth with healthy but decreased periodontium where mobility is increased.
- Tooth with increased mobility that patient finds uncomfortable during function.

It is very easy to design splints that are impossible for patients to keep clean, as all additions to the natural tooth surface will increase plaque retention. A wide range of different techniques and materials have been described, including orthodontic wire fastened to teeth by resin composite, resin-composite alone, fixed bridges, partial prostheses, acid-etch retained splints, and, more recently, fiber-reinforced resin-composite splinting.

1 J. Waerhaug 1970 *J Periodont* **50** 355.

2 F. A. Carranza 2002 *Carranza's Clinical Periodontology*, **9**, p. 359, Saunders.

3 L. F. Rose 2004 *Periodontics: Medicine, Surgery and Implants*, p. 29, Elsevier Mosby.

4 S. C. Miller 1950 *Textbook of Periodontia* **3** p. 125.

Perio-endo lesions

Given the relative frequency of both periodontal disease and periapical pathology, it is not surprising that both may occur together, which can result in diagnostic confusion. In addition, the periodontic–endodontic lesion often presents a diagnostic and treatment dilemma. In fact, there is little evidence to support the popular notion that periodontitis leads to pulp necrosis. However, there is no doubt that pulpal pathology can exacerbate periodontal problems and vice versa.

Diagnosis[1]

There are several signs and symptoms of pulpal and periodontal lesions that allow them to be distinguished. These include pain; swelling; periodontal probing; tooth mobility; percussion on palpation; pulp tests, including thermal, electric, and preparation of the test cavity; and radiographic interpretation.

Pulpal problems

Acute pulpitis See p. 228.

Non-vital pulp (p. 228) may cause asymptomatic periapical lesion or periapical abscess.

Lateral canal and/or non-vital pulp may mimic a periodontal abscess, as can a root perforation following endodontic therapy.

Vertical root fracture and/or non-vital pulp can lead to periodontal inflammation and may mimic periodontal abscess.

Horizontal root fracture may mimic a periodontal abscess.

Periodontal pathology and its effect on the pulp

Deep pocketing may encroach on lateral canals in the apical 1/3 of the root, but is otherwise unlikely to cause direct pulpal necrosis.

Gingival recession is directly associated with hypersensitivity of root dentine.

Root planing and furcation treatment that remove cementum and underlying dentine may lead to hypersensitivity and chronic pulpitis through bacterial penetration of dentinal tubules.

Differential Diagnosis

	Primarily periodontal	Primarily pulpal
History	No preceding toothache	Often toothache
Percussion	TTP, especially lateral	TTP, especially vertical
Probing	Pocketing always	May be no pockets
Probing sinus	May lead to pocket	May lead to apex
Vitality test	Usually vital	Non-vital
Radiographs	Vertical bone loss	Apical area

---

1 L. F. Rose 2004 Periodontics: Medicine, Surgery, and Implants, p. 773, Elsevier Mosby.

Combined perio-endo lesions

These may be either

- coexisting, but separate from each other, in which case standard endodontic and periodontal therapy are used as indicated, or
- interconnected, in which case probing both pocket and sinus will reach the apex. This can be confirmed by taking a periapical film with a GP point inserted into the pocket.

Treatment First, resolve the acute infection and inflammation by drainage and/or antibiotics, then treat with orthograde RCT (the greater the pulpal component the better the prognosis). The apparent periodontal lesion will often be seen to resolve to a substantial degree over a period of months. The decision to carry out surgery should be deferred. Combined apicoectomy and periodontal surgery is quite feasible but carries a poor long-term prognosis. The worst prognosis applies to those teeth where the periapical/pulpal pathology has been due entirely to apical extension of the periodontal pocket. These are often diagnosed after the fact, when endodontics completely fails to resolve the lesion.

Furcation involvement

The extension of periodontal disease into the bi- or trifurcation of multi-rooted teeth is known as furcation involvement. The earlier the clinician recognizes furcation involvement, the simpler the treatment required to manage the problem. Bowers reported that 81% of all furcation entrance diameters measure <1 mm, with 58% <0.75 mm.[1] Since commonly used curettes have blade face widths ranging from 0.75 to 1.10 mm, it is unlikely that proper instrumentation of furcations can be achieved with curettes alone.[1] In addition, the possibility of pulpal pathology is increased in teeth with furcation involvement, and vitality testing is essential.

Diagnosis Not counting the third molars, 24 potential furcations exist, and diagnosis is best made through the use of radiography and clinical probing (Nabers probe). Diagnosis is made more difficult by certain anatomic factors. Furcation entrances for maxillary molars are located 3.6, 4.2, and 4.8 mm apical to the CEJ on the mesial, facial, and distal surfaces, respectively.[2] The mesial furcation of maxillary molars is located in the palatal third on the tooth, therefore can be approached only from the palate. The distal furcation is usually detected from the buccal. Booker found mesial concavities in 100% of 50 maxillary first premolars evaluated, and the average cementoenamel junction (CEJ) to furcation distance was 7.9 mm.[3]

Etiology
- Periodontal disease
- Local anatomic factors that affect the deposition of plaque or hamper its removal (cervical enamel projection, root form variation, root trunk lengths, etc.)
- Dental caries
- Iatrogenic
- Factitial injury

Classification[4]

Grade I   Incipient involvement into flute or furcation with suprabony pockets and no interradicular bone loss
Grade II   Any involvement of the interradicular bone without through-and-through probability
Grade III   Through-and-through loss of interradicular bone
Grade IV   Through-and-through loss of interradicular bone, with total exposure of the furcation due to gingival recession

Therapeutic management of furcation involvement[5]

Treatment selection varies according to the following considerations:
- Size, shape, and divergence of roots
- Length of root trunk
- Crown/root ratio
- Amount of remaining bone support

Scaling and root planing (for Grade I furcation) is used for incipient lesions having no interradicular bone involvement but suprabony pockets.

Furcation plasty (for Grade I and early Grade II furcation) involves raising a mucoperiosteal flap to provide access to the furcation area, and combining scaling and root planning, osteoplasty (reshaping nonsupporting bone), and odontoplasty (reshaping of tooth) to open the furcation to allow the patient access to clean and maintain the area. The flap is repositioned and sutured to ↑ access postoperatively. There is a risk of pulpal damage and postoperative dentine sensitivity.

Tunnel preparation (for Grade II and Grade III furcations) involves surgical exposure of the entire furcation. This procedure is suitable for long and divergent roots and is generally indicated for the mandibular molars. There is a high risk of postoperative caries, dentine sensitivity, and pulpal exposure, making this a method to be used with caution. In many cases considered for furcation plasty or tunneling, it may be more sensible to proceed to a more radical approach such as root resection.

Root resection involves amputation of one (or even two) of the roots of a multirooted tooth. It is important to ensure that the root to be retained can be treated endodontically, is in sound periodontal state with good bony support, is restorable, and will be a viable tooth in the long term. The ideal tooth has long roots that have adequate divergence and a narrow root trunk. Resection of the root with a high-speed bur is followed by smoothing, recontouring, and restoration of any residual pulp cavity. It is sometimes not possible to proceed with root resection, despite apparently favorable radiographs, especially in maxillary molars. Patients should be informed of this preoperatively. At the end of the procedure the patient needs to be able to clean the whole circumference of the root to maintain good periodontal status and prevent caries.

Hemisection involves dividing a two-rooted tooth in half to give two smaller units each with a single root. Again, RCT is necessary preoperatively and the divided crown must be restored postoperatively.

Extraction Although molars with advanced Grade II or Grade III furcation involvement may be maintained for significant periods by frequent instrumentation, they should be removed before allowing the development of bony deformities that would require major surgical repair or preclude routine prosthesis.[6]

Bone grafts and GTR Resorbable and nonresorbable membrane along with bone grafts (autografts, allografts, xenografts, and alloplastic materials) may be used to treat molar furcation defects. The GTR procedure is technique sensitive and requires more than average clinical skills. It is most successful in the intrabony portion of the defects and is best applied to Class II furcations. It is least successful in Grade III or Grade IV furcation.

1 R. C. Bower 1979 *J Periodontol* **50** 23.

2 M. E. Gher 1985 *J Periodontol* **56** 39.

3 B. W. Booker 1985 *J Periodontol* **56** 666.

4 I. Glickman 1958 *Clin Periodontol* 693.

5 E. S. Cohen 1989 *Atlas of Cosmetic and Reconstructive Periodontal Surgery* **2** 369, Williams & Wilkins.

6 L. F. Rose 2004 *Periodontics: Medicine, Surgery, and Implants*, p. 553, Elsevier Mosby.

Restorative dentistry

Relevant pages in other chapters: Caries diagnosis, p. 26; amalgam,
p. 594; resin composite, p. 596; the acid-etch technique, p. 600;
dentine adhesive systems, p. 602; glass ionomers, p. 604; cermets,
p. 607; cements, p. 610; impression materials, p. 612; casting alloys,
p. 615; acid-etch tip, p. 104.

Principal sources and further reading: H. Shillingburg, et al. (eds.) 1997 Fundamentals of Fixed Prosthodontics 3rd ed., Quintessence. T. Roberson et al. (eds.) 2006 Sturdevant's Art and Science of Operative Dentistry, 5th ed., Mosby. Operative Dentistry. Dental Update. B. G. N. Smith 1998 Planning and Making Crowns and Bridges (3rd ed.), Martin Dunitz. P. A. Brunton 2002 Decision Making in Operative Dentistry, Quintessence. J. L. Gutmann et al. 1997 Problem Solving in Endodontics, 3rd ed., Mosby. E. A. M. Kidd et al. 2003 Pickard's Manual of Operative Dentistry, 8th ed., OUP. S. J. Davies and R. J. Gray 2002 A Clinical Guide to Occlusion, British Dental Association. J. M. Whitworth 2002 Rational Root Canal Treatment in Practice, Quintessence.

Attempting to resolve the problem of caries by preparing and restoring teeth is comparable to trying to resolve the problem of poliomyelitis by manufacturing more attractive and better quality crutches, more quickly and more cheaply.

Treatment planning

A proper treatment plan can only result from a thorough patient assessment, which must include a history, an examination, relevant special tests, and, ultimately, a diagnosis.

Under ideal circumstances an integrated treatment plan is formulated for each patient at the start of every course of treatment. Very often, however, the treatment plan will need to be revised in light of clinical findings as the treatment progresses, e.g., patient cooperation, response to periodontal therapy, investigation of teeth of doubtful prognosis, etc. When dealing with patients with a range of problems it is therefore wise to formulate a treatment plan, which has a number of achievable goals, and then focus on completion of this to reassess the patient and decide on what, if any, further treatment is necessary.

Sequence of treatment

This list is obviously an oversimplification, but it should serve as a general guide to the order in which treatment should be carried out.
- Relief of pain.
- Control of active disease and achievement of stability:
  - OHI, dietary advice, topical fluoride, and initial periodontal therapy;
  - extraction of unrestorable teeth;
  - treatment of large and active carious lesions;
  - consideration of definitive prosthesis design;
  - remaining simple restorations;
  - RCT.
- Reassessment of success of initial treatment, OH, periodontal condition, and prognosis of teeth
- Definitive treatment: crowns, bridges, and dentures
- Maintenance and review

Practical points

- The priority of items of treatment must be taken into account when formulating a treatment plan, which may lead to deviations from the scheme described above. For example, in an apprehensive patient it would be more appropriate to complete small restorations before dealing with the large ones.
- Explain to the patient what the treatment plan involves and the role they will have to play in controlling their dental disease. Success is dependent on patient compliance, ∴ time spent discussing their expectations, treatment options, time involved, cost implications present and future, and their role in maintenance is never wasted. Furthermore, without such a discussion consent is by definition not informed.
- If necessary, check medical history with patient's primary care physician or refer patient to a specialist, and allow sufficient time to elapse before arranging to carry out any treatment dependent on the outcome.
- It is important to bear in mind subsequent items on a treatment plan, e.g., the design of a partial upper denture (P/-) may influence the choice of material and contour of restorations.

- For complex cases, several short treatment phases, each ending with a reassessment, are more logical and efficient than one long one that keeps changing.
- When formulating a treatment plan, group items together into appointments to form a visit plan. Decide how long you will need for each visit.
- Although it is usually advantageous to complete as much work as possible at each visit, in some patients (or if carried to an extreme in any patient) this can be counterproductive. If in doubt about how much treatment to do at a visit, discuss this with the patient.
- Regularly reinforce the OH throughout the treatment (e.g., while waiting for LA to take effect).
- Record keeping is very important. At the end of each visit carefully note what has been done and the materials used (including sizes and shades). Check that item off the treatment plan and adjust the patient's chart. Note what is to be done at the next visit; this will save time.
- It is important to recognize your own limitations; when appropriate, refer patient for care by a specialist.

Stabilization or caries control In patients with multiple carious lesions it may take several weeks or months to complete the permanent restorations necessary to secure OH. In these cases it may be advisable to prevent any asymptomatic large lesions from increasing in size by placing temporary restorations. The cavities should be rendered caries-free at the margins and temporarily restored with strong temporary, restorative materials, e.g., traditional or resin-modified GI cement.

Dental pain

When a patient complains of a toothache, pain may be arising from a variety of different structures and may be classified as follows:

- Pulpal pain
- Periapical/periradicular pain.
- Nondental pain.

Dental pain can be very difficult to diagnose, and the clinician must first gather as much information as possible from the history, clinical and radiographic examinations, and other special tests (see Chapter 1).

Pulpal pain

The pulp may be subject to a wide variety of insults, e.g., bacterial, thermal, chemical, and traumatic, the effects of which are cumulative and can ultimately lead to inflammation in the pulp (pulpitis) and pain. The dental pulp does not contain any proprioceptive nerve endings, ∴ a characteristic of pulpal pain is that the patient is unable to localize the affected tooth. The ability of the pulp to recover from injury depends on its blood supply, not the nerve supply, which must be kept in mind when vitality testing is carried out (p. 14).[1] It is impossible to reliably achieve an accurate diagnosis of the state of the pulp on clinical grounds alone; the only 100% accurate method is histological section.

Although numerous classifications of pulpal disease exist, only a limited number of clinical diagnostic situations require identification before effective treatment can be given.

Reversible pulpitis

Symptoms Fleeting sensitivity or pain to hot, cold, or sweet with immediate onset. Pain is usually sharp and may be difficult to locate. Quickly subsides after removal of the stimulus. Spontaneous pain is not present.

Signs Exaggerated response to pulp testing. Carious cavity/leaking restoration.

Rx Remove any caries present and place a sedative dressing (e.g., ZOE) or permanent restoration with suitable pulp protection.

Irreversible pulpitis

Symptoms Spontaneous pain that may last several hours, be worse at night, and is often pulsatile in nature. Pain is elicited by hot and cold at first, but in later stages heat is more significant and cold may actually ease symptoms. A characteristic feature is that the pain remains after the removal of the stimulus (the lingering effect of pain). Localization of pain may be difficult initially (due to lack of proprioceptive nerve fibers in the pulp), but as the inflammation spreads to the periapical tissues, the pain is localized to the tooth as it becomes more sensitive to percussion.

Signs Application of cold results in prolonged, lingering pain (generally +15 sec). Application of heat (e.g., warm GP) also elicits pain that may linger. Affected tooth may give no or a reduced response to electric pulp tester.

1 A. H. R. Rowe 1990 *Int Endod J* **23** 77.

Rx Complete extirpation of the pulp (full pulpectomy) and RCT is the treatment of choice if the tooth is to be saved. If time is short, partial removal of the pulp (partial pulpectomy) and placement of a calcium hydroxide dressing in the chamber and the canals can often control the symptoms until the remaining pulp can be extirpated at the next appointment. The partial pulpectomy procedure requires enlarging the canals to a size of at least 20–25 .02 taper file. Stabbing the pulp with smaller size files without completely removing it can potentially result in more inflammation and pain after the procedure.

Dentinal hypersensitivity

This is pain arising from exposed dentine in response to a thermal, tactile, or osmotic stimulus (but not all exposed dentine gives rise to symptoms). According to the hydrodynamic theory, the discomfort is caused by dentinal fluid movement in the dental tubules, stimulating pulpal pain receptors. Prevalence is ~1:7 adults, with a peak in young adults, then decreases with age.[1] Diagnosis is made by elimination of other possible causes and by evoking symptoms.

Rx involves addressing the etiological factors (i.e., OHI, possibly including tooth-brushing technique and intrinsic and extrinsic dental erosion) and by reducing the permeability of dentinal tubules (e.g., by toothpaste containing strontium and/or fluoride; placement of varnishes, dentine desensitizers, dentine adhesive systems, or, if indicated, a restoration).

Cracked tooth syndrome

Symptoms Sharp pain on biting—short duration, unexpected and not in a consistent manner.

Signs are often relatively few, diagnosis is difficult. Tooth often has a large restoration. Crack may not be apparent at first but transillumination with fiber optics and possibly removal of the restoration and visualization with the aid of a microscope or high-magnification loops may be helpful. A positive response to vitality testing and pain can normally be elicited by getting the patient to bite with the affected tooth on a cotton roll. A tooth sleuth biting test on each cusp tip may also be helpful in diagnosing the affected cusp. Crack may be associated with bruxing habit.

Rx An adhesive resin-composite restoration may be appropriate in teeth minimally restored, but in some cases a cast restoration with full occlusal coverage will be needed. Occasionally RCT may be required if clinical tests correspond to irreversible pulpitis or if conservative therapy does not address the discomfort.

Periapical/periradicular pain

Progression of irreversible pulpitis ultimately leads to death of the pulp (pulpal necrosis). At this stage the patient may experience relief from pain and thus may not seek attention. If neglected, however, the bacteria and pulpal breakdown products leave the root canal system via the apical foramen or lateral canals and lead to inflammatory changes and potential pain. Characteristically, the patient can precisely identify the affected tooth, as the periodontal ligament, which is well supplied with proprioceptive nerve endings, is inflamed.

1 P. Dowell 1985 *BDJ* **158** 92.

Pulpal necrosis with periapical periodontitis

Symptoms Variable, but patients generally describe a dull ache exacerbated by biting on the tooth.

Signs Usually no response to vitality testing, unless one canal of a multi-rooted tooth is still vital (in this situation, the clinical vitality testing results are inconsistent, but not normal). The tooth will be TTP. Radiographically the apical PDL may be widened or there may be a periapical radiolucency (granuloma or cyst).

Rx RCT or extraction.

Acute periapical abscess

Symptoms Severe pain, which will disturb sleep. Tooth is exquisitely tender to touch.

Signs Affected tooth is usually extruded, mobile, and TTP, and may be associated with a localized or diffuse swelling. Vitality testing may be misleading, as pus may conduct stimulus to apical tissues. Radiographic changes can range from a widening of the apical PDL space to an obvious radiolucency. It is important to differentiate this condition from a periodontal abscess.

Rx Drain pus and relieve occlusion, if indicated. Drainage of pus can often be achieved by entering the pulp chamber with a high-speed diamond bur. The tooth should be steadied with a finger to prevent excessive vibration. After drainage has been achieved, it is preferable to prepare the canal and place a temporary dressing. Leaving the tooth on "open drainage" should be avoided if possible, but if absolutely necessary, for <24 h, as after this time further contamination of the root canal by anaerobic bacteria makes subsequent RCT very difficult. If a fluctuant swelling is present in the soft tissues, this should be incised to achieve drainage. Antibiotics should be prescribed if there is systemic involvement (pyrexia, lymphadenopathy) or if the infection is spreading significantly along tissue planes. When the acute symptoms have subsided, RCT must be performed or the tooth extracted.

Chronic periapical abscess

This is often symptomless, possibly associated with persistent sinus. Presentation may be coincidental or acute exacerbation.

Lateral periodontal abscess

Symptoms are similar to periapical abscess with acute pain and tenderness, and often an associated bad taste.

Signs Tooth is usually mobile and TTP, with associated localized or diffuse swelling of the adjacent periodontium. A deep periodontal pocket is usually associated, which will exude pus on probing. Radiographs normally show vertical or horizontal bone loss, and vitality testing is usually within normal limits, unless there is an associated endodontic problem (perio-endo lesion).

Rx Debride the pocket and achieve drainage of pus. Irrigate with a chlorhexidine solution. If there is systemic involvement or it is a recurrent problem, prescribe antibiotics (metronidazole or amoxicillin).

Nondental pain

When no signs of dental or periradicular pathology can be detected, then nondental causes must be considered. Other causes of pain that can present as toothache include
- TMPDS (p. 470);
- sinusitis (p. 384);
- psychological disorders (atypical odontalgia) (p. 454);
- tumors (pp. 382 and 420).

Isolation and moisture control

Isolation is required to aid visibility, prevent contamination during moisture-sensitive techniques, maintain a relatively aseptic environment, and protect the patient from caustic materials or aspiration of foreign material.

High-volume suction e.g., an aspirator.

Low-volume suction e.g., a saliva ejector. Many designs are available—the most useful are (a) flanged metal type to keep tongue at bay when working in the lower arch, and (b) disposable plastic type for working on upper teeth.

Compressed air This tends to redistribute the moisture to somewhere else (e.g., your eye) rather than remove it. It should be used with care in deep preparations as prolonged use can cause pulpal damage, let alone displace adhesive materials when the solvent is being evaporated prior to curing. Compressed air should be used when either a suction tip or an absorbing material (such as a cotton roll) is present to minimize splashing of water, saliva, and debris.

Absorbents
- Cotton rolls. Insert with a rolling action away from the alveolus. Moisten before removal to prevent tearing mucosa.
- Paper pads
- Carboxymethylcellulose pads (Dry Tips). Very effective if inserted the correct way round with the impermeable plastic against the tooth.

Rubber dam
This provides effective isolation and also improves access to the operating site. It is indicated where moisture control and airway protection are essential, e.g., RCT (RCT without a rubber dam is considered negligent), bonding technique. With practice, the rubber dam can be applied quickly and often saves time in the long run. The dam must be secured to the teeth; several methods are available:
- Rubber dam clamps. These consist of two metal jaws linked by one or more bows. They are commonly used for posterior teeth.
- Floss ligatures
- Wedges
- Pieces of rubber dam, worked through contact points
- By pinching dam between a tight contact point.

Types of dam **1** Sheet grade, 6-inch square (15 cm), which is supported with a frame. Moderate to thicker gauges are preferable. **2** Mask type, which is supported by a paper margin and looped over ears with elastic. Increasingly, latex-free rubber dams are available and arguably should be used routinely.

Placement Several regimens have been described; the following is popular:
- Place cotton roll in sulcus beside tooth for treatment.
- Mark position of center of each tooth to be included with a ball pen while dam is held stretched. Or preferably, use an ink stamp to indicate tooth position.
- Punch holes cleanly in the rubber dam that correspond to tooth size.

- Try-in clamp (with floss tied to it).
- Fit clamp into appropriate hole, with bridge distally, and using forceps place clamp and dam onto tooth.
- Position dam on other teeth, using floss to ease through contact points.
- Secure dam anteriorly using one of the methods above.
- If a frame is required, position.
- Put napkin on patient's chin under dam. A saliva ejector will add to the patient's comfort.

If using caustic materials, a rubber dam sealer (e.g., Oraseal) should be used.

Removal

- Take away clamps and ligatures, etc.
- Stretch dam, carefully cut interdental septa with scissors, and remove.

Protection of the airway Mandatory when fitting crowns, bridges, inlays, and carrying out RCT. It is best provided by a rubber dam, but if this is not possible a butterfly sponge or gauze can be used.

Gingival retraction ↓ gingival exudate and exposes subgingival preparations prior to impression taking. Some retraction cords are impregnated with substances such as adrenalin to ↓ bleeding. The cord should be gently placed into the gingival crevice with a flat plastic instrument (leaving no tag hanging out) prior to impression taking and temporization. Braided cords are better than twisted. Bleeding from the gingival margin can be ↓ by applying an astringent. Aluminum chloride provides for retraction and hemorrhage control.

Electrosurgery May be indicated where a margin extends subgingivally and gingival overgrowth is hampering restoration placement or impression taking. It is also for crown-lengthening procedures, although bone removal is required too.

Principles of tooth preparation

Why restore?

- To restore function
- To prevent further spread of an active lesion not amenable to preventive measures
- To preserve pulp vitality
- To restore aesthetics

However, these reasons need to be evaluated with regard to the patient and the rest of the dentition. For example, there is little point in attempting restoration of a nonfunctional third molar.

Preparation design With caries prevalence declining, emphasis has changed from extension for prevention, to minimizing removal of tooth tissue. Tooth preparation should be based on the morphology of the carious lesion and the requirements of the restorative material being used.

General principles of tooth preparation

- Gain access to caries.
- Remove all caries at DEJ (to prevent spread laterally).
- Cut away all significantly unsupported enamel.
- Extend margins so that they are accessible for instrumentation and cleaning.
- Shape preparation so that remaining tooth tissue and restorative material will be able to withstand functional forces.
- Shape preparation so that restoration will be retained, i.e., undercut for amalgam, none required for resin composite or bonded amalgams.
- Check that preparation margins are appropriate for the restorative material. Small areas of unsupported enamel may be left if a resin - composite restoration is being placed.
- Remove remaining caries unless indirect pulp cap to be carried out.
- Wash and dry preparation.

Helpful hints

- While care must be exercised not to overprepare, do not limit access by insufficient preparation so that caries removal is compromised by poor visibility.
- Mark centric stops with articulating paper prior to tooth preparation and try to preserve if possible, or place the preparation margins past the occlusal contact areas.
- Avoid crossing marginal ridges.
- In removing caries a tactile appreciation of the hardness of dentine is important, ∴ use slow-speed instrument excavators. The use of caries detection materials may also be beneficial.
- The base of the preparation should not be flattened, as this runs the risk of pulp exposure.
- Unless caries dictates, margins should be supragingival.
- All internal line angles should be rounded to ↓ internal stresses. Removing caries with a large-diameter round bur automatically produces the desired shape.
- In a proximal box, the margin should extend below the contact point because this is where the caries is!

Amalgam[1] *(see also p. 594)*

- Amalgam is brittle, ∴ an amalgam cavo-surface margin of at least 70°, preferably 90°, is required to prevent ditching. Also avoid leaving amalgam overlying cavity margins and overcarving.
- Accepted minimal dimensions for amalgam are 1.5–2 mm occlusally, 0.1–0.2mm into dentin, and 1 mm elsewhere.
- In deep preparations, sealers and/or liners are required to seal the dentine and prevent ingress of bacteria.

Resin composite *See p. 596.*

Glass ionomer *(see also p. 604)*

- Wear precludes their use in load-bearing situations except for primary teeth, management of root caries, temporary restorations, and the atraumatic restorative technique.

Gold

- Relies on minimally divergent walls and cement lute for retention.
- A preparation margin of >135° is advisable to give good marginal fit to restoration and to allow burnishing.

It would be foolish to think that experience in tooth preparation can be adequately assimilated from the written text. The purpose of the following pages is to give the reader some practical tips on how to do the procedures considered, as well as to describe recent innovations and techniques.

Nomenclature

Black's classification of cavities is now not widely used. It has been replaced by the following:

Occlusal (Class I)	Cavity in pits and fissures
Proximal (Class II or III)	Cavity in proximal surface(s) of any tooth
Incisal (Class IV)	Proximal in an anterior tooth, but including incisal edge
Cervical (Class V)	Cavity in cervical third of buccal or lingual surface of any tooth.

1 P. B. Robinson 1985 *Dental Update* **12** 357.

Occlusal (Class I)

Amalgam

Amalgam is still the most widely used material for occlusal cavities, probably because it is more forgiving of technique than some of the newer materials. It is now widely accepted, however, that resin composite placed in conjunction with minimal preparation techniques has a role in initial lesion management. If enamel margins are cut to an angle of 90° (or, if cusps steeply inclined, >70°) the resultant preparation will be adequately retentive.

Lining Recently, emphasis has changed, with linings being used to seal the underlying dentine for moderate to deep cavities. Light-cured GIs (e.g., Vitrebond) are now recommended. A preparation sealer (Gluma Desensitizer) can be used in minimal preparations.

Resin composite

The controversy surrounding posterior resin composites is dealt with on pp. 238 and 598. A technique that has gained more widespread acceptance is described below.

Preventive resin restoration Introduced by Simonsen (then by others as the minimal resin-composite restoration!). Preparation is limited to caries removal and the resultant preparation restored using fissure sealant alone if small, or resin composite followed by sealant if larger. Alternatively, GI can be used instead of resin composite. The rationale of this approach is that adjacent fissures are sealed for prevention. It is particularly useful for investigating any suspect areas of a fissure, a technique that is often referred to as an enamel biopsy (obviously coined by an academic). This involves exploring the area with a small bur, and if no caries is found further preparation can be aborted and sealant placed. If carious, a PRR can be carried out. It is often possible to complete preparation of a PRR without LA; however, if the cavity appears larger than originally thought, LA can then be given. If the preparation extends significantly into load-bearing areas, conventional tooth preparation should be carried out and the tooth restored with resin composite.

Technique for medium-sized cavities

- Assess whether LA required. If not, ask patient to signal if tooth becomes sensitive.
- Isolate tooth (preferably with rubber dam).
- Gain access to caries with a small bur at high speed.
- Use a small round bur run at slow speed to remove caries. Only remove as much enamel as required for access.
- Apply a dentine adhesive system.
- Restore preparation with resin composite placed and cured in increments, but don't overfill.
- Paint sealant over occlusal surface and cure.
- Check occlusion.

Where possible a related sealant and resin composite should be used to ensure a good bond.

Hints for resin composite restorations
- Use etchant gel in a syringe to aid placement. Many newer adhesive systems do not have a separate etch stage, however, and rely on the use of acidic primers often used in conjunction with bonding resins or as a separate stage.
- Additions are generally easy as new resin composite will bond to old.
- Avoid eugenol-containing cements with resin-composite restorations.
- Resin composite must be cured incrementally, with increments being no deeper than 2 mm.

Proximal (Class II)

▶ Avoid the creation of an overhang at the cervical margin and ensure a good contact point with adjacent tooth with a well-contoured matrix band and wedges.

Amalgam In practice, preparation size is determined by the size of the carious lesion and extension beyond this should be minimal. Proximal box preparations comprise a proximal box with vertical grooves. The preparation should only extend occlusally if there is evidence of caries in the occlusal fissures. Retention from occlusal forces is derived from a 2–5° divergence of the walls toward the floor in both parts of the preparation. The margins of the box should extend just outside the contact area unless caries dictates a wider position.

Amalgam restorations are prone to # at the isthmus in restorations extended occlusally, ∴ sufficient depth must be provided in this area. The width of the isthmus should not be overcut (ideally 1/5 to 1/4 intercuspal width). If the cusps are extensively undermined or missing they should be replaced with a bonded restoration (p. 280). A chisel can be used to plane away unsupported enamel from the margins of the completed preparation to produce a 90° butt joint. In molar teeth with mesial and distal caries it is preferable to try and cut two separate cavities, but often a confluent MOD preparation is unavoidable. Increasingly, the use of resin composite placed in conjunction with a dentine adhesive system is advocated for the restoration of small to moderate proximal preparations in premolar and molar teeth.

Tunnel preparations A "tunnel" approach to interproximal caries has been described, although it is not recommended.[1] Access to the caries is made through either the occlusal or buccal surfaces, leaving the marginal ridge intact. This approach is only suitable for small lesions, as when preparation is completed at least 2 mm of marginal ridge must remain. The access cavity may need to be widened buccolingually to complete caries removal. A caries indicator may have a place here to ensure complete caries removal. A piece of mylar strip wedged into place will act as a matrix. A resin-modified glass ionomer composite (RMGIC) is used to fill the bulk of the preparation and the occlusal access cavity restored with a posterior resin composite. In view of the difficulty of accurately removing all the caries, let alone the incidence of marginal fracture, this technique is rarely used.

Resin composite Posterior resin composites should be used predominately to restore posterior teeth, but the technique is more demanding, taking ~50% longer. In addition, it is difficult to establish adequate contact points and occlusal stops. Polymerization shrinkage can cause cuspal flexure, post-operative pain, and marginal gaps. Posterior resin composites are best avoided in the following situations:
• Cusp replacements
• Poor moisture control

1 J. W. McLean 1988 *BDJ* **164** 293.

- Restorations with deep gingival extensions, although a bonded base approach can be adopted
- Bruxism or heavy occlusion
- If the restored area is a primary occlusal centric stop

If a resin composite is to be used, then a hybrid material with >75% filler is advisable. Pre-wedging one but not both proximal contacts aids creation of a contact point. Resin composite should be placed, and cured, incrementally. If possible, centric stops should be preserved on sound tooth tissue or the restorative material, but never on the marginal interface of the restoration.[1]

1 R. W. Bryant 1992 *Aust Dent J* **37** 81.

Proximal (Class II)—resin composite and inlays

Resin composite and porcelain inlays These inlay techniques appear to overcome some of the problems associated with direct resin-composite restorations. When used in conjunction with a bonding technique, existing tooth tissue can be reinforced. Curing resin composite outside the mouth with the addition of heat (110° for 5 min) or pressure overcomes polymerization shrinkage and possibly ↑ strength. Because the inlays are bonded to the tooth with an adhesive, parallel walls are less important, but undercuts must be removed or blocked out with an RMGIC. In general, porcelain inlays offer improved aesthetics, surface finish, and bond in comparison to resin-composite inlays; however, placement and adjustment can be more difficult.

Technique: preparation

- The preparation should have slightly divergent walls, rounded line angles, and a slight bevel of the enamel margins, but not occlusally. For onlays, a minimum 1.5 mm reduction of cusps is necessary.
- Block out any undercuts with RMGIC.
- Take an impression of the preparation and opposing arch and, if necessary, make an interocclusal record.
- Choose shade.
- Make and place temporary with a resin-based temporary material (e.g., Fermit).

Technique: cementation

- Place rubber dam.
- Remove temporary and clean tooth.
- Try-in inlay, and carefully check marginal fit and adjust as necessary. Do not adjust the occlusion at this stage.
- Polish any adjusted areas.
- Remove inlay and clean with alcohol. For porcelain only, place layer of silane coupling agent on bonding surface.
- Apply dentin and enamel bonding agent following manufacturer's instructions.
- Apply dual-cure resin composite luting cement to prep and inlay and carefully seat.
- Cure for 10sec and then remove any excess resin composite.
- Complete light-curing (dual-cure resin composite will finish setting chemically under inlay in ~6 min).
- Trim any excess cement and polish.
- Check occlusion and adjust.

Proximal (Class III), incisal (Class IV), cervical (Class V), and root surface caries

Anterior proximal

Resin composite is the most widely used material for anterior interproximal restorations (Class III).

Access should be gained from either the lingual or facial aspect, depending on the position of the lesion. As resin composite is adhesive, the preparation is just extended sufficiently to remove all peripheral caries. Some unsupported enamel can be retained labially, but the margins should be planed with chisels to remove any grossly weakened tooth structure. Tooth preparation can be completed almost entirely with slow-speed burs and hand instruments. Margins may be beveled to enhance shade blending between tooth and composite material. A slight excess of material should be molded into the preparation with a mylar strip, wedged cervically. Once the material is set, the excess can be removed. After checking the occlusion, the restoration can be polished with one of the proprietary products (e.g., Soflex discs, Enhance).

Incisal

The restoration of choice is resin composite, the so-called acid-etch tip (p. 104); however, for large incisal cavities in the adult patient, a dentine-bonded crown or porcelain veneer may give better retention and esthetics.

Cervical

Although cervical cavities are seen less frequently in younger patients, they are an ↑ problem in older age groups with gingival recession. Resin composite, compomer, or RMGIC are the preferred materials in this situation. Amalgam is acceptable for use in the treatment of Class V cervical lesions.

Once caries have been removed, the occlusal margin should be beveled. The cervical margin should not be beveled as it has been shown to ↑ microleakage. The materials are ideally placed incrementally under rubber dam isolation.

Root surface caries

Gingival recession is a prerequisite to root caries; it occurs predominantly in the >40 age group. Dentine, which has a critical pH below that of enamel, is thus directly exposed to carious attack. It is sometimes seen secondary to ↓ saliva flow (which reduces buffering capacity and may alter dietary habits) caused by salivary gland disease, drugs, or radiation. Long-term sugar-based medication may also be a factor. Rx requires, first, control of the etiological factor, and for most patients this involves dietary advice and OHI. Topical fluoride varnishes and 1.1% NaF prescription toothpaste (5000 ppm) may aid remineralization and prevent new lesions from developing. However, active lesions require restoration, typically with composite. Traditional or RMGIC are also viable alternatives. See also rampant caries (severe early childhood caries), p. 89.

Management of the deep carious lesion

Assessment

- Is the tooth restorable and is restoration preferable to extraction?
- Is the tooth asymptomatic? If not, what is the character and duration of the pain?
- Test vitality and percuss the tooth (before LA!).
- Take radiographs to check extent of lesion and if apical pathology.

Management depends on a guesstimate of pulpal condition (p. 228).

Irreversible pulpitis/necrotic pulp Rx: RCT (p. 284) or extraction.

Reversible pulpitis/healthy pulp Aim is to maintain pulp vitality by selective removal of carious dentine without pulp exposure. If in doubt, treat as reversible pulpitis. You can always institute RCT later.

Indirect pulp cap Ideally, tooth preparation should involve the elimination of all caries, but where this would risk pulp exposure and the tooth is vital, it may be more prudent to carry out an indirect pulp cap. This involves leaving a small amount of softened (affected but uninfected) dentine at the base of a deep cavity with the aim of arresting further bacterial spread and maintaining pulpal health.

Rationale

- Softening of dentine precedes bacterial invasion.
- Pulpitis does not occur until bacteria are within 0.5–1 mm of the pulp, therefore if a vital tooth is asymptomatic the softened dentine closest to the pulp is unlikely to contain bacteria.
- Prognosis for continuing vitality of healthy pulp is better if exposure avoided.
- Materials with antibacterial properties help decrease bacterial activity.
- Bacteria sealed under a restoration are denied substrate, therefore lesion arrests.

Sequence of treatment for vital pulp

- Use LA.
- Apply rubber dam to decrease risk of further bacterial contamination.
- Prepare the tooth, removing caries from DEJ and cut back unsupported enamel.
- Cautiously remove softened dentine from floor. If possible, complete removal, but if likely to result in exposure and dentine only slightly softened, stop.
- Apply hard-setting calcium hydroxide to floor.
- Cover with traditional composite or RMGIC (e.g., Vitrebond).
- Adjust margins and restore.
- Warn patient that some sensitivity should be expected initially, but to return if symptoms occur after that.
- Follow-up for at least 1 yr.

If it is necessary to leave dentine that is probably infected, place hard-setting calcium hydroxide and a traditional GI cement dressing. Leave tooth for 3 months before re-entering to complete caries removal. If the tooth is asymptomatic it would be prudent to cut back the GI cement dressing and place a resin-composite restoration, as it is likely that the caries has burnt out.

Exposure

- If traumatic, small, and uncontaminated, perform direct pulp cap with hard-setting calcium hydroxide and restore.
- If carious exposure, and continued pulp vitality is doubtful, RCT will be required. If time is short, you can dress tooth with calcium hydroxide and a traditional GI cement, and extirpate pulp at next visit.

Pulpotomy is removal of coronal part of pulp to eliminate damaged or contaminated tissue. It is indicated for teeth with immature apices, as continued vitality of apical pulp will allow root formation to proceed. Once the apex has closed, conventional RCT can be carried out. The pulp is amputated to the cervical constriction, dressed with non-setting or hard-setting calcium hydroxide or MTA (mineral trioxide aggregate), and the tooth temporarily restored.

Materials used in the management of pulp vitality

Calcium hydroxide has a pH of 11, which makes it bacteriostatic and promotes the formation of a calcific barrier. When calcium hydroxide comes into contact with the pulp, a zone of pulpal necrosis is formed. This is subsequently mineralized with calcium ions from the pulp. It is the material of choice for direct pulp caps, particularly the hard-setting type.

Survival and failure of restorations

Survival of restorations

The results of Elderton's study into the durability of routine restorations placed in the General Dental Services in Scotland provided both a shock and a stimulus to the profession, as he found that 50% lasted for less than 5 yr.[1] This led to debate over both clinical technique and the profession's readiness to replace restorations. It has been reported that 60% of practitioners' time is spent replacing restorations. It is also interesting to note that those patients who change dentists frequently are more at risk of replacement restorations than those who are loyal to the same dentist.[2] In order to increase longevity we need to consider the reasons for the failure of restorations and diagnosis of secondary caries.

Reasons for failure of restorations

- Incorrect diagnosis and treatment planning—e.g., pulpal pathology; caries of another surface; extraction of tooth for another reason
- Poor understanding of the occlusion
- Incorrect preparation—e.g., caries left at DEJ; incorrect margin preparation; inadequate retention; preparation too shallow; weakened tooth tissue left unprotected
- Incorrect choice of restorative material—e.g., inadequate strength or resistance to wear for situation
- Incorrect manipulation of material—e.g., inadequate moisture control; over- or undercontouring

Before replacing a failed restoration it is important to identify the cause of failure and decide whether this can be dealt with by replacement or repair. When making this decision, bear in mind that cavity size is increased on average by 0.6 mm each time a restoration is removed.[3]

Secondary caries

Unfortunately, placement of a restoration does not confer caries immunity upon a tooth. When caries occurs adjacent to a restoration it is called secondary or recurrent caries. More correctly it is defined as a new lesion that just happens to be adjacent to an existing restoration, and it should be managed in its own right. While secondary caries is an accepted phenomenon, we as a profession have perhaps been a little too ready in the past to diagnose and treat it. Ditched amalgam margins are not a reason for replacement per se, and active intervention is only required if caries can definitely be demonstrated as active. Secondary caries is difficult to diagnose, but careful observation (clinically and radiographically) rather than intervention, is now advocated. Intervention is only indicated when the lesion is in dentine and there is evidence of progression and/or cavitation is present. To prevent secondary caries it is important to not only educate the patient to reduce their caries rate, but also examine our restorative technique, to ensure good long term-restorations.

1 R. J. Elderton 1983 *BDJ* **155** 91.
2 J. A. Davies 1984 *BDJ* **157** 322.
3 R. J. Elderton 1979 *Proc Br Paedodont Soc* **9** 25.

Occlusion—1

In a book of this size it is (thankfully) not possible to consider all aspects of occlusion; therefore we will try to concentrate on the practical aspects and leave the more esoteric considerations to other texts. We also suggest that significant occlusal adjustment is rarely indicated and should only be attempted by a specialist.

Definitions[1]

Ideal occlusion Anatomically perfect occlusion—rare.

Functional occlusion The contacts of the maxillary and mandibular teeth during mastication and swallowing.

Balanced articulation (occlusion) The bilateral, simultaneous, anterior, and posterior contact of teeth in centric and eccentric positions.

Group function Multiple contact relations between the maxillary and mandibular teeth in lateral movements on the working side whereby simultaneous contact of several teeth acts as a group to distribute occlusal forces.

Canine protected articulation (occlusion) A form of mutually protected articulation in which the vertical and horizontal overlap of the canine teeth disengage the posterior teeth in the excursive movements of the mandible.

Hinge axis (transverse horizontal axis) An imaginary line around which the mandible may rotate within the sagittal plane. The axis of rotation of the condyles during the first few millimeters of mandibular opening.

Centric relation (CR) Maxillomandibular relationship in which the condyles articulate with the thinnest avascular portion of their respective disks with the complex in the anterior-superior position against the shapes of the articular eminences. This position is independent of tooth contact. This position is clinically discernible when the mandible is directed superior and anteriorly.

Centric occlusion (CO) The occlusion of opposing teeth when the mandible is in centric relation. This may or may not coincide with the maximal intercuspal position.

Maximal intercuspal position (MIP) The complete intercuspation of the opposing teeth independent of condylar position, sometimes referred to as the best fit of the teeth regardless of the condylar position— also called maximum intercuspation.

Physiologic rest position The mandiblular position assumed when the head is in an upright position and the involved muscles, particularly the elevator and depressor muscles, are in equilibrium in tonic contraction, and the condyles are in a neutral, unstrained position.

Interocclusal rest space (freeway space) The difference between the vertical dimension of rest and the vertical dimension while in occlusion.

---

1 Glossary of Prosthodontic Terms, eighth ed. (GPT-8) 2005 *J Prosthet Dent* **94** 10.

Centric stops Opposing cuspal/fossae contacts that maintain the occlusal vertical dimension between the opposing arches.

Supporting or functional cusps The cusps or incisal edges of teeth that contact in and support maximum intercuspation. Usually buccal cusps of the mandibular posterior teeth, the maxillary palatal cusps, and the incisal edges of the mandibular anterior teeth.

Non-supporting (guiding) cusps The cusps that do not occlude with the opposing teeth. Usually buccal on upper and lingual on lower.

Deflective occlusal contacts A contact that displaces a tooth, diverts the mandible from its original path of action into a different path of motion, or is capable of disturbing the relation between a denture base and its supporting tissues.

Interferences Any tooth contacts that interfere with or hinder harmonious mandibular movement.

Occlusal vertical dimension (VDO) The distance measured between two points when the occluding members are in contact (facial height)

Do occlusal factors play a role in temporomandibular joint (TMJ) dysfunction?

Temporomandibular disorder (TMD) is recognized as being of multifactorial etiology (p. 470). The evidence would suggest that occlusal interferences usually cause either subclinical or no dysfunction because they lie within the adaptive capacity of the patient's neuromusculature. However, this may be lowered by stress and emotional problems so that in susceptible patients occlusal interferences can result in muscle hyperactivity at certain times. It is important, therefore, to ensure that iatrogenic interferences are not introduced during restorative procedures.

Occlusion—2

Occlusal examination

Prior to carrying out restorative treatment the dentist should examine the patient's occlusion. Occlusal contacts can be identified with a 13 μm (.0005 inch) metal foil (shim stock Artus Corp.) and marked using thin articulating paper (20 μm). Important features to look for are:

- Number and distribution of occluding teeth
- Overeruption, tilting, rotation, etc.
- Presence or absence of centric stops.
- The CO and any slide between CO and MIP.
- Anterior guidance—look for disclusion of posterior teeth on protrusion.
- Lateral excursions—?group function, ?canine guidance—check for non-working interferences.
- TMJs and muscles of mastication

The clinical examination can only reveal a limited amount of information and in some circumstances (such as prior to crown and bridgework or in patients with TMD) a more detailed occlusal examination is required. This is called an *occlusal analysis* or a *diagnostic mounting*, and is done by mounting study models on an adjustable articulator (see below) to facilitate examination of the features above.

Occlusal considerations for restorative procedures

In most situations restorations are made to conform to the patient's existing occlusion and the main consideration is to prevent the introduction of iatrogenic occlusal interferences. This approach to treatment is known as the *conformative* or *physiologic approach*. In some circumstances the conformative approach is not appropriate and a new occlusal scheme must be planned. This is often the case when extensive crown and bridgework is required, such that the patient's existing occlusion will be effectively destroyed by the preparations. A new occlusion is established, free of interferences and with the patient occluding in centric relation, which is the only reproducible position. This approach to treatment is called the *reconstructive* or *rehabilitative approach;* further consideration of this line of treatment is beyond the scope of this book.

For simple intracoronal restorations there is generally no need to employ any complex methods, but care must be taken to ensure that the correct occlusal scheme is reproduced. Before preparing a tooth it is worthwhile marking the centric stops with articulating paper and trying to preserve them if possible. On completion of the restoration it must be checked in centric occlusion to ensure that it is not high, but also to ensure that it has re-created the centric stops, because if it is out of occlusion overeruption will occur (which may produce interferences). The restoration should then be checked in all mandibular excursions to ensure that no interferences have been introduced.

One or two units of extracoronal restorations can again be constructed in a relatively simple manner. This is usually done in the laboratory using hand-held models to reproduce the occlusion. Again, great care must be taken at the try-in stage to check the occlusion as above. This technique should be used with care when restoring the most distal tooth in the arch, as it is very easy to introduce errors in this situation; it may be more appropriate to use an occlusal record (transfer coping technique— see later) and mount the models on an articulator.

More complex laboratory-made restorations need to be constructed with the models mounted on an articulator. This allows the restorations to be constructed in harmony with the patient's occlusion in all mandibular positions, which should minimize the amount of time spent adjusting the restoration at the try-in stage. Also, if any changes to the patient's occlusion are planned, they can be made on the articulator in a controlled fashion.

An articulator is a device that holds the models in a particular relationship and simulates jaw movements. Numerous types of articulators are available but only certain types are appropriate for use in crown and bridgework, (e.g., the Denar Mark 2 and the Hanau Wide-Vue Arcon 183-2, which are semi-adjustable articulators). The articulator must accurately reproduce mandibular movements, and to do this the casts must be mounted in the correct relationship to the TMJs; this is achieved by taking a facebow record. In a physiologic or conformative approach, casts should be related in MIP for restoration.

Occlusal records

Occlusal records are required to mount the models on an articulator in a particular position. Two positions are commonly used for the mounting, the MIP and the CR. A wax "squash bite" has commonly been used to record MIP; however, it is inaccurate, as the mandible can be deviated as the teeth "bite" through the wax. It is far better not to use any record and to mount the models to the position of "best fit." After the preparations have been carried out, it can be difficult to locate the working model to this position of best fit; in this situation the *transfer coping technique* can be used. In this technique pattern acrylic material (e.g., Duralay or Pattern Resin) copings are constructed on the working dies, which are taken to the clinic and seated in place on the preparations; they are then adjusted to ensure that they are clear of the occlusion. A further mix of pattern acrylic is applied to the occlusal surface of the coping and the patient is asked to close together. This produces an indent of the opposing tooth in the resin and provides a very accurate occlusal registration.

When the models are to be mounted in CR, the position of the mandible on the retruded arc of closure is recorded just before tooth contact occurs. This is termed a *centric occlusal record* and is generally registered with a relatively hard wax (Moyco Dental Wax). The record is constructed on the maxillary model and trimmed flush with the buccal surfaces of the teeth. It is then softened and seated on the maxillary teeth and the mandible manipulated onto the retruded arc of closure to indent the wax, without allowing tooth contact to take place. The registration can be refined by using a low-viscosity material (e.g., Temp Bond) in the wax record.

Alternatively, a proprietary interocclusal registration material (e.g., Jet Bite, Blu-mousse) may be used to record the space between prepared teeth and their opponents.

Anterior crowns for vital teeth—1

▶ Defer preparation of any crowns until the patient can attain good OH. Not only will this help to increase their motivation, but also healthy gingiva is necessary for correct placement of preparation margins and accurate impressions.

Preliminary treatment

- Assess the tooth: Check vitality, take a periapical radiograph to check for apical pathology, health of supporting tissues, and anatomy of pulp.
- If any doubt, institute RCT first.
- Get study models. A trial preparation and diagnostic wax-up on a duplicate model can be helpful (especially for the less confident operator). This helps to anticipate any complications and can also be used for fabrication of a temporary crown.
- Record the shade so that it can be checked at subsequent visits.
- Examine the occlusion.

Porcelain jacket crown (PJC)

This was previously the first choice for aesthetics in cases where occlusal loading was not a problem. It has been superseded by newer ceramic systems.

All-ceramic crown

This provides better aesthetics and increased strength compared with PJC (e.g., Inceram, Empress II, Procera, Katana).

Principles

- Sufficient tooth reduction to permit adequate thickness of crown for strength (1.5–2 mm)
- Reduction should follow tooth contours. **Note:** two-plane reduction on labial face, of incisor teeth
- Chamfer preparation: 1.5 mm labial (just into gingival crevice) and palatal (supragingival)
- 5° taper of opposing walls for retention

Preparation

Check shade in natural and artificial light with the help of the dental assistant and patient. Alternatively, use a shade-matching system such as Crystaleye (Olympus) to acquire shade data as images to send to the dental laboratory.

Interproximal Use a long, tapered chamfer bur. Walls should have 5° taper and converge lingually.

Labial With the same bur, first place three depth grooves and then remove intervening tooth tissue. Extend 0.5 mm subgingivally.

Lingual If possible, carry out under direct vision. Continue interproximal shoulder round to form cingulum wall, supragingivally. The remainder of the palatal surface should be prepared to have 1.0 mm clearance from opposing teeth.

Incisal A reduction of 1.5–2 mm is required.

Finishing Finishing burs should be used to round off line angles.

Fabricate temporary crown (p. 278) next, for if time runs out, impressions can be deferred, but a temporary crown cannot.

Impressions (p. 614) The opposing arch can be recorded in alginate (cheaper), interocclusal record, and facebow, if required.

Crown insertion Protect airway. Remove temporary crown. Check marginal fit, contact points, and occlusion. If any adjustments are required, polish with porcelain polishing wheels. Make sure patient is happy before you cement crown.

Anterior crowns for vital teeth—2

Porcelain fused to metal (PFM) crown increases strength, but increases labial reduction (some ceramic crowns can be more destructive than PFMs) and decreases esthetics. Preparation requires 0.5 mm reduction of lingual surface with chamfered margin and labial reduction of 1.2–1.5 mm, with shoulder. The transition from shoulder to chamfer is on the proximal surface. The junction between porcelain and metal must not be in an area of contact with the opposing teeth. Occlusal contacts are most frequently on porcelain. This requires adequate tooth preparation for the restorative material being used.

Common problems with anterior crowns

- *Preparation likely to expose pulp* Consider veneer as interim measure.
- *Completed crown does not seat* Check **1** that there is no temporary cement left on preparation; **2** interproximal contacts with floss, and if too tight, adjust; **3** that there are no undercuts on preparation; if present, correct preparation and repeat impressions; **4** ? distorted impression; **5** if die overtrimmed, leading to overextension of margin, cut back crown margin.
- *Core material showing through crown* Need to reduce preparation so that sufficient bulk of enamel and dentine porcelain can be built up over core, and remake.
- *Color not right* If a technician is handy, see if surface stains will give sufficient improvement. If not, re-choose shade and remake.

Removing old crowns (Protect airway)

A crown-removing instrument can be used to try and remove a crown without destroying it. If the crown is to be replaced, cut a longitudinal groove in labial surface of crown. Insert a flat plastic instrument and twist. Diamond burs are best for cutting porcelain and all ceramic cores, while tungsten-carbide burs are best for cutting metal.

Anterior post and core crowns

In root-filled anterior teeth it may be necessary to insert a post and core prior to the placement of a crown. Post and cores provide support and retention; however, as the placement of a post makes further orthograde endodontics difficult, it is important to check first that the root-filling and apical condition are satisfactory. If in doubt, repeat RCT.

Preliminary preparation The first step is to prepare the crown of the tooth to receive the appropriate coronal restoration. The appropriate reductions and margin preparations are carried out with the intention of retaining as much coronal dentine as possible. Grossly weakened tooth substance is removed, but the root face should *not* be flattened off. The retention of a core of tooth substance is important, as it effectively ↑ the length of the subsequent post; obviously in some cases this will not be possible, e.g., if the tooth has fractured at gingival level. The coronal GP is removed with a heated instrument or Gates-Glidden bur, taking care not to disturb apical seal. The root canal is then prepared according to the particular technique being used. As a general guide, the post should be at least equal to the anticipated crown height, but a minimum of 4 mm of well-condensed GP should be left. A periodontal probe is helpful to check prepared canal length.

Types of post and core system

Many different types of post system are available, and they can be classified in numerous ways:

Prefabricated or custom-made Prefabricated posts obviously have the advantage of being cheap and quick, however, they lack versatility and many of the systems require all coronal dentine to be removed. Custom-made techniques are preferred as they are more versatile, but they are also more expensive and require an additional laboratory stage.

Parallel-sided or tapered Parallel-sided posts are generally preferred to tapered as they provide greater retention and do not generate as much stress within the root canal. Tapered posts, however, are less likely to perforate in the apical region and are better for small, tapered roots, e.g., lateral incisors.

Threaded, smooth, or serrated Threaded posts provide greater retention than smooth-sided ones; however, they will ↑ stress within the root canal and are ∴ C/I. Serrated posts do not concentrate stress but simply ↑ the surface area for retention. Other design features include antirotational components and cementation vents.

Examples

Custom-made The cast post and core is a popular choice. First, the root canal is prepared using parallel-sided twist drills, and an antirotation groove is placed in the coronal dentine. The post and core can then be constructed by either a *direct technique* or an *indirect technique*.

In the direct technique a pattern is fabricated in the mouth using either inlay wax or a burn-out resin (e.g., Duralay), which is then sent to the laboratory for casting. For the indirect technique, which is more widely used, an impression is taken using a matched plastic impression post placed in the prepared post space. When using this technique it is generally inadvisable to have the post and subsequent crown constructed on the same impression.

Preformed These are available in various different forms:
   Parallel, serrated e.g., Parapost.
   Parallel, threaded e.g., Radix, Kurer.
   Tapered, threaded e.g., Dentatus screw. These are the poorest design in terms of stress production and, in the authors' opinion, should not be used. If they are used in small tapered roots they should be cemented "passively."

Some of these systems have a prefabricated core on the post, while with others it must be built up around the neck using resin composite. For most crowns choice is one of personal preference. However, no one system will be versatile enough to cover every eventuality, so it is wise to be familiar with more than one method. Tooth-colored posts based on ceramic or fiber-reinforced resins (Lightposts, Paraposts, Fibrewhite, and Snowposts) are increasingly available and the results are mixed.

Anterior post and core crowns—practical tips

Some problems and possible solutions

- *Subgingival tooth loss* Either extrude tooth orthodontically or use cast post and core method, extending post into defect in the form of a diaphragm. In these cases, a crown-lengthening periodontal procedure may be required.
- *Insufficient space for separate core and PJC* Construct post crown in one piece with porcelain bonded to labial face.
- *Extensive tooth loss and calcified canal* (e.g., dentinogenesis imperfecta, severe toothwear) Use dentine pins (plus dentine adhesive system) to retain pinned resin composite core for porcelain-bonded crown or consider crown-lengthening surgery.
- *Perforation of root by post* Apical 2/3—if the post can be removed it is worth trying to encourage the laying down of a calcific barrier by dressing with calcium hydroxide. If successful, re-prepare post hole to correct alignment. Alternatively, this will need a surgical approach to cut back excess post and seal perforation with GI or MTA. Coronal 1/3—incorporate perforation into diaphragm preparation and make new cast post and core.
- *Loss of post* Check **1** Is length adequate? If not, remake with increased length. **2** Loose fit or too much taper? Try sandblasting post and re-cementing with adhesive cement, e.g., Panavia 21. Alternatively, correct and remake. **3** Perforation? Take radiographs in parallax to check, and see above. **4** Root # ? Extract.
- *Apical pathology* If post and core crown is satisfactory, arrange apicoectomy. If not, remove and carry out revision endodontic therapy and place new post and crown.

Causes of failure in post and core crowns A survey of failed posts showed that most failed within 1 yr, but that a post crown that has survived satisfactorily for 3 yr has a good chance of lasting for 10 yr. Common causes of failure were caries, root #, and mechanical failure of the post.[1]

Removing old posts and cores Unretentive posts may be removed by grasping with Spencer-Wells forceps and twisting. Post removers are available (but C/I for threaded posts) that work by drawing out post using the root face as anchorage, e.g., the Eggler post remover. Some proprietary kits, e.g., Masseran, can be used to cut a channel around the post to facilitate removal. In some cases an ultrasonic scaler tip can be used to vibrate the post loose, but heat generation can be a problem.

---

1 R. Lewis 1988 *BDJ* **165** 95.

Veneers

Indications Mild discoloration (can increase success by bleaching first), hypoplasia, fractured teeth, toothwear lesions, closing space, or modifying shape (within limits). Veneers are particularly useful in adolescents, where more extensive tooth preparation may risk exposure.

Contraindications Large existing restorations, severe discoloration, insufficient tooth substance to bond restoration to, and parafunction. Overlapping teeth, pencil-chewing, or nail-biting are relative C/I.

Types

Acrylic laminate veneers No longer used.

Resin-composite resin Useful for the treatment of adolescent patients. Can be made directly or, more commonly, indirectly. Problems are shrinkage, staining, and wear. Average life span ~4 yr.[1]

Porcelain Better performance and aesthetics than resin composite and long-term follow-up is now available.[2] In addition, porcelain is less plaque retentive. They are made indirectly in the laboratory and roughened on their fitting surface by etching or sandblasting. This surface is treated with a silane coupling agent prior to bonding to the tooth structure with a bonding agent and a resin-composite luting cement.

Technique for porcelain veneers

Tooth preparation The veneers are usually 0.5–0.7 mm thick, ∴ unless deliberate overbuilding is required, the tooth needs to be reduced labially. To guide reduction depth, cuts of 0.5 mm are advisable. A definite chamfered finishing line will make the technician's job considerably easier and this should be established first. If the tooth is discolored, the margin should be subgingival, otherwise keep slightly supragingival. The finishing line is extended into the embrasures but kept short of the contact points. Incisally, the veneer can be finished to a chamfer at the incisal edge or wrapped over onto the palatal surface (see opposite).

An impression of the preparation is taken using an elastomeric impression material in a stock tray and the shade taken with a porcelain shade-guide. Temporary coverage may not be required (see p. 278).

Try-in Careful handling is necessary so as not to contaminate the fitting surface of the veneer. Do not check the fit of the veneer on the stone cast. The prepared tooth should be cleaned and isolated and then the veneer tried in wet (to ↑ translucency). Minor adjustments are best deferred until after cementation to ↓ risk of #. The effect of different shades of resin composite and/or opaquers and tints can be tried prior to etching to get the best color match. If several veneers are to be fitted, check them individually and then together to work out the order of placement.

1 J. S. Clyde 1988 *BDJ* **164** 9.
2 F. J. Shaini 1997 *J Oral Rehabil* **27** 553.

Placement The fitting surface of the veneer is cleaned with alcohol, dried, and then coated with a thin layer of silane coupling agent followed by bonding resin. The tooth is re-isolated and cellulose acetate strips used to separate from adjacent teeth. After preparing the tooth surface for bonding, a dentine adhesive system is used. Numerous cementation systems are available, e.g., Calibra, Nexus, Variolink. The resin composite luting cement is placed thinly on the fitting surface of the veneer and the veneer carefully positioned. Excess luting cement should be removed with a brush dipped in bonding resin before curing. Adjustments are made with flame-shaped diamond or multiblade tungsten carbide bur before polishing. The patient should be instructed in the use of floss.

Porcelain slips are veneered corners or edges used to restore # incisors or close spaces by building out the tooth mesially or distally. They are now rarely used, as direct placement of resin composite is preferred.

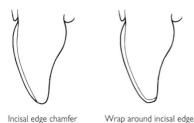

Incisal edge chamfer   Wrap around incisal edge

Porcelain veneer preparations.

Posterior crowns

Posterior crowns are indicated as bridge abutments, to restore endodontically treated teeth, and for repair of tooth substance lost due to caries,
wear, or #. Tooth loss due to these causes should first be restored using
a suitable plastic restorative material. Prior to preparation any doubtful
restorations should be replaced, let alone the vitality of the tooth
checked, and a preoperative radiograph taken.

Full gold crown

Principles
- Remove enough tooth substance to allow adequate thickness of gold,
  i.e., 1.5 mm on functional cusp, 1 mm elsewhere, following original
  tooth contours.
- Use wide bevel on the functional cusp (normally buccal—lowers,
  palatal—upper) for structural durability.
- Convergence of opposing walls should be <10°.
- Keep height of axial walls as great as possible (without compromising
  occlusal reduction).
- Chamfer finishing line.
- Where possible, margins should be supragingival and on sound tooth
  substance.

Preparation

Occlusal Using a short diamond fissure bur, reduce the cusp height, maintaining the original anatomy.

Buccolingual With a torpedo-shaped bur, eliminate undercuts, retaining 5°
taper in cervical 2/3, but usually remaining 1/3 will converge occlusally.

Interproximal Using a fine tapered diamond bur within the confines of the
tooth, eliminate undercuts at an angle of 5°.

Finishing Round axial line angles and cusps. Check that there are no undercuts and smooth preparation with fine diamonds.

Impressions, p. 614, and temporary coverage, p. 278.

Porcelain fused to metal crown

This is used where a combination of strength and aesthetics is important.
The preparation is similar to that for the full veneer gold crown except
that where porcelain coverage is required, more tooth substance must
be removed. The amount of porcelain coverage must be decided before
the preparation is commenced and the patient consulted at this stage to
make sure that they are happy.

Occlusal reduction If an all-porcelain occlusal surface will be used, 2 mm
will need to be removed from the supporting cusps and 1.5 mm from the
nonsupporting cusps. Careful preparation is necessary to avoid compromising retention in teeth with short clinical crowns, let alone the vitality
of the tooth.[1] If a metal occlusal surface will be used, reduction can be
limited to 1.5 mm.

1 W. P. Saunders 1988 *BDJ* **185** 137.

Buccal reduction 1.5 mm should be removed to provide enough room for the metal and porcelain.

Margins A porcelain tooth margin requires 1.5 mm deep shoulder. If it is acceptable to the patient to have a metal-to-tooth margin, it will necessitate a narrow collar of metal around the gingival margin. In this case, the finishing line should be a deep chamfer, a modified, or beveled shoulder. Where no porcelain coverage is needed, a chamfer finishing line is produced, as for the full veneer gold crown.

Three-quarter gold crown
The preparation is as that for a full veneer gold crown except:
- The buccal surface is left unprepared.
- Retention grooves are placed on the mesial and distal surfaces—these must both be parallel to the line of withdrawal of the preparation.
- A groove or "occlusal offset" is prepared along the occlusal surface between the two retention grooves, just inside the tips of the buccal cusps. This serves to ↑ structural durability of the restoration, which can be quite weak in this region.
- For maxillary teeth a minimal buccal overlay is prepared. In mandibular arch the buccal cusps are the supporting cusps, ∴ an off-cut bevel is cut to ↑ strength of casting.

Crowns for endodontically treated posterior teeth
Single-rooted posterior teeth can be treated as anterior teeth (p. 254). In multirooted teeth the major problem is the divergence of the root canals. The two most commonly used methods of solving this problem are described below.

Direct method Preformed posts are cemented into one or more canals. Amalgam may also be packed into the coronal aspect of the root canals and an amalgam core built up, which is the preferred technique. Resin-modified GI or resin composite may also be used. These materials have the advantage that the preparation can be completed at the same visit. A dentine adhesive system should be used with resin composite to enhance retention.

Indirect method A sprue is placed in the least divergent canal and a lubricated post (e.g., SS wire) positioned in the more divergent. A wax pattern (or Duralay) is then built up to form a core. The lubricated post is removed before the pattern is sent to the lab for casting. The cast post (for the least divergent canal) and core is cemented in position, then either stainless steel post or SS wire is cemented through the hole in the casting into the more divergent canal.

With either technique a gold or porcelain fused to metal crown can be used for the final restoration.

All ceramic crowns

These new systems (e.g., Inceram, Empress I and II, Procera, Katana) are built on high-strength alumina or Zriconia cores and may be used for posterior crowns. However, few long-term clinical studies of these crowns have been completed; although 5-yr data for Procera are good.[1]

Problems with post and core crowns in multirooted teeth

- Short or very curved canals: use a sandblasted metal post in conjunction with a metal adhesive system, e.g., Panavia 21.
- Subgingival tooth loss: use preformed post(s) with amalgam core that is well-condensed into region of defect. Some corrosion between the dissimilar metals may be preferable to extending preparation and impressions below level of amalgam. A crown-lengthening periodontal procedure may be required to enable adequate ferrule of the new restoration.

1 P. A. Brunton 1999 *BDJ* **186** 430.

Fixed dental prosthesis

Definitions[1]

Fixed dental prosthesis (bridge) Any dental prosthesis that is luted, screwed or mechanically attached or otherwise securely retained to natural teeth, tooth roots, and/or dental implant abutments that furnish the primary support for the dental prosthesis.

Abutment A tooth or a portion of a tooth, or that portion of a dental implant that serves to support and/or retain a prosthesis

Retainer Any type of device used for the stabilization or retention of a prosthesis.

Pontic An artificial tooth on a fixed dental prosthesis that replaces a missing natural tooth, restores its function, and usually fills the space previously occupied by the clinical crown.

Connector That portion of a fixed dental prosthesis that unites the retainer(s) and the pontic(s). May be rigid or non-rigid.

Units Number of units = number of pontics + number of retainers.

Retention That quality inherent in the dental prosthesis acting to resist the forces of dislodgment along the path of placement.

Support The foundation on which a prosthesis rests.

Resistance Prevents dislodgement of the restoration by forces directed in an apical or oblique direction and prevents movement of the restoration under occlusal forces.

Types of bridge

Fixed–fixed The pontic is anchored to the retainers with rigid connectors at either end of the edentulous span. Both abutments provide retention and support. Both preparations must have a single line of draw.

Fixed–movable The pontic is anchored rigidly to the major retainer at one end of the span and via a movable joint to the minor retainer at the other end. The major abutment provides retention and support while the minor abutment provides support only. This design allows some independent movement of the minor abutment and has the advantage that the preparations need not be parallel.

Direct–cantilever Pontic is anchored at one end of the edentulous span only.

Resin-bonded Retained by resin composite (p. 274).

Removable Can be removed by dentist for maintenance.

Types of retainers
- Full coverage crown
- Three-quarter crown
- Post-retained crown
- Onlay
- Inlay

1 Glossary of Prosthodontic Terms, eighth ed. (GPT-8) 2005 *J Prosthet Dent* **94** 10.

All of the above restorations have been used as retainers in conventional bridgework. They are listed in order from most retentive to least retentive. Wherever possible one of the first two should be used, as the failure rate of the last three is much higher.

Selection of abutment teeth

When selecting abutment teeth general factors must be taken into account, such as caries status and existing restorations, but there are two other considerations that specifically relate to bridgework—retention and support.

Assessment of retention

The factors that affect the amount of retention offered by a potential abutment tooth are the clinical crown height and the available surface area. Obviously, the larger teeth offer more retention and should be chosen in preference to the smaller ones. The teeth of both arches are listed below in order of the amount of retention offered (if a full coverage restoration is used).

	Greatest	→	→	→	→	→	Poorest
Maxilla	3/14	2/15	5/12	4/13	6/11	8/9	7/10
Mandible	19/30	18/3	20/2	21/28	22/27	23/26	24/25

Assessment of support

Three factors are important:

Crown–root ratio ideally should be 2:3 but 1:1 is acceptable. Because bone is lost the lever effect on the supporting tissues is ↑.

Root configuration Widely splayed roots provide more support than fused ones.

Periodontal surface area The more root that is attached to the bone via the PDL the greater the support offered. At one time this factor was given great significance and it formed the basis of Ante's law (1926), which states that the combined pericemental area of all abutment teeth supporting a fixed dental prosthesis should be equal to or greater in pericemental area than the tooth or teeth to be replaced.

Ante's law has no scientific basis and no longer has a place in contemporary bridgework design. It does not take into account that we are dealing with a biological system—because the load is ↑ on the abutment teeth a biofeedback mechanism operates to cause a reduction in this load.

The teeth of both arches are listed below in order of the amount of support offered, assuming that the periodontal tissues are intact.

	Greatest	→	→	→	→	→	Poorest
Maxilla	3/14	2/15	6/11	5/12	4/13	8/9	7/10
Mandible	19/30	18/31	22/27	20/29	21/28	23/26	24/25

Taper and parallelism
- Opposing walls of abutments should have 5° taper.
- For most designs abutments should be prepared with a common line of draw.
- To checking parallelism use direct vision, with one eye; survey mirror with parallel lines inscribed. Study models of prepared teeth may also be useful.
- For management of tilted abutments, see p. 269.

Types of pontic

Modified ridge lap As the name suggests, this type of pontic should make (minimal) contact with buccal aspect of ridge. It provides good aesthetics and is the most popular type.

Hygienic Does not contact residual ridge, ∴ easy to clean. Unaesthetic, ∴ limited to molar replacement.

Conical Makes point contact with tip of ridge.

Ovate A round-end design used where aesthetics is a concern. The tissue contact area is rounded and set into a depression in the tissue that is created by allowing a temporary restoration partially extending into the extraction socket at the time of the extraction.

Saddle Extends over ridge buccally and lingually, ∴ difficult to clean; should not be used.

Fixed dental prosthesis—treatment planning and design

Treatment planning

First consider whether benefits of replacing missing teeth (improved aesthetics, occlusal stability, mastication, and speech) outweigh disadvantages (↑ oral stagnation, tooth preparation, cost). Do not forget to consider implants or shortened dental arch therapy. If replacement is indicated ? fixed or removable prosthesis. A number of factors affect this decision:

General	Local
Patient's motivation condition	OH and periodontal health
Age	Number of missing teeth
Health	Position of missing teeth
Occupation	Occlusion
Cost	Condition of abutments
	Length of dentulous ridge/s
	Degree of resorption

These factors need to be favorable if expensive and complex fixed prosthetics is required. Removable prostheses are indicated if general or local factors are less than ideal (p. 302). Remember that removable prostheses can be more harmful than fixed partial dentures.[1]

Designing fixed prostheses

- Assess prognosis of all teeth in vicinity to reduce risk of another tooth requiring extraction in the near future.
- Assess possible abutment teeth (check restorations, vitality, periodontal condition, mobility, and associated periradicular pathologies and take periapical radiographs).
- Select design of retainers, e.g., full or partial crown. Full coverage is preferred.
- Consider pontics and connector types.
- With this information compile a list of possible designs for prosthesis.
- Consideration of the advantages and disadvantages of each design combined perhaps with a diagnostic wax-up should help to narrow down the choice.

Specific design problems

Periodontally involved abutments First assess periodontal status and treat disease. Then ? if fixed prosthesis indicated. Fixed–fixed type of design is preferable to splint teeth together.

Pier abutments This is the central abutment in a fixed prosthesis that supports pontics on either side, which are in turn anchored to the terminal

---

1 Budtz-Jorgensen 1990 *J Prosthet Dent* **64** 42.

abutments. In this situation the pier abutment can act as a fulcrum, and when one part of the bridge is loaded the retainer at the other end experiences an unseating force that can lead to cementation failure. To overcome this problem, the fit of the prosthesis framework must be excellent. To obtain the best fit possible, the framework may require soldering at the try-in stage.

Tilted abutments This occurs most commonly following loss of a molar. There are several approaches:
- Orthodontic treatment to upright abutments
- Two-part bridge, e.g., fixed–movable
- Telescopic crowns—placement of individual gold shell crowns on abutments, over which telescopic sleeves of bridge fit
- Partial veneer preparations in which pins or slots are prepared to compensate for slight alignment discrepancies of abutments (least satisfactory)
- Precision attachments—a precision screw and screw tube can be incorporated into a two-part bridge. After cementation the screw is inserted, which effectively converts the bridge to a fixed–fixed design.

Canines The canine is often the keystone of the arch, and is a very difficult tooth to replace. The adjacent teeth are poor in terms of the amount of retention and support that they offer and the canine is often subject to enormous stresses in lateral excursion (in a canine-guided occlusion). If a canine is to be replaced with a bridge, the occlusal scheme should be designed to provide group function in lateral excursion rather than canine guidance.

Fixed dental prosthesis—practical stages

- Take a **history** —Why is a fixed prosthesis necessary? When and why was tooth lost? Remember the dental history, social history, and medical history.
- Carry out a **clinical examination** —*extraoral* and *intraoral*. Extraorally look for signs of TMJ dysfunction. Intraorally look at the general condition of the mouth, the length of edentulous span, the condition and position of the potential abutment teeth. Carefully examine the occlusion and try to formulate some initial ideas on possible prosthesis designs.
- *Special tests*—Radiographs of the potential abutments are mandatory along with vitality (sensibility) tests, accepting their limitations.
- *Diagnostic mounting*—Take accurate impressions of both arches and a facebow record and have the models mounted on an adjustable articulator. The mounting can be carried out either in MIP (best fit) or in CR. If a rehabilitative approach to reconstruction is being considered, or if the clinical examination has revealed significant occlusal interferences, a CR mounting should be performed. Carefully examine the occlusion and consider what occlusal consequences the proposed restoration will have.
- *Diagnostic waxing*—In effect, this is a mock-up of the final restoration on the mounted models. Wax can be added to the teeth to simulate the effect that the restoration will have on the final occlusion and aesthetic result. In the anterior part of the mouth a denture tooth can be used. In addition to assessing aesthetics and occlusion, the diagnostic wax-up can serve as a template from which the temporary bridge can be constructed. An impression is taken of the wax-up in silicone putty and saved for later. At this stage the design of the prosthesis must be finalized.
- *Preparations*—Before the preparations are carried out, any suspect restorations in the abutment teeth are replaced. Preparations are carried out in accordance with basic principles (p. 234) and care is taken to ensure that a single path of insertion is established. When checking for parallelism one eye should be kept closed and the use of a large mouth mirror is very helpful. Custom-made paralleling devices can be used, but they are very cumbersome.
- *Temporary bridge*—This is normally constructed with the matrix that has been formed from the diagnostic wax-up; in this way the temporary prosthesis should reproduce the aesthetics and occlusion of the final fixed prosthesis (if the wax-up was done properly!). The matrix is filled with one of the proprietary temporary crown and bridge resins and seated over the preparations. After it has set it is removed, trimmed, polished, and cemented with temporary cement (e.g., Temp bond).
- *Impressions*—An impression is taken using an elastomeric material. Ideally, all of the preparations should be captured on one impression, but this can be very difficult if multiple preparations are involved.

If difficulties are encountered in this respect, they can often be overcome by using the transfer coping technique. In this technique acrylic (Duralay) copings are made on dies of the preparations for which a successful impression has been achieved. These are then taken to the mouth and seated on the appropriate tooth, and the impression is repeated to capture the other preparations. On removal, the coping will be removed in the impression and the dies can be reseated in the copings and a new model poured around them.

- *Occlusal registration*—Under most circumstances the models will be mounted in MIP in the position of best fit. Where numerous preparations have been carried out and it is difficult to locate this position, some form of interocclusal record will be necessary. A popular technique is described in the section on occlusion (p. 249).
- *Metal framework try-in*—If a porcelain fused to metal prosthesis is being constructed it is advisable to try in the metal work before the porcelain is added. At this stage, the fit of the framework can be evaluated and the occlusion adjusted. On occasions it will be found that one retainer seats fully while the other does not. This can occur if there has been some minor movement of the abutments since the impression was taken or if a deformation occurred during the impression-making process. If this is the case, the framework should be sectioned, and perhaps both retainers will then seat. The two parts are then secured in their new position with acrylic resin (Duralay) and sent back to the lab for soldering.
- *Trial cementation*—The finished prosthesis is tried in and any necessary adjustments made. The bridge should then be temporarily cemented (with modified Temp bond) for a period of a month or so. The advantage of a trial cementation period is that if any further adjustments are necessary they can be carried out outside the mouth and the restoration polished and glazed. The patient is instructed in how to clean the prosthesis (use of Superfloss).
- *Permanent cementation*—After the period of trial cementation the bridge is re-evaluated and the patient questioned to check that they are happy with it. If all is well, the prosthesis is removed and cemented with permanent cement (usually GI cement).
- *Follow-up*—Arrangements are made to recall the patient to check that the prosthesis is still functioning satisfactorily.

Fixed dental prosthesis failures

Most common reasons

- Loss of retention
- Mechanical failure, e.g., # of casting
- Problems with abutment teeth, e.g., secondary caries, periodontal disease, loss of vitality

Management of failures

Depending on type and extent of problem:

- Keep under review.
- Adjust or repair *in situ*.
- Replace.

Replacement

Before replacement of a fixed prosthesis is embarked upon, a careful analysis of the reasons for failure is necessary. Minor problems in an otherwise satisfactory prosthesis should be repaired if at all possible. Fractured porcelain can be repaired with one of the specialized repair kits available (e.g., Cojet). Secondary caries or marginal deficiencies, if small, can be restored with traditional GI cement.

A survey of fixed bridges placed by general dentists in Sweden found that 93.3% were still in service after 10 yr.[1] The most common reason for failure was loss of vitality. This is not necessarily an indication for removal of the prosthesis because RCT can often be carried out through the retainer of the abutment.

Removing old fixed prostheses

To remove intact, try a sharp tap at cervical margin with a slide hammer. Orthodontic band-removing pliers can also be used, but these require a small hole to be cut in the occlusal surface. If only one retainer is loose, support bridge in position while trying to remove it so that it does not bind.

Retainers can be cut through (p. 252), but this will destroy the prosthesis.

1 S. Karlsson 1986 *J Oral Rehab* **13** 423.

Resin-bonded fixed prosthesis

This prosthesis is also known as a Maryland bridge. This technique involves bonding a cast metal framework, carrying the pontic tooth, to abutment teeth using an adhesive resin. This type of bridge is almost exclusively used for cantilever adhesive bridgework, i.e., one abutment and one pontic. Fixed–fixed designs have been problematic, with one retainer debonding being a common clinical finding. The resin bonds to the abutment tooth and to the metal framework by mechanical and/or chemical means using a composite-based cement and a bonding system.

Classification by:

1 Position	Anterior or posterior	
2 Retention	Macromechanical	(a) Perforated (Rochette)
		(b) Mesh (Klettobond)
		(c) Particular (Crystalbond)
	Micromechanical	(a) Electrolytically etched (Maryland)
		(b) Chemically etched
	Chemical	(a) Sandblasted
		(b) Tin-plated

Chemical retention to a sandblasted metal surface is now used virtually exclusively. A dual-affinity cement (Panavia 21) is used, which chemically bonds to both enamel and nonprecious alloys.

Indications	Advantages
Short span	Cheaper than conventional bridge
Sound abutment teeth	Minimal tooth reduction
Favorable occlusion	No LA required
	Disdvantages
	Tendency to debond, especially if tooth preparation is poor
	Metal may show through abutments

Treatment planning is the same as for conventional fixed prosthetics. If orthodontic treatment is needed to localize space or upright adjacent teeth, it is advisable to retain with a removable retainer for at least 3 months prior to bridge placement.

Tooth preparation is required to:
- Give a single path of insertion by providing near-parallel guiding planes that eliminate undercuts, which allows coverage of maximal surface area for bonding.
- Provide space in occlusion to accommodate bridge. Need at least 0.5 mm for wings.
- ↑ retention, e.g., using a wrap-around design (covering >180° of tooth circumference) to resist lateral displacement.

- Mesial and distal grooves enhance resistance form.
- Prevent gingival displacement. A minimal chamfer is recommended.
- Provide axial loading of the abutments—prepare cingulum or occlusal rests. **Note:** Tooth preparation should usually be confined to enamel, and the framework should be designed with maximal coverage (to ↑ surface area available for bonding).

Technique (chemical method using Panavia 21) Following tooth preparation an elastomeric impression of the abutment teeth is taken plus an alginate impression of the opposing arch. At the try-in stage, the bridge should be assessed for fit, aesthetics, occlusion, etc., and then the bonding surface thoroughly cleaned with alcohol. Contamination of the bonding surface with saliva must be avoided and cementation is best done under rubber dam. Following etching and washing of the abutment(s) and placement of a dentine adhesive system, the wings of the bridge are coated with Panavia 21 and the bridge seated into place and held firmly until set. Use of acetate strips and Superfloss at this stage will clear most of the excess cement and prevent it from adhering to the adjacent teeth. The cement must then be covered with a substance known as Oxyguard, which prevents O_2 inhibition of the surface layer. After 5 min or so the rubber dam is removed and any excess cement removed.

Problems

- *Dentine exposed during preparation* Use a dentine adhesive system.
- *Metal shining through abutments* Cut wings away incisally before cementation or use a more opaque cement. You may have to consider a conventional fixed prosthesis or placing veneer on labial surface.
- *Debonds* If one flange only, you can usually detach the other one by a sharp tap with a chisel or by using ultrasonic scaler tips. If this is a persistent problem, consider conventional fixed prosthesis. The trend is for these bridges to be used for cantilevered bridgework and fixed–fixed adhesive bridgework is usually to prescribed because of problems with unilateral debonding.
- *Caries occurring under debonded wings* Remove bridge, treat carious lesion, and consider the design of a new fixed bridge solution or placement of an implant.

Attrition, abrasion, and erosion

As these rarely occur individually, the term *toothwear* is preferred. This is also called *non-carious tooth tissue loss* or *tooth surface loss*, but this is often an understatement!

▶ Some toothwear during life is inevitable, but where it has resulted in an unsatisfactory appearance, sensitivity, or mechanical problems, the condition warrants investigation and treatment.

Abrasion is physical wear of a tooth caused by an external agent. Classically, toothbrushes are blamed for the characteristic cervical notches, but it is now believed that other factors may also be operating.[1] Abfraction lesions are now typically thought to be due to flexure of teeth under excursive occlusal loading, possibly coupled with some form of stress corrosion.

Attrition is physical wear caused by movement of one tooth against another. It affects interproximal and occlusal surfaces. ↑ in more abrasive diets and in bruxism. It is often assumed that attrition is greater in patients with reduced posterior support, but no evidence exists to support this.[2] Bruxism ↓ with ↑ age.

Erosion is loss of tooth substance from nonbacterial chemical attack. The incidence of erosion appears to be ↑, but this may be the result of an ↑ awareness of the problem. As the presence of acid results only in demineralization, for loss of tooth substance to occur erosion must act in conjunction with attrition, abrasion, or both. Erosion will be enhanced if the buffering capacity of the saliva is ↓, e.g., in dehydration secondary to alcoholism. Classically, one sees smooth plaque-free surfaces with proud restorations, regardless of whether the acid is industrial (rare), dietary, or gastrointestinal in origin. The latter may be caused either by gastric reflux, which can be asymptomatic, or vomiting (e.g., bulimia, p. 501, or pregnancy). Such conditions warrant referral.

Diagnosis From the clinical picture and history. Because toothwear may be due to a factor that no longer operates, it may be necessary (tactfully) to delve into the patient's past. In a proportion of cases, the etiology will remain obscure and this will complicate prevention. It is important to establish whether the toothwear is ongoing. If teeth are sensitive, probably yes; however, sequential study models will provide definitive evidence.

Toothwear indices are only of value if reproducible, i.e., used regularly. If interested, see study by Smith.[3]

Management[4]

- Prevention requires an understanding of the etiology. However, an explanation of possible exacerbating factors to the patient may help to limit loss even if the exact etiology is unknown.

---

1 B. G. N. Smith 1989 *Dental Update* **16** 204.
2 A. F. Kayser 1985 *Community Dent Health* **2** 285.
3 B. G. N. Smith 1984 *BDJ* **156** 435.
4 E. A. M. Kidd 1993 *Dental Update* **20** 174.

- Monitoring. Take study models and photos to allow rate of wear to be monitored. Intervention is indicated in cases with an unsatisfactory appearance, sensitivity, or functional problems.
- GI or resin composite restorations may help improve appearance and ↓ sensitivity, but if toothwear is progressive, full-coverage crowns are preferable. A nightguard is reccommended to prevent fracture and wear of placed restorations.
- If toothwear is excessive it may not be possible to provide esthetic crowns without ↑ VDO. The patient's tolerance to this should normally be tested first with an acrylic splint. Most patients seem to cope with an ↑ of <5 mm.
- Overdentures may be indicated in cases of excessive toothwear, but are aesthetically less satisfactory.
- Referral to a physician (gastrointestinal problems), psychiatrist (bulimic patient), or prosthodontist (complicated restorative problem) may be necessary.

Temporary restorations

Indications
- Protection of pulp and palliation of pulpal pain
- Restoration of function
- Stabilization of active caries prior to permanent restoration
- Aesthetics
- Maintenance of position of prepared and adjacent teeth
- To prevent overeruption of opposing teeth and migration of teeth
- To prevent gingival overgrowth

Temporary dressings Choice of material depends on the main purpose of the dressing, i.e., therapeutic or structural, but the dressing must also be capable of promoting a good seal and being readily removed. For palliation of pulpal pain ZOE is indicated; for caries control, a calcium hydroxide liner and traditional GI cement. If the remaining tooth tissue requires support, a copper ring or an orthodontic band can be used. The interim seal during RCT is very important, ∴ a relatively strong material that prevents microleakage (e.g., GI) should be used.

Temporary crowns There are three main types.

Preformed **1** Polycarbonate crown, which is trimmed to correct shape and customized by lining with an acrylic or bis-acryl material (e.g., Protemp). **Note:** roughen the inside of the crown to facilitate retention. **2** Soft metal alloy crowns.

Laboratory made Advisable if preparing multiple crowns or if temporary crown needs to last for several months while other aspects of treatment are completed. This is the preferred method for temporary bridges.

Chairside This is a versatile technique. Crowns are custom-made using an alginate or a silicone impression of the tooth taken prior to preparation as a mold. When the preparation is completed, any undercuts should be blocked out with carding wax to prevent the temporary crown material from locking in the mouth. The material for the crown is then syringed into the impression around the preparation and re-seated in the mouth. When the initial set has been reached, the impression is removed and the temporary left to finish curing before being polished. Suitable materials are acrylics (e.g., Trim, Jet, Tep-Art) or bis-acrylics (e.g., Pro-temp, Versa-Temp, Integrity, Luxatemp). Care must be taken when using acrylics because of the heat of exothermic reactions on curing. An alternative technique is to make a duplicate model of the diagnostic waxing. This approach is useful for multiple crowns or where changes are being made to occlusion/aesthetics. It is applicable to both anterior and posterior crowns, however bis-acrylic materials are more brittle than acrylics and therefore may not be as suitable for bridges.

If preparing several adjacent teeth, consider linking temporary crowns to aid retention.

Temporary post and core crowns Some systems (e.g., Para post) come complete with temporary posts, otherwise they can be made at the chairside with a suitably sized piece of wire. The length of the post should be adjusted so that it protrudes 2–3 mm out of the canal without interfering with the occlusion. A one-piece temporary post and crown is made either by the chairside method described above or with a polycarbonate crown-former and acrylic.

Temporary bridges The best type is made in the laboratory in acrylic and relined at the chairside. Alternatively, make a chairside bridge using the diagnostic waxing.

Veneers These provide temporary coverage by tacking a temporary composite veneer to the prepared surface by etching two small areas of enamel.

Temporary inlays A light-cured temporary material (e.g., Fermit) has been introduced for this situation.

Temporary cements The preferred material is Temp bond or similar.

Pin-retained restorations

Extensive loss of the crown of a tooth leads to problems with retention of subsequent restorations. In posterior (and occasionally anterior) teeth these can be alleviated by the use of dentine pins, although their use is ↓. Pin retention may also be necessary to support the cores of full coverage crowns. Pins ↓ the compressive and tensile strength of amalgam and ∴ should not be overprescribed. A rule of thumb is one pin per missing cusp. Now virtually all pins used are of the self-threading variety, where the pin is carried to the prepared channel in a handpiece. They are usually self-shearing when the correct depth (usually 2 mm) is reached. Pins have largely been replaced by bonding of amalgam coupled with use of auxiliary forms of retention such as boxes and slots, circumferential grooves.

Retention can be ranked: self-threading >> friction lock > cemented.

▶ Care is required to avoid perforation into the pulp or PDL. Place pins in the transitional line angle areas.

Technique (self-shearing threaded pin system)
- Complete tooth preparation and place lining.
- Choose pin site: 1 mm away from dentinoenamel junction and clear of bi- or trifurcation areas. A radiograph may be helpful.
- Use a small round bur to indent chosen site.
- Pin channel is then cut parallel to root surface and bur removed while still running, then reintroduced to full depth and removed.
- Line up pin with channel and insert. Pins usually shear off when base of channel is reached. If not, move handpiece back and forth until it does.
- Check occlusion and, if necessary, bend pin inward. An old chisel with a groove cut in it is a suitable instrument.
- Fit matrix band and condense amalgam (or resin composite).

Problems and their management
- Pin perforates into pulp: isolate to prevent contamination with saliva; place hard-setting calcium hydroxide and seal with resin-modified GI cement (e.g., Vitrebond). Monitor vitality of pulp.
- Pin perforates into PDL: monitor; extend preparation margin to include defect and carefully re-site pin (!); or try to smooth off if accessible in gingival crevice.

Pin retention in anterior teeth Following the introduction of the acid-etch and other bonding techniques, pins are rarely required in anterior teeth. Pins used to retain resin composite restorations may show through, detracting from the aesthetics, and are rarely indicated. Gold veneer pinledge preparations are occasionally used as bridge abutments. They rely on pins (which are an integral part of the gold casting) for retention and avoid proximal involvement necessary for 3/4 crown.

Bleaching

Bleaching provides a conservative solution for mild to moderately discolored vital or root-filled teeth. Take photos as a preoperative record or note shade of tooth using a porcelain shade-guide. Alternatively, capture the shade of the tooth with a spectrophotometer such as the Crystaleye to compare shade after bleaching.

Vital bleaching

Two methods have been described.

In-office bleaching Carbamide or hydrogen peroxide (30–35%) is used as the bleaching agent. It is caustic, ∴ protective eyewear and care are required. Dental curing lights or specially designed light sources are commonly used to activate the bleaching agent.[1] It is likely, however, that no activation is required.

Home bleaching A gel of 10–15% carbamide peroxide in a soft splint has also been advocated for "home bleaching." This is worn for a few hours, typically 2–8 h each day for several weeks, usually 2 weeks, and is the preferred technique.

In-office bleaching technique

- Record teeth shade and get patient approval of the base shade.
- Polish teeth with pumice.
- Apply Orabase to gingiva prior to placing rubber dam over teeth to be treated or use a light-cured resin dam material (e.g., OpalDam).
- Etch enamel, wash, and dry, although the need to etch has been questioned.
- Apply the bleaching agent according to the manufacturer's instructions. Use a light source if indicated by manufacturer.
- Wash teeth with copious amounts of water.
- Repeat the process if indicated by manufacturer and wash teeth with copious amounts of water again.
- Remove rubber dam and polish teeth.
- Compare new shade to the one selected at the beginning of the treatment.
- Advise patient to avoid tea, coffee, red wine, cigarettes, etc., for 1 week and that some sensitivity may occur.
- Process can be repeated as required after a few days.

Home bleaching technique

- Record teeth shade and get patient approval of the base shade.
- Take an impression.
- Ask the laboratory to make a bleaching tray.
- Fit the tray, and show patient how to dispense the carbamide peroxide (10%) in it, and give instructions.
- Advise 2–8 h treatment per day.
- Review weekly to compare new shade to the one selected at the beginning of the treatment.
- Avoid overbleaching.

Non-vital bleaching

This provides a conservative alternative to a post-retained crown for the discolored root-filled tooth. However, it usually only achieves an improvement in shade. There is a tendency for the discoloration to recur over time, ∴ warn the patient and overbleach. Interestingly, it has been shown that the degree and duration of discoloration and the age of the patient do not affect the prognosis for a successful result.[1]

Walking bleach technique

- Place Orabase around gingiva of tooth to be treated and isolate with rubber dam.
- Open access cavity and remove root filling to 2 mm below gingival margin (a periodontal probe is a useful guide).
- Place thin layer of GI cement over the root canal filling to prevent leakage of the bleaching material into the root and potential root resorption.
- Remove any stained dentine within pulp chamber.
- Clean access cavity with etchant on a cotton palette and then repeat with alcohol. Wash and dry.
- Mix together sodium perborate with water to a paste and place in the access cavity.
- Seal with a cotton palette and GI.
- Review patient after 1–2 weeks for shade improvement and repeat (up to two times) if necessary.
- Seal access cavity permanently with a light shade of resin composite.

Thermocatalytic techniques, where the hydrogen peroxide is heated within the pulp chamber, should no longer be used, as they are associated with the development of cervical resorption lesions.

1 R. A. Howell 1980 *BDJ* **148** 159.

Root canal therapy

Root canal therapy involves the removal of pulpal remnants and cleaning and obturation of the root canal space to prevent bacterial proliferation within this space. Resolution of apical pathology is dependent on separation of invading microorganisms and their products from the host's defense reactions.

Indications

- Pulp irreversibly damaged and/or evidence of periapical disease
- Crown of tooth requires extensive modification, e.g., requiring a post

Those patients at risk from bacteremia should be protected with prophylactic antibiotic coverage (p. 528) prior to endodontic treatment and for acute periapical conditions regardless of whether the pulp is necrotic. This is primarily due to the mandatory need for rubber dam placement prior to performing any endodontic therapy. Antibiotic coverage is based on The American Heart Association (AHA) recommendations.

Anatomy

The apical foramina are usually sited 0.5–0.7 mm away from the anatomical and radiographic apex. The apical constriction usually occurs 0.5–0.7 mm short of the foramina. These distances increase with age due to deposition of secondary cementum. Root filling to the constriction provides a natural stop to instrumentation, thus the working length should be established. 5–2 mm from the radiographic apex.

	Central inc.	Lateral inc.	Canine	Premolars	First m.	Second m.
Maxilla	21	20	25	19	19	18.5
Mandible	19	19.5	24	20	19.5	18.5

Average working lengths (in mm):

The average tooth lengths and canal numbers may differ ethnographically. Most canals are flattened mesiodistally (ribbon shaped in cross section), but become more rounded in the apical 1/3. Lateral canals are branches of the main canal and occur in 17–30% of teeth. There are more dentinal tubules coronally than there are apically. The character of apical dentin is more amorphous.

Remember:

Maxillary
1st PM   >90% have two canals or more.
2nd PM   75% have 1 canal with 1 foramina.
Molars   >80% have 4 canals. Assume that these teeth have 4 canals
          (2 MB; 1 P; 1 DB) unless second MB canal cannot be found
          after thorough search under magnification and illumination.

---

1 European Society of Endodontology 1994 *Int Endodont J* **27** 115.

Mandibular

Incisors   ~30% have 2 canals, but most join with one apical exit.

Premolars ~5% may have 2 canals, with separate foramina. The incidence may vary by race. Multiple canals are more common in the African-American population than in whites.

Molars   Generally have 3 canals (MB; ML; D), but ~30% have 4 canals (2 in D root).

Some endodontists are using a technique involving maintenance of apical patency (having an open apex) and others prefer an apical stop. There is evidence supporting both techniques.

Assessment

- Check if there is no doubt about which tooth requires root canal treatment (if there is doubt, due to diffuse pain, wait for symptoms to localize). Do not begin treatment unless a proper diagnosis is at hand.
- Is tooth restorable following RCT?
- Good radiographs are essential. Minimum requirements are (1) preop assessment (preferably two, one straight shot and one with an angle to check for additional canals; an additional bite wing may be of help for access and periodontal assessment); (2) check working length; (3) check obturation and provide baseline for follow-up. In addition, a radiograph of the master point prior to obturation is taken if indicated. Radiographs are information pieces. Don't hesitate to take all necessary radiographs, as they improve the predictability of case outcome.

Root canal therapy—instruments

It is helpful to make up RCT sterile kits containing the commonly used instruments, e.g., front surface mirror, perio probe, DG-16 type endo explorer, Locking pliers, long-shanked spoon excavator, Glick or Woodson type plastic instrument/condenser, root-canal spreaders and condensers, rulers, and rubber dam isolation instruments and materials (clamps, forceps, dam, frame, etc.).

Broaches These are either smooth for exploring or barbed for pulp extirpation (some practitioners prefer the rotary instruments instead of the barbed broaches).

Reamers Hand reamers are rarely used today because of their inflexibility with larger sizes. Hand reamers have basically been replaced with k files.

Files These are used either with a longitudinal rasping or a rotary action (e.g., wrist-watch action).[1] The main types of file available are as follows:

K-type-file Made by twisting a square metal blank.

Hedstrom file Made by machining a continuous groove into a metal blank. More aggressive than a K-file. It must never be used with rotary action as it is prone to break.

K-flex file Similar to K-file but made by twisting a rhomboid shape blank in alternating blades with acute and obtuse angles. It is more flexible than a K-file but becomes blunt more quickly.

Flex-o-file Looks similar to a K-type-file but is made from a triangular blank of a more flexible steel. The file also has a blunt tip, which means that it decreases the chance of transportation and perforation. This file is more flexible than K-types and is now becoming a popular replacement.

Greater taper (GT) Hand files made from nickel titanium (NiTi). They have increasing tapers (0.06–0.12) with matched GP cones.

Hand files have traditionally been made from steel, but newer varieties made of NiTi are gaining popularity as they are much more flexible. Larger-sized files can be sterilized and reused more than the smaller sizes. All instruments should be examined regularly and discarded if there are any signs of damage. It is good practice to dispose smaller files after one use. In the future files may all be single use (disposable). NiTi rotary instruments (Profile) reduce creation of blocks, ledges, transportations and perforations by remaining centered within the natural path of the canal. They are useful for curved canals but have a higher risk of breakage. Prior to use check for patency/pilot-path up to the full working length with a size 10 file.

NiTi rotary files Nickel titanium files are now available as engine-driven, rotary files. These files operate at designated RPMs (depending on file design), with the aid of an electric or air-driven handpiece. Many systems are available in United States and several more in Europe. In the United States, the EndoSequence (BrasselerUSA), Profile, Protaper, and GT files (Tulsa Dentsply), and K3 (Kerr Sybron) are the more popular ones. Each product has its own obturation system.

1 W. P. Saunders 1997 *Dental Update* **24** 241.

Rotary files have improved the efficiency of endodontic treatment. Some of the procedural errors that were commonplace with hand files (transportation and zipping) are less frequent when using rotary files. On the negative side, NiTi files are prone to failure if used inappropriately. Excessive torque and cyclic fatigue are the two common causes of file failure. Cyclic fatigue results from overuse of a file (multiple usage of the same file). Excessive torque results if too much pressure is exerted on the file during instrumentation. File failure can be reduced by single use of instruments and avoiding excessive pressure on file during instrumentation.

Spiral root fillers These may be used to deposit paste materials within the canal but are liable to breakage; the inexperienced operator should use them by hand. A preferred alternative is to coat a file with paste and spin it by hand in a counterclockwise direction to deposit paste in the canal.

Gates–Glidden burs These are bud-shaped with a blunt end and are used, at slow speed (about 2500 RPM), for preparing the coronal 2/3 of the canal. A new instrument, Orifice opener, is an NiTi file of greater taper and works in the same fashion.

Rubber stops These indicate the working length on RCT instruments. Some have a notch to indicate the direction of a curvature.

Finger spreaders/pluggers These are used to condense the cones of GP during canal obturation. They come in various sizes.

Other equipment Sterile cotton pellets and paper points will be required for drying canals, and a syringe and needle for irrigating them.

Root canal therapy—materials

Irrigants These are required to flush out debris and lubricate instruments. Various concentrations of sodium hypochlorite (NaClO; household bleach) are generally considered best for irrigation of the root canal. NaClO is bacteriocidal and dissolves organic debris. Concentrations between 1–6% are generally used for irrigation. The most common concentration is about 2.5% NaClO. Chelating agents that soften dentine by their demineralizing action are particularly helpful when trying to negotiate calcified or blocked canals (e.g., EDTA paste, File Eze, RC Prep).

Canal medication The emphasis in RCT should be placed on thorough chemomechanical debridement of the canals rather than trying to sterilize their contents (which is impossible!). Canal medicaments therefore play an important but generally secondary role in RCT. Strong antiseptics, such as phenolic compounds, have been used in RCT, but they are potentially toxic and their effects appear short-lived, so their use is not recommended. For routine cases it is normal practice to leave the root canal empty, but in certain situations a medicament is helpful. Two types are worthy of consideration:

- *Non-setting calcium hydroxide paste* (see below) can be very effective in treating an infected canal where there is a persistent inflammatory exudate from the periapical tissues. This is calcium hydroxide powder (Sultan) mixed with water or, better yet, diluted sodium hypochlorite (~2%).
- *Iodine-containing pastes* are useful in retreatment cases, as certain organisms are resistant to calcium hydroxide.

Filling materials Gutta perch cones, which are composed of a mixture of 70% zinc oxide and a 15% GP rubber extracted from tropical trees, come the closest to meeting the requirements of an ideal filling material. It is supplied in cones that come in various tapers and diameters. Some GP cones are sized according to ISO standards and others have nonstandard tip sizes and tapers (fine, medium, large, etc.). Greater-taper GP cones (.04 and .06 tapers) are becoming increasingly popular as the they match the shape of the root canals instrumented and are prepared with their corresponding size NiTi rotary files (.04 and .06 taper files).

Sealers A wide variety is currently available. The eugenol-based sealers (e.g., Sealapex, Kerr PCS, and Roth) are currently the most commonly used in the United States. GI sealers (Active GP Sealer), epoxy resin sealers, (AH-Plus), and resin-based sealers, however, are rapidly gaining popularity.

Calcium hydroxide This is considered separately, because it has a wide range of applications in endodontics because of its antibacterial properties and ability to promote the formation of a calcific barrier. The former is thought to be due to a high pH and to the absorption of carbon dioxide, whose metabolic activities are required by many root-canal pathogens. It is also proteolytic. Indications for the use of calcium hydroxide include the following:

- To promote apical closure in immature teeth
- In the management of perforations (if unable to seal immediately)
- In the treatment of resorption
- As a temporary dressing for canals where filling has to be delayed. In the management of recurrent infections during RCT.

In RCT, a suspension of calcium hydroxide in carboxy-methyl cellulose (e.g., Hypo-cal) is useful. Alternatively, a suspension of (powder) calcium hydroxide and sterile water or diluted sodium hypochlorite can be made up in-house. This mixture could be loaded into a CR syringe and injected into the root canal. The mixture of calcium hydroxide and water/sodium hypochlorite does not set hard. Therefore, it can be removed easily with a file and irrigation from the canal.

Canal preparation—1

Aims of preparation Described as cleaning and shaping.

Cleaning The aim is to remove bacteria and organic debris from the root canal.

Shaping The aim is to produce the ideal shape for obturation of the root with the root filling material. Because the filling material of choice is normally GP, the shape should be a continuously tapering cone with its narrowest diameter at the apical constriction and its widest diameter in the coronal region. This shape results in the best mechanical obturation of the canal.

Preparation of tooth Prior to starting RCT, all caries must be removed from the crown of the tooth. Once caries are removed, should the tooth lack structural bulk to hold a rubber dam clamp, a bonded, reinforced, composite core material can be used to build the tooth up prior to isolation. This stabilizes the clamp, prevents ingress of bacteria from the mouth, and provides a stable reference point for measurement of working length.

Isolation This is required to maintain an aseptic environment, protect the patient from toxic materials, and prevent inhalation of small RCT instruments. Use of rubber dam is mandatory. Failure to use a rubber dam during root canal therapy is considered negligence.

Access The outline form of access preparations helps in discovering the root canal orifices. The roof of the pulp chamber, including pulp horns, must be removed for proper access. The access cavity in anterior teeth should be midway between incisal edge and the cingulum, and in posterior teeth will vary according to anatomy of the pulp chamber. Lining up a bur with the preoperative radiograph will help in gauging the depth of preparation. A high-speed turbine handpiece should be used to gain initial access, reverting to slow speed for removal of the roof of the pulp chamber and subsequent preparation. The use of piezoelectric ultrasonics under magnification is invaluable in searching for new canals and removing chamber calcification to find canal orifices. When completed, the access cavity should have a smooth, funnel shape. Long-shanked burs are helpful, as are safe-ended diamond burs.

Extirpation of the pulp This is achieved using a barbed broach or nickel titanium rotary files. Often the pulp remnants are necrotic and copious irrigation is required for complete removal.

Working length[1] This is defined as the distance from a fixed reference position on the crown of the tooth to the apical constriction of the root canal. Remember that the apical constriction is normally 0.5–2 mm short of the radiographic apex of the tooth. There are two methods of establishing the working length: (a) radiography and (b) an electronic device known as an apex locator. The radiographic technique is the most commonly used one and is described below. Apex locators work by

1 C. J. R. Stock 1994 *BDJ* **176** 329.

measuring electrical impedance or frequency ratio between two electrodes. With one electrode attached to a file in the root canal, when the file tip reaches the apical foramen it emits an audible or visible signal. Arguably the use of an apex locator reduces the number of radiographs taken for RCT. However, the combined use of radiographs and apex locators can improve the accuracy of working-length determination.

Common errors in canal preparation

- *Incomplete debridement.* Working length is short, missed canals.
- *Lateral perforation.* often occurs as a result of poor access.
- *Apical perforation.* makes filling difficult and can cause postoperative pain.
- *Ledge formation:* can be very difficult to bypass.

Apical transportation (zipping) A file will tend to straighten out when used in a curved canal and straightening can transport the apical part of the preparation away from the curvature. The use of flexible files reduces the likelihood of this happening.

Elbow formation When apical zipping happens, a narrowing often occurs coronal to this in the canal such that the canal is hourglass in shape. This narrowing is termed an *elbow.*

Strip perforation This is a perforation occurring in the inner or furcal wall of a curved root canal, usually toward the coronal end.

Techniques of canal preparation

Numerous techniques have been described.

Stepback technique The apical part of the root canal is prepared first and the canal is then flared from apex to crown. Blockage of canals may occur using this technique, and irrigation can be difficult.

Stepdown technique (AKA the *crowndown technique*) This (along with several others) is used to prepare the coronal part of the canal before preparing the apical part. This technique has advantages (see below) and is the preferred technique.

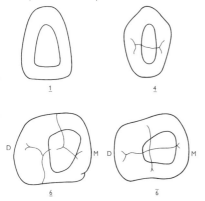

Access cavity preparations.

Balanced force technique This involves using blunt-tipped files with a counterclockwise rotation while applying an apically directed force. It requires practice to master but is particularly useful when preparing the apical part of severely curved canals.

Anticurvature filing This was developed to minimize the possibility of creating a "strip" perforation on the inner walls of curved root canals. It is used in conjunction with other techniques or preparation, and the essential principle is the direction of most force away from the curvature.

To avoid confusion we have tried to provide a simplified guide to preparation of root canals. The recommended techniques are described on p. 293.

Canal preparation—2

Technique for preparation of large, relatively straight root canals with hand files (modified crown-down technique)

1 Obtain a good-quality preoperative radiograph. Identify the root canal.
2 Place a rubber dam and prepare the access cavity. Prepare the outline first (remembering your pulpal anatomy) with a high-speed bur and then change to a slow-speed round bur. Remove the roof of the pulp chamber in its entirety, leaving no ledges or overhangs. A piezoelectric ultrasonic tip can be useful to finish the fine exploring and troughing for additional canals and facilitating straight-line access into the orifice and the apical 1/3 of the root.
3 Irrigate the pulp chamber, and identify the root canal with an explorer or fine file.
4 Estimate 2/3 length of canal from preoperative X-ray. Check for patency with a size 15 file. Widen to form gradual coronal flare with Gates–Glidden bur 2, then 3, then 4 at successively shorter lengths.
5 Take diagnostic radiograph to confirm working length. Prepare apical region to three sizes larger than the size of the first file that binds at the working length. Irrigate well between each file.
6 The remainder of the canal is now flared by "stepping back." Take a file one size larger than the master apical file and insert it to a length 1 mm short of the working length. Work this file with a circumferential filing motion. Continue this enlarging procedure with successively larger size files, each 1 mm shorter than the previous, to complete the preparation. After each file is used it is important to reinsert the master apical file to the full working length (recapitulation) and irrigate thoroughly to ensure that the canal does not become blocked.

Technique for preparation of fine and curved root canals with hand files

1 Same as above.
2 Same as above.
3 Irrigate the pulp chamber and identify the root canals using a fine file. Use the grooves in the floor of the pulp chamber as a guide to their location. Pass a fine instrument down the canals to ensure their patency.
4 Go back to your preoperative radiograph and, for each canal, estimate the distance (in millimeters) from an occlusal reference position to the beginning of the canal curvature. This will vary depending on the tooth in question. Widen to form gradual coronal flare with Gates–Glidden bur 2, then 3, then 4 at successively shorter lengths. Copious irrigation must be used to prevent the canal from becoming blocked.
5 The working length is now determined for each canal. It is important that this is not done before orifice enlargement, as the reference point on the crown will move as the coronal part of the canal is straightened. Remember to use the preoperative radiograph to estimate the working length prior to taking the radiograph.

6 The next step is to prepare the apical stop. This is done with files, using a longitudinal filing motion and copious irrigation. It is permissible to use a quarter turn with the finer files at this stage to help engage the dentine. As a general guide, the apical stop should be prepared three sizes larger than the first file that binds at the full working length, but it must also be at least a size 25 (preferably a 30). Remember that when using this technique in curved canals the larger files (generally 25 and above) will need to be precurved; this is done by bending around a mirror handle. When using precurved files try to use very short cutting strokes; long ones will produce an incorrect canal shape. The *balanced force* or modified double-flared techniques[1] can be very effective at this stage in curved canals, provided the operator is experienced in the technique.

7 The rest of the root canal is now flared by "stepping back" in the conventional manner. This procedure is made much easier as the coronal part of the root has already been enlarged.

Technique for preparation of fine and curved root canals with rotary NiTi instruments (crown-down technique)

Since there are multiple NiTi rotary file systems with different instruments for use, it is advised that you consult the instruction manual for the system you currently use. In general, the rotary files follow the same crown-down technique. Discussion of all techniques is beyond the scope of this handbook. The technique for a the EndoSequence file (BrasselerUSA) in a small canal is described here.

1 Same as above.

2 Same as above.

3 Same as above.

4 Use the Expeditor File in the canal. The Expeditor is a screening file used in this system. It tells you which package file you need to open (canals are divided into small, medium and large sizes). If the Expeditor does not go into the canal or it goes in half way, then you have a small canal and need the Small Procedural Pack (this pack contains the following files: 30/.06, 25/.06, 20/.06, 15/.06).

5 Estimate the canal length on the basis of preoperative radiograph and deduct 3–4 mm from this length (e.g., if canal is estimated to be 20 mm, use 17 mm as initial length). Use a size 15/.02 hand file and check for patency of this length. If unable to reach that length, use small Gates-Glidden drills (size 2–3) or orifice shapers coronally and smaller hand files apically until the 15/.02 can fit loosely at about 3 mm from the estimated working length.

6 Use a size 30/.06 taper EndoSequence file to resistance or to the point 3 mm short of the estimated working length, whichever comes first! Do not push the file! Allow the root canal to guide the file and back off immediately when resistance is met.

7 Use a size 25/.06 EndoSequence file (paying attention again to stop at least 3 mm short of the working length or when resistance is met, whichever comes first!).

1 C. J. R. Stock 1995 *Color Atlas and Text of Endodontics* p. 95 Mosby.

8 Stop and measure the root length with a radiograph, an apex locator, or preferably both.

9 Use the 20/.06 taper file in the same manner as above (use until resistance is met or full working length is achieved, whichever comes first!)

10 Follow with size 15/.06. Use same principle as above.

11 Go back to the same crown-down sequence of sizes 30 → 15 sequentially, paying attention not to force any files down until the master apical file reaches the apex. In molars the canal has to be enlarged to at least a size 20/.06 or preferably larger.

In some cases, especially those with thin, long roots, or teeth with severely curved canals, it maybe best to use the .04 taper Procedural Pack vs. the .06 taper files. The decision is based on planning before the procedure by evaluating the preoperative radiograph. Occasionally the .06 files may need to be switched with .04 files during the procedure, if excessive torque is put on the files because of the narrow geometry of the root canal.

Advantages of orifice enlargement

- It allows straight-line access to the apical 1/3 of the canal, eliminating excessive pressure on files as the file is used apically. This reduces the likelihood of apical transportation (zipping).
- It allows improved access for the flow of irrigation solution within the root canal system.
- It reduces the likelihood of apical extrusion of infected material, as most of the canal debris is removed before apical instrumentation takes place. This is particularly important because most of the bacteria in an infected root canal are in the coronal region.

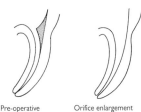

Pre-operative   Orifice enlargement

Completed canal

Diagram of stages of canal preparation.

Canal obturation

Purpose To provide a three-dimensional hermetic seal to the root canal that will prevent the ingress of bacteria or tissue fluids, which might act as a culture medium for any bacteria that remain in the root canal system. In the past, the critical factor was considered achievement of an apical seal, but now it is realized that coronal seal is also important. For this reason, the whole of the root canal must be filled, and techniques that only seal the apical region (e.g., silver points) have fallen from favor.

Techniques

Numerous techniques have been described; all of those mentioned here use gutta percha (GP).

Cold lateral condensation This is a commonly taught method of obturation and is the gold standard by which others are judged. The technique involves placement of a master point chosen to fit the apical section of the canal. Obturation of the remainder is achieved by condensation of smaller accessory points. The steps involved are as follows:

- Select a GP master point to correspond with the master apical file instrument. This should fit the apical region snugly at the working length so that on removal a degree of resistance, or "tug-back," is felt. If there is no tug-back, select a larger point or cut 1 mm at a time off the tip of the point until a good fit is obtained at the working length. The point should be notched at the correct working length to guide its placement to the apical constriction.
- Take a radiograph to confirm that the point is in correct position if you are in any doubt.
- Coat walls of canal with sealer using a small file.
- Insert the master point, covered in cement/sealer.
- Condense the GP laterally with a finger spreader to provide space into which accessory points can be inserted until the canal is full.
- Excess GP is cut off with a hot instrument and the remainder packed vertically into the canal with a cold plugger.

Warm lateral condensation Same as above, but a warm spreader is used after the initial cold lateral condensation. Finger spreaders can be heated in a flame, or a special electronically heated device (Touch & Heat) can be used.

Vertical condensation In this technique the GP is warmed by a heated instrument and then packed vertically. A good apical stop and proper resistance form (in the shape of an appropriate taper and cone fit) is necessary to prevent apical extrusion of the filling, but with practice a very dense root filling can result. Following the down-pack of GP, the coronal canal space can be filled with thermoplastic GP guns such Obtura (Spartan), Element (Sybron), or Calamus (Tulsa Dentsply).

Thermomechanical compaction This involves a reverse turning (e.g., McSpadden compactor or GP condenser) instrument that, like a reverse Hedstrom file, softens the GP, forcing it ahead of and lateral to the compactor shaft. This is a very effective technique, particularly if used in conjunction with lateral condensation in the apical region, but it requires much practice to perfect.

Thermoplasticized injectable GP (e.g., Obtura, Ultrafil) These commercial machines extrude heated GP (150–200°C) into the canal. It is difficult to control the apical extent of the root filling, and some contraction of the GP occurs on cooling. This method is useful for irregular canal defects, e.g., following internal root resorption and C-shaped canal anatomy.

Coated carriers (e.g., Thermafil) Metal or plastic cores are coated with GP and heated in an oven. They are then pushed into the root canal to the correct length. The core serves to push the softend GP into canal irregularities. The core is then severed with a bur. A dense filling results, but again apical control is poor and extrusions are common. They are expensive and difficult to retreat or to do apical surgery on in case of root canal retreatment.

Resin based (Epiphany) The use of polyester-based resin sealers and cones to replace GP is a recent development in endodontics. The resin bond is primer dependent. The challenge is getting primer down the canal. The bond is mechanical. These sealers may prevent coronal leakage through the conceptual form of a monoblock. The fill can be done with thermoplastic obturation, vertical compaction, lateral condensation, or single cone, and is retreatable.

Sealer based (Active GP) The use of GI sealers has the advantage of a chemical bond to the tooth structure that is stable over time. Active GP (BrasselerUSA) has GP with coated glass particles that chemically bond to GI sealer, which in turn bonds chemically to the dentin. This technique may also produce a monoblock and prevent coronal leakage.

Once the root filling is in place, the tooth will need to be permanently restored, provided the follow-up radiograph is satisfactory. Fillings that appear inadequate radiographically are best retreated for a more satisfactory fill (if possible). Otherwise they should be reviewed regularly, depending on the clinical circumstances.

Follow-up Ideally, the tooth should be reviewed radiographically after 6 months and thereafter annually for up to 4 yr. Failure of endodontic treatment may present as pain, swelling, a draining sinus tract, or radiographically as an enlargement of a periapical radiolucency. Following effective RCT, most radiolucent periapical lesions show signs of resolution within 2 yr.

Coronal seal This is now recognized as very important for success in endodontics. Too often good endodontic therapy is jeopardized by a poor restoration that does not provide a good coronal seal.[1] Exposure of GP to saliva can potentially reinfect the root canal system, requiring retreatment or extraction.

---

1 W. P. Saunders 1994 *Endod Dent Traumatol* **10** 105.

Some endodontic problems and their management

Acute periapical abscess Relief of symptoms requires drainage of the abscess and where possible. This should be obtained through the tooth. Open the pulp with a diamond bur in a turbine handpiece while supporting the tooth to prevent vibrations. Deep, regional anesthesia and occasionally sedation may be required. Once opened, the canal is irrigated with sodium hypochlorite and, if at all possible, resealed. It may be necessary to see the patient again in 24 h, but this is more labor saving over the long term than leaving the tooth on open drainage. Relieve any traumatic occlusion.

If a fluctuant abscess is associated with the tooth, this should be incised. If drainage can be obtained through the tooth and there is no evidence of cellulites, then antibiotics are not required (p. 372).

Pain following instrumentation This is usually due to instruments, irrigants, or canal debris being forced into the apical tissues. Occasionally, an acute flare-up of a previously asymptomatic tooth occurs following initial instrumentation—this is called a *phoenix abscess*. Loss of face is saved by warning patients that this can happen. Affected teeth should be opened and irrigated and, if possible, resealed. This may need to be repeated after 24–48 h.

Recurrent symptoms or intractable infection If thorough cleaning and repeated dressing of the canal with calcium hydroxide are unsuccessful, it may be necessary to do an apicoectomy (p. 366). Do not routinely turn to surgery for failed cases—consider retreatment in the first instance.

Calcified canals As the incidence of pulp necrosis following canal obliteration is only 13–16%, elective RCT is not warranted.[1] However, where pulp death has occurred, finding the canal orifice may be difficult.

If careful exploration with a small file is unsuccessful, investigation of the expected position of the canal entrance with a small round bur may help. Once the canal is found, a No. 8 or 10 file should be used to try and negotiate it, using EDTA, File Eze, or RC Prep as a lubricant, and the canal prepared and filled conventionally. Success rates of 80% have been reported for canals that were hairline or undetectable on radiographs.[1] Occasionally, a total blockage of the canal is encountered, in which case the filling is placed to this level and/or an apicoectomy done, provided an apical infection is present.

Pulp stones in the pulp chamber can usually be flicked out. Ultrasonic instruments are useful to shatter such calcifications in the pulp chamber. If calcifications and stones occur in the root canal the use of EDTA or other chelating agents may be warranted.

Fractured instruments Sometimes it is possible to get hold of the fractured portion with a pair of fine mosquitoes or Stieglitz forceps. The use of piezoelectric ultrasonics for separated file removal is essential. Fine ultrasonic tips can help loosen and dislodge the instrument provided that

---

1 J. O. Andreasen 1994 *Textbook and Colour Atlas of Traumatic Injuries to the Teeth*, Munksgaard.

straight-line access can be gained to the fractured instrument tip. If not, insertion of a fine file beside the instrument may bypass and dislodge it; should this be unsuccessful a Masseran kit or Ruddle Kit (p. 256) may be required. Should the fractured piece be lodged in the apical portion of the canal and deemed irretrievable, the canal can be filled conventionally and the tooth should be kept under observation over the next 6 months. Should symptoms arise, an apicoectomy can be performed with good success, provided that the root is surgically accessible, adequate root length will remain after an apicoectomy, and the root canal is otherwise cleaned and well obturated. The endodontic patient should always be informed about the separated instrument for medicolegal reasons.

Immature teeth with incomplete roots See p. 112.

Removing old root-fillings If a single-point technique or a root-filling paste has been used, removal is straightforward. If a well-condensed GP filling is present, this may be softened with a heated probe or Gates-Glidden burs to gain purchase for a fine file to be inserted. Use of Xylol or other lipid solvents may aid softening and removal. Use of a NiTi rotary instrument at about 1000 RPM with very gentle touch can help to remove the GP once the solvent has been introduced into the canals. Apical silver points or amalgam will require an apicoectomy to achieve a satisfactory apical seal if pathology is present. However, using the surgical operating microscope, removal of such canal obstructions through nonsurgical retreatments has also been reported.

Perforations can be iatrogenic or caused by resorption (p. 112). In the latter case, dressing with non-setting calcium hydroxide may help to arrest the resorption and promote formation of a calcific barrier. Increasingly MTA is being used for the repair of perforations and in surgical endodontics as a retrograde filling material, with excellent results.[1] Management of traumatic perforations depends on their size and position:

Pulp chamber floor Can also be repaired with MTA followed by coronal sealing with GI. But if large, hemisection or extraction may be necessary.

Lateral perforation If this occurs near the gingival margin, it can be incorporated in the final restoration of the crown. If in the middle 1/3, the remainder of the canal may be cleaned by passing instruments down the side of the wall opposite the perforation. Then the canal can be filled with GP, using lateral or vertical condensation technique to try and occlude the perforation as well. Use of GP to fill the canal apical to the perforation and MTA to fill the rest of the canal has also been reported in such cases. In case of failure in multirooted teeth, hemisection or extraction may be unavoidable.

Apical 1/3 It is usually worth trying a vertical condensation technique to attempt to fill both the perforation and the remainder of the canal. If this is unsuccessful, an apicoectomy will be required.

Ledge formation If this occurs, return to a small file curved at the apex to the working length and use this to try and file away the ledge, using EDTA or RC Prep as lubricants.

Perio-endo lesions See p. 218.

1 M. Torabinejad 1999 *J. Endod* **25** 197.

Four-handed dentistry

Working in a seated position is now the norm for all dentists. This has resulted in the dental assistant taking a more active role by working closely with the dentist. The development of four-handed dentistry is credited to Ellis Paul.[1]

Advantages and disadvantages
- ↑ comfort for dentist and assistant
- ↑ efficiency
- ↑ patient comfort
- ↑ operator visibility
- ↓ backache
- ↑ professional satisfaction for the dentist and dental assistant

Seating the patient Except for the elderly, infirm, or pregnant patient, a supine position is preferable. Remember to warn the patient that you are about to position them backward.

Seating the dentist The aim is a relaxed, undistorted, and comfortable posture, with good vision of the teeth to be treated. Adjust the dentist's stool so that the top of their thighs slope at 15° to the floor. Position the dental chair so that, with the operator's back straight, the patient's mouth is at the dentist's focal distance (just above elbow level). Forearms should slope upward to this point. The operator's location is between 10 and 11 o'clock (1 and 2 o'clock if you are left handed) relative to the patient's head. Ensure that the patient's head is at the top of the headrest.

Seating the dental assistant The dental assistant must also be seated comfortably with a straight back, with eye level 4 inches higher than the dentist's for maximum vision. The dental assistant's normal working environment is at between 2 and 3 o'clock (9 and 10 o'clock if working with a left-handed dentist), within easy reach of the instruments and equipment to be used.

Role of the dental assistant
- Receive, seat, and look after the patient.
- Place bib and protective glasses on patient.
- Position dental light.
- Retract patient's lips and protect their soft tissues.
- Suction fluids—hold suction in right hand.
- Hold air and water syringe in left hand while suctioning.
- Pass instruments to the operator.

Instrument transfer The transfer zone is just in front of, and slightly below the patient's mouth, not over their eyes. There are several techniques that enable the dental assistant to pass and receive instruments effectively from the dentist. All require practice. Each dental team needs to choose adapt, practice, and perfect a system that safely achieves instrument transfer.[2]

1 J. E. Paul 1991 *Team Dentistry*, Dunitz.
2 J. E. Paul 1997 Fact File: Occupational Back Pain, BDA.

Removable prosthodontics

Relevant pages in other chapters: Fixed dental prosthesis—treatment planning and design, p. 268; occlusion, p. 246; acrylic and other denture materials, p. 622; casting alloys, p. 615; impression materials, p 612.

Principal sources and further reading: Glossary of Prosthodontic Terms, eighth ed. (GPT-8) 2005 *J Prosthet Dent* **94** 1–92. A. Carr, G. McGivney, D. Brown 2005. *McCracken's Removable Partial Prosthodontics* 11th ed. 2005 Mosby. G. Zarb, C Bolender, et al. 2003 *Prosthodontic Treatment for Edentulous Patients*, 12th ed. Mosby. M. R. Y. Dyer 1989 *Notes on Prosthetic Dentistry*, Wright. J. C. Davenport 1988 *A Colour Atlas of Removable Partial Dentures*, Wolfe. J. F. McCord 2002 *Missing Teeth: A Guide to Treatment Options*, Churchill Livingstone. D.W. Bartlett 2004 *Clinical Problem Solving in Prosthodontics*, Churchill Livingstone.

Treatment planning

Reasons for prosthetic replacement of missing teeth

- Restore aesthetics
- ↑ masticatory efficiency
- Improve speech
- Preserve or improve health of the oral cavity by preventing unwanted tooth movements
- Improve distribution of occlusal loads
- Space maintenance
- Prepare patient for complete dentures

Disadvantages of prosthetic replacement

- ↑ plaque accumulation and changes in composition.
- Damage to soft tissues and remaining teeth, due either to poor denture design or lack of patient care

Treatment options for the partially edentulous patient

- No replacement of missing teeth. If the benefits of a prosthesis do not outweigh the disadvantages, then replacement is C/I. An occlusion with first premolar to first premolar present in each jaw (shortened dental arch) is usually functionally adequate. Poorly controlled epilepsy is a C/I to dentures.
- Bridges (p. 264) are preferable for short bounded spans in well-motivated patients.
- Removable partial dentures are indicated for patients with satisfactory OH and whose remaining teeth have an adequate prognosis, or as a training or interim appliance prior to full upper and lower dentures (F/F).
- Complete immediate dentures are indicated for patients who have already mastered wearing a partial denture and/or whose remaining teeth have a poor prognosis.
- Extraction of the remaining teeth and provision of a denture after healing has occurred should be avoided if possible, as considerable guesswork is involved in the subsequent denture and the chances of the patient coping successfully are ↓.
- In the older, partially dentate patient, it is important to assess whether the patient is likely to retain some functional teeth for the remainder of their lifespan. If this is improbable, treatment could be aimed toward providing F/F dentures while the patient is still young enough to adapt, according to some authors.

Treatment planning for partial dentures

▶ It is important to inquire about previous denture history (just because a patient is not wearing a denture does not mean that they have not had one) and assess the reasons for failure or success. If a patient produces an extensive collection of unsuccessful dentures, unless there is an obvious and easily remedied fault, it is probably wiser to assume that you are unlikely to succeed where so many have failed and refer the patient to a prosthodontist for treatment.

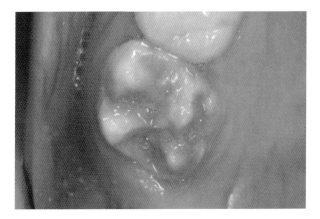

Plate 1(a) Upper first permanent molar in a patient with molar incisor hypomineralization prior to restoration.

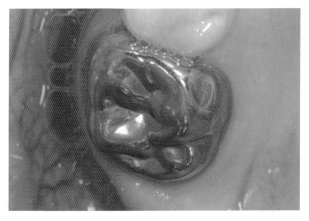

Plate 1(b) The same tooth following placement of a stainless steel crown.

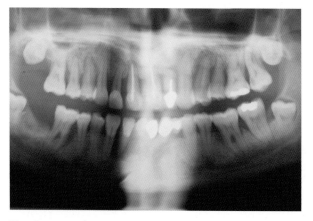

Plate 2 Panoramic film of a diabetic smoker aged 35 with chronic periodontitis.

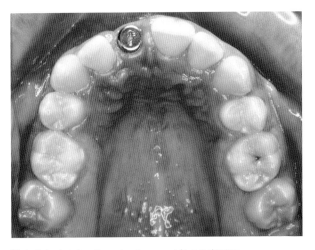

Plate 3 Implant placed to replace the upper right central incisor.

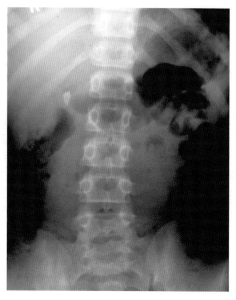

Plate 4 Chest X-ray showing inhaled tooth. This is a mandatory investigation for an inhaled tooth. Refer immediately for removal.

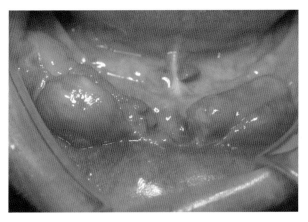

Plate 5 "Denture" hyperplasia. These soft irritation-induced masses are benign.

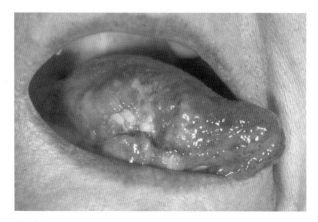

Plate 6 Squamous cell carcinoma of the tongue. This has a typical appearance *and* a typical "feel." Always palpate the lesion.

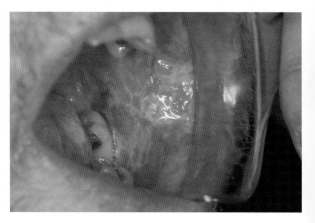

Plate 7 Lichen planus showing a typical reticular (lacy, white lines) pattern.

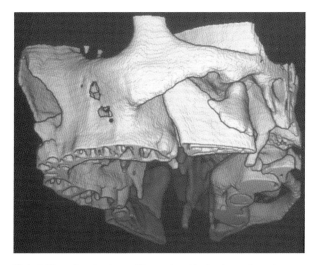

Plate 8 Three-dimensional scan of fractured condyle showing overlap and displacement.

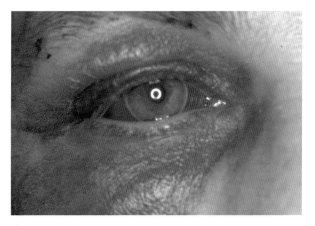

Plate 9 Black eye. The combination of circumorbital ecchymosis with medial *and* lateral subconjunctival hemorrhage means this is a much more substantial injury than it first appears.

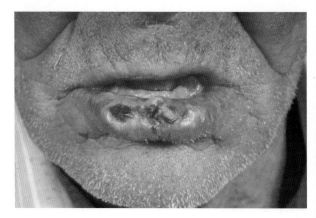

Plate 10 Squamous cell carcinoma of the lip showing a typical position and appearance.

- Relief of pain and any emergency treatment
- History and exam, including a thorough clinical and radiographic assessment of remaining teeth and edentulous areas
- Unless immediate dentures are planned, extract any teeth with poor prognosis.
- OH and periodontal treatment
- Preliminary design of partial denture
- Carry out restorative treatment required.
- Modify design if necessary and begin prosthetic treatment (p. 312).

Treatment planning for complete dentures
- Relief of pain and any emergency treatment, including temporary modification of existing dentures, if indicated
- History and exam including a thorough clinical and radiographic assessment of remaining teeth and edentulous areas
- Investigation and treatment of any systemic problems
- Removal of pathological abnormalities (e.g., retained roots) and pre-prosthetic surgery, if necessary
- ? rebase (p. 326), copy (p. 334), or fabricate new dentures (p. 316).

▶ Discussing with the patient the limitations of dentures prior to their fabrication is more likely to be viewed as explanation, whereas leaving it until after inserting the dentures will be seen as making excuses!

Principles of removable partial dentures

Definitions[1]

Denture base The part of a denture that rests on the foundation soft tissues.

Major connector The portion of a removable partial denture that unites its components.

Minor connector The components of a removable partial denture that serve as a connecting link between the major connector and clasp, rests, and indirect retainers.

Support The foundation area on which a dental prosthesis rests. With respect to dental prostheses, the resistance to displacement toward the basal tissue or underlying structures.

Retainers Any type of device used for the stabilization or retention of a prosthesis.

Indirect retention The effect achieved by one or more indirect retainers of a partial removable denture prosthesis that reduces the tendency for a denture base to move in an occlusal direction or rotate about the fulcrum line.

Fulcrum line A theoretical line around which a removable dental prosthesis tends to rotate.

Bracing The resistance to horizontal components of masticatory force.

Guiding planes Vertically parallel surfaces on abutment teeth or/and dental implant abutments oriented so as to contribute to the direction of the path of placement and removal of a removable dental prosthesis.

Survey line A line produced on a cast by a surveyor marking the height of contour in relation to the planned path of placement of a restoration.

Classification

Kennedy classification of removable partial dentures

Class I Bilateral edentulous areas located posterior to the remaining natural teeth

Class II Unilateral edentulous area located posterior to the remaining natural teeth

Class III Unilateral edentulous area with natural teeth located both anterior and posterior to it.

Class IV A single bilateral edentulous area located anterior to the remaining natural teeth. Any additional edentulous areas are referred to as modifications (except Class IV), e.g., Class I modification 1 has posterior bilateral edentulous areas and a bilateral edentulous area anterior to remaining natural teeth.

---

1 Glossary of Prosthodontic Terms, eighth ed. (GPT-8) 2005 *J Prosthet Dent* **94** 1–92.

Acrylic versus metal dentures

Most of the removable partial dentures provided in the United States have a metal framework with an acrylic denture base and teeth. Metal frameworks are generally preferred, because the greater strength of metal permits a more hygienic design. An acrylic base is indicated for the following:

- Temporary replacement, e.g., following trauma or in children
- Where there is inadequate support from the remaining teeth for a tooth-borne denture
- When additions to the denture are likely in the near future

However, where financial constraints C/I a metal framework, attention to the following factors may avoid production of a prosthesis that may be damaging to oral structures:

- Broad mucosal coverage to provide maximum suppor
- Keep base clear of the gingival margins wherever possible.
- No interproximal extensions of acrylic
- Point contact and wide embrasures between natural and artificial teeth
- Labial flanges for extra retention and bracing
- Additional support from wrought SS rests

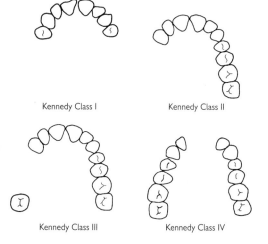

Kennedy Class I

Kennedy Class II

Kennedy Class III

Kennedy Class IV

Components of removable partial dentures

Denture base can be made entirely of acrylic or have a subframework of metal overlaid by acrylic.

Rests The components of the removable partial denture that function as a vertical support. They are an extension of the denture onto a tooth. Occlusal rests are used on posterior teeth over either the mesial or distal marginal ridge and fossa at an angle of <90°. They should be as long as they are wide, triangular in shape, and at least 2.5 mm for molars and premolars. Cingulum or incisal rests are used on anterior teeth.[1] Rests may be wrought or cast; the latter is preferred for strength and fit.

Clasps provide direct retention by engaging the undercut portion of a tooth. The action of a clasp must be resisted either by a nonretentive clasp arm above the height of contour of the tooth or by a reciprocal arm. Clasps can be classified by their position (occlusally approaching or gingivally approaching) or by their construction and material.

Cast (chrome cobalt) clasps are stiff, easily distorted, and liable to #. However, provided they are generally limited to undercuts of 0.25 mm, the advantage of being able to cast them as an integral part of a denture framework offsets the drawbacks. Clasp flexibility is a function of length, diameter, and cross-sectional shape.

Wrought clasps are usually attached by insertion into the acrylic of a denture base. Stainless steel is the most commonly used alloy, but gold clasps are more flexible and easily adjusted (and distorted).

The stiffer the wire the smaller the undercut that can be engaged. This can be offset by reducing the diameter of the wire to ↑ flexibility (but ↑ the likelihood of #) or by increasing the length of the clasp arm (e.g., gingivally approaching clasp). Cast chrome cobalt can be too stiff for occlusally approaching clasps on premolar teeth. The actual design used depends on the following:

- Depth of undercut: 0.25 mm—cast cobalt chrome; 0.5 mm—SS wire; <0.75 mm—wrought gold
- Position of undercut on tooth and relative to denture base, e.g.,
  - High survey line: gingivally approaching clasp or modify tooth shape by grinding
  - Diagonal survey line (a) sloping down from denture base: gingivally or occlusally approaching ring or reverse c-clasp; (b) sloping up from denture base: gingivally or occlusally (circumferential) approaching clasp
  - Medium survey line: as above
  - Low survey line: modify tooth shape, e.g., with surface recontouring
- Position of tooth. Gingivally approaching clasps are less conspicuous and are ∴ preferred for anterior teeth.
- Occlusion: adequate interocclusal space should be present or created for a clasp arm to cross a contact point between two natural teeth, to prevent occlusal disruption.

1 A. Carr 2005 *McCracken's Removable Partial Prosthodontics*, 11th ed., Mosby.

- Shape of vestibular sulcus: frenal attachments and alveolar undercuts may prevent use of gingivally approaching clasps.
- Periodontal health: reduced periodontal support deserves more flexible clasps to avoid overload of individual teeth.
- Material of denture base. Cast clasp arms are easily cast as part of the framework, but for acrylic dentures wrought clasps are more common.

Major connectors

In addition to joining parts of the denture together, the connector can also contribute to support and retention.

P/– connectors

	Patient tolerance	Indirect retention	Support	Comments
Ant. Bar	–	+	–	Useful for Kennedy IV
Mid. Bar	+	–	++	C/I torus
Post. Bar	++	+	–	Need mucocompression
Ring	–	++	+	
Plate	+	++	++	Less hygenic
Horseshoe	+	+	++	Useful with multiple denture bases

–/P connectors

- *Lingual bar* should only be used if there is >7 mm between floor of mouth and gingival margin to give 3 mm clearance from gingiva. Does not contribute to indirect retention. Usually cast. C/I if incisors are retroclined. If insufficient space, use sublingual bar.
- *Sublingual bar* lies horizontally in anterior lingual sulcus, but opinions differ as to patient tolerance. More rigid than lingual bar.
- *Lingual plate* is well tolerated and provides good support, bracing, and indirect retention if used in conjunction with rests but covers gingival margins. Can be made of cast metal or acrylic.
- *Continuous clasp* is really a bar that runs along the cingulae of the lower anterior teeth and is usually used in conjunction with a lingual bar. It is poorly tolerated.
- *Dental bar* is similar to continuous clasp, but of ↑ cross-sectional area and without lingual bar. Useful for teeth with long clinical crowns. Provides support and indirect retention. It may not be well tolerated.
- *Buccal/labial bar* is indicated when the lower incisors are retroclined.

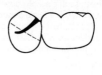

Occlusally approaching circumferential (three-arm) clasp.

One arm is the bracing reciprocal arm.
Oone arm is the retentive component.
One arm is the occlusal rest.

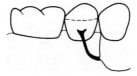

Gingivally approaching T bar (clasp).

The two most commonly used types of bars.

Removable partial denture design

Partial upper and lower denture (P/P) design is carried out after assessment of the patient and with reference to any previous dentures. A set of accurately articulated study models is essential.

Surveying

A dental surveyor should be used to determine heights of contour with a common path of insertion.

Objectives

- Establish path of insertion.
- Define those undercuts that may be used to retain denture.
- Define those undercuts that require blocking out prior to finish.

If the path of insertion is at 90° to the occlusal plane insertion of the denture will be straightforward; however, where the teeth are tilted or few undercuts exist, an angulated path of insertion may be advantageous. Which path provides more resistance to displacement during function is controversial.

A survey line can then be marked on the teeth to indicate their height of contour in the plane of the path of withdrawal.

Design

1. Outline denture bases Usually straightforward. If <1/2 tooth width or if in doubt about the need to replace a missing tooth, omit.

2. Plan support Support can be tooth only, mucosa only, or both. Tooth-born support (occlusal and cingulum rests) should be used wherever possible, as teeth are better able to withstand occlusal loading and support will not be compromised following resorption. Tooth and mucosa support are inevitable with large or distal extension edentulous areas and where plate designs are used. Tissue-only support should be used when no suitable teeth are available,and is less damaging in the maxillary than the mandibular arch, because of the palatal vault.

The role of the denture, length of the denture base, amount of support required (? denture opposed by natural or artificial teeth), and potential of remaining teeth to provide support (root area in bone) need to be assessed before a final decision is made.

3. Obtain retention Retention can be:

Direct e.g., clasps, guide planes, soft tissue undercuts, or precision attachments. Of these, clasps are the most commonly used. The best arrangement is to use three clasps as far away from each other as possible. Guide planes help to establish a precise path of insertion and withdrawal. They only need to be 2–3 mm in length, reducing reliance on clasps.

Indirect This is derived by placing components so as to resist "rocking" of the denture around direct retainers, e.g., by the position of clasps and rests and the type of connector. This is particularly important with free-end and large anterior denture bases.

4. Assess bracing required Bracing is provided by the connector, maximum denture base extension, and the reciprocal arms of clasps. Elimination of occlusal interferences ↓ need for bracing.

5. Choose connector after consideration of the above. Is there space in the occlusion to accommodate the chosen connector? Where possible the connector should be cut away from the gingival margins.

6. Reassess ? as simple as possible ? aesthetic.

Instructions to technician should include written details and a diagram drawn on a duplicate stone model. Where some confusion may arise over the precise position of a component, it is helpful to mark this directly on the cast.

Some design problems

The mandibular Kennedy Class I (bilateral free-end saddle) This presents a particular problem because of a lack of tooth support and retention distally, small denture base area compared to force applied, and distal leverage on abutment tooth in function (which ↑ with resorption). Possible solutions include the following:

- Maximize indirect retention by placing rests and clasps on mesial aspect of the abutment tooth and using lingual plate design.
- Use a mucocompressive impression of the edentulous area to ↓ displacement in function. Use the altered cast technique.
- Use fewer, smaller teeth and maximize denture base extension.
- RPI system for distal abutment teeth. Mesial rest, distal guiding plate, and mid-buccal I bar. During function the denture base moves tissue-ward and rotates around the mesial rest. The plate and I bar are constructed in such a way as to disengage from the tooth and avoid potentially harmful loading.
- Stress-breaker design (advantages are more theoretical than practical)
- Use precision attachments (beware of overloading abutments).

Class IV Can sometimes avoid unsightly clasps by use of the following:
- A flange engaging a labial alveolar undercut
- A rotational path of insertion[1] using rigid minor connectors that are rotated into proximal undercuts anteriorly
- Interproximal undercuts, which may allow minimal display of clasps—"hidden clasps"

Multiple Class III areas A horseshoe design, which uses guide planes for retention, may be indicated.

---

1 T. W. Chow 1988 *BDJ* **164** 180.

Clinical steps for removable partial dentures

1. Assessment and treatment plan See p. 302.

2. Prelimary impressions These are usually taken using alginate in a stock tray. For distal extension edentulous areas (Kennedy Class I and II), modify the tray first with compound or silicone putty.

3. Occlusal record If MIP is obvious, the occlusion can be recorded conventionally (p. 249) at the same visit as first impressions. If MIP is not obvious, occlusal rims (wax record blocks) will be required, as will a separate visit. Where there are no teeth in occlusal contact, the steps involved are the same as for recording the occlusion for F/F (p. 320). If there is an occlusal stop but insufficient standing teeth to produce a stable relationship of the casts, the procedure is as follows:
- Determine the VDO and mark the position of two index teeth with pencil.
- Define the arch form and occlusal plane using the occlusal rim on which this is easiest, e.g., tooth to tooth, tooth to retromolar pad.
- Check the occlusal rim in the mouth, using the mark on the index teeth as a guide, and adjust blocks if necessary.
- Record occlusion with bite-recording paste or wax.
- Check that the relationship of the index teeth on the articulated casts corresponds to that in the mouth.

4. Survey mounted casts and design denture See p. 310.

5. Tooth preparation may be required to:
- Accommodate rest seats. Rests need to be >1 mm for strength, ∴ if insufficient room in occlusion to accommodate this bulk, tooth reduction is required.
- Establish guide planes
- Modify unfavorable survey line, e.g., ↓ height of contour

6. Final impressions using a custom tray. Alginate is the most commonly used material, but elastomers are preferable for deep undercuts. It is helpful to have a wax try-in before the framework is made. This enables you to confirm tooth position so that the retentive elements for the acrylic are placed appropriately.

7. Framework try-in
- Check extension, adaptation, and position of clasp, and rests. If casting does not fit, use of correcting fluid or a fit checking material (e.g., Fit-Checker) may reveal which areas to relieve.
- Check upper and lower separately for VDO and occlusion, and then together.
- Major faults: repeat final impressions.
- Minor faults: adjust at finish.
- Make new occlusal record, if required.
- Select tooth mold and shade.
- Use altered cast technique, if required.

8. Wax try-in
- Check position of denture teeth.
- Check flange extensions/thickness.
- Check VDO, arch form, occlusal plane and occlusion.
- Check aesthetics with patient and only proceed when patient is satisfied.
- Prescribe post-dam relief areas and management of undercuts.

9. Finish Once any fitting surface roughness is eliminated, the dentures are tried in separately, adjusting undercuts and contacts as required. The extension, occlusion, and articulation are then adjusted if necessary. Give the patient written and verbal instructions, and a further appointment.

Rebasing P/P

Acrylic mucosa-born dentures can be rebased at the chairside with self-cure materials, but difficulty may be experienced in removing the denture in the presence of undercuts, and the materials are generally inferior to the original denture base. Alternatively, P/P can be rebased in the laboratory by means of a technique similar to that used for F/F (p. 326). Alternatively, make a new denture. For cast metal dentures an impression can be recorded of the edentulous area using an elastomer or ZOE, while holding denture by the framework. In all cases care must be taken to avoid the introduction of occlusal errors, e.g., ↑ VDO.

Immediate complete dentures

When the remaining teeth have a poor prognosis, management depends on whether the patient is already a partial-denture wearer or not.

Rx alternatives for patients with no previous denture experience

- Extract remaining teeth, wait 6 months for resorption to slow, and then construct F/F dentures. A recipe for disaster!
- Provide partial denture and allow patient to adapt before progressing to an immediate complete denture. The best solution.

Rx alternatives for partial denture wearer

- A partial denture to which teeth are added as required. This allows a gradual progression toward edentulism and is preferable for the elderly patient.
- Immediate complete denture. This has the advantage that the form and position of the natural teeth can be copied and is said to promote better healing and reduce resorption, but frequent adjustments and early replacement are necessary.
- Overdenture (p. 336).

Clinical procedures

- *Assessment* Warn the patient about the effects of resorption and the need for early rebasing and replacement.
- *Preliminary impressions* (as for P/P, p. 318).
- *Final impressions* ZOE or elastomeric impression material.
- *Occlusal record* Where there are sufficient posterior teeth remaining a wax wafer should suffice, and this can be taken at the same visit as impressions are recorded. Otherwise, occlusal rims will be required.
- *Wax try-in* This will be limited to those teeth that are already missing. Check fit, extension, and stability, etc. In addition, you need to prescribe any proposed changes in position of anterior artificial teeth compared to natural teeth.
- *Extraction* of remaining teeth with alveoloplasty if necessary to remove undercuts or areas of excessive bone that may prevent complete seating of the denture.
- *Finish* Repeated removal and insertion of the denture should be avoided, therefore adjustments should be limited to making the patient comfortable. They should be instructed not to remove the denture before the postoperative appointment in 24 h.
  - *Review.* The fitting and occlusal surfaces are adjusted as required. If dentures are not retentive they will require a temporary reline (see below).
  - *Recall.* Regular inspection of immediate dentures is important, as rapid bone resorption means that they will require rebasing early. However, this should be deferred, if feasible, for at least 3 months after the extractions. A possible regimen is 1 week, 1 month, 3 months, 9 months, and then yearly.

Laboratory procedures

These are similar to those for F/F except that the teeth are removed from the stone cast and the area is trimmed and smooth before final processing.

Surgical procedures See p. 353 and 388.

Problems

- *Poor denture retention* Use a temporary reline material (e.g., Lynal, Coe-Soft) and replace it regularly to tide patient over the initial 3 months. Subsequently, reline the denture base with heat-cured acrylic.
- *Gross occlusal error* Adjust occlusal surface of one denture until even contact is attained. This denture can then be replaced after initial healing and resorption have occurred.

Principles of complete dentures

Definitions[1]

Retention The resistance of a denture to dislodgement. Dependent upon **1** peripheral seal; **2** contact area between denture and tissues; **3** close fit; and **4** viscosity/volume of saliva. Neuromuscular control has more to do with stability than retention.

Retromylohyoid space An anatomic area in the alveololingual sulcus just lingual to the retromolar pad bounded anteriorly by the mylohyoid ridge, posteriorly by the retromylohyoid curtain, inferiorly by the floor of the alveololingual sulcus, and lingually by the anterior tonsillary pillar when the tongue is in a relaxed position.

Stability The ability of the denture to resist displacing forces during function. Stability is influenced by forces acting on polished and occlusal surfaces, as well as the form of the supporting tissues.

Neutral zone The potential space between the lips and cheeks on one side and the tongue on the other; that area or position where the forces between the tongue and cheeks or lips are equal.

Ways to optimize retention and stability
- Maximum extension of denture base (as far as the surrounding musculature will allow). The maxillary denture should extend distally over the tuberosities and onto the compressible tissue just anterior to the vibrating line on the palate. The mandibular denture should extend the full depth and width of the retromylohyoid space, and halfway across the retromolar pad. **Note:** Overextension will result in a denture that is displaced in function.
- Have as close an adaptation of denture base to mucosa as possible, to maximize the surface tension effects of saliva.
- Placement of the teeth in the neutral zone. More important in -/F. The better retention of F/- often allows some latitude in this respect.
- Correct shape of the polished surfaces so that muscle action tends to reseat the denture.
- A good border seal. This is achieved by ensuring that the flanges fill the entire sulcus width and by placing a post-dam on compressible tissue.
- Balanced occlusion free from interfering contacts

Patient assessment should include the following:
- Previous dental history, including when they became edentulous, number and degree of success of previous dentures, and their opinion of present F/F.
- Extraoral examination of skeletal pattern and biological age.
- Intraoral examination for signs of any pathology, and an assessment of ridge form, compressibility of mucosa, tongue size, tonicity of the lips, and the volume and viscosity of saliva.
- An evaluation of their present F/F—what to copy and what to correct.
- Personality

---

1 Glossary of Prosthodontic Terms, eighth ed. (GPT-8) 2005 *J Prosthet Dent* **94** 1–92.

Common denture faults are, in order of decreasing prevalence:[1]
- Lack of interocclusal rest space
- Failure to reproduce closely enough the features of previous successful dentures
- Occlusal errors
- Incorrect adaptation and extension
- Incorrect vertical dimension
- Incorrect occlusal plane
- Incorrect arch form
- Esthetics—teeth look "too perfect"

1 R. Yemm 1985 *BDJ* **159** 304.

Impressions for complete dentures

▶ Tissues must be healthy before final impressions are recorded. If
necessary, use tissue conditioner in present F/F (p. 326).

Classically, two sets of impressions are recorded of the edentulous
mouth. The purpose of the first is to record sufficient information for a
custom tray to be made in which to record the final (master) impression.
In practice, some use the first impression recorded in a stock tray for
construction of the denture. This technique this may suffice for some
patients, but especially for those with retention problems, second impressions in a custom tray are advisable.

Preliminary impressions

These are recorded using an (edentulous) stock tray and alginate, elastomer (both preferable for undercut or flabby ridges), or (modeling
compound impression plastic) compound. A line should be marked on
the impression to indicate to the technician the desired extension of the
special tray. In the maxilla, the posterior limit should be the hamular
notches and the vibrating line, and in the lower, the retromolar pads.

Custom trays can be made in self-cure or light-cure acrylic. The space left
for the impression depends on the material to be used: ZOE = 0.5 mm;
elastomer = 0.5–1.5 mm (depending on viscosity); plaster = 2 mm;
alginate = 3 mm. For trays with >1 mm space use stops to aid positioning.

Final impressions

The aim of these is to record the maximum denture-bearing area and to
develop an effective border seal the functional width and depth of the
sulcus. The special tray should be modified by reducing any overextension and border molding the peripheries adapted by the addition of stick
compound. It is important that the trays are not perforated and that you
can demonstrate a peripheral seal with the upper tray before you take
your impression. Gently manipulate the patient's soft tissues and ask
them to slightly protrude their tongue to imitate functional movements.

Mucocompressive versus mucostatic A mucocompressive impression technique is sometimes advocated to give a wider distribution of loading
during function and to compensate for the differing compressibility of the
denture-bearing area, thus preventing # due to flexion. ZOE or composition are used. However, dentures made by this method are less well
retained at rest, which is the greater proportion of time. Alginate and
plaster are said to be more mucostatic. Tissue adaptation following a
period of use probably reduces the clinical difference between the two
techniques.

Special techniques

Neutral zone impression technique This is used for recording the neutral
zone in patients with limited natural retention for -/F.
• Record final impressions and the maxillomandibular relation.
• A fully extended acrylic baseplate is made on the lower cast, with
  wire loops added that do not extend above the occlusal plane.

- The upper trial denture or occlusal rim is inserted.
- Tissue conditioner is placed on the baseplate and around loops, and inserted.
- The patient is asked to swallow, purse lips, and say "Ooh" and "Eee."
- The impression is removed and trimmed down until it can be fitted onto the articulator to replace the lower occlusal rim.
- A mold of the impression is made into which wax is poured.
- The wax is cut away so that each denture tooth can be positioned within the zone recorded to make the trial denture. The polished surfaces should replicate the impression.

Flabby ridge Classically occurs under a F/- opposed by natural lower teeth. If mild, then an impression recorded with alginate or elastomer in a tray perforated over the flabby area may suffice. For more severe cases, a two-stage technique is required, using a custom tray with a window cut out over the flabby tissue. First, an impression is recorded in the tray with ZOE and the paste trimmed away from the flabby area. This is then reseated and low-viscosity elastomer or impression plaster placed into the window to complete the impression. **Note:** Combination-type cases should have the dentures constructed on a semi-adjustable articulator to minimize occlusal displacing forces.

Functional impression Tissue conditioner is placed inside the patient's existing denture. After several days of wear, a functional impression is produced.

Common impression problems and faults

- A feather edge indicates underextension. This can be corrected by the addition of greenstick to the tray and repeating.
- Tray border shows through impression material. The tray should be reduced in the area of overextension and the impression repeated.
- Air bubbles. If small, they can be filled in with a little soft wax. If large, retake the impression.
- Tray not centered. This is often at least partially due to using too much material so that it is difficult to see the placement of the tray. Remember to line up the tray handle with the patient's nose (except for ex-boxers).
- Gagging and vomiting. A calm and confident manner is necessary for successful impressions. Gain the patient's confidence by attempting the lower first and use a fast-setting, viscous material. Distraction techniques may help, e.g., wriggling the toes on the left foot and the fingers of the right hand at the same time (the patient, not the operator!).
- Patient with dry mouth: ZOE is C/I; use elastomer instead.
- Areas where tray shows through in otherwise good impression can be overcome by prescribing a tin-foil relief when dentures are being processed.

Recording the occlusion for complete dentures

When recording the occlusion the aim is to provide the technician with the following information for constructing trial dentures.

Vertical dimension The interocclusal rest space (freeway space [FWS]) is the difference between the vertical dimension at rest and the vertical dimension in occlusion. In most patients it is 2–4 mm. The VDO for an edentulous patient can ∴ be determined by measuring their resting face height and subtracting a FWS. Resting face height is assessed using

- A Willis gauge, to measure the distance between the base of nose and the underside of the chin. It is only accurate to ±1 mm.
- Spring dividers or a marked tongue blade, to measure the distance between a dot placed on both the chin and the tip of the patient's nose. This method is less popular with patients and is C/I for bearded gentlemen (or ladies!).
- The patient's appearance and speech

Position of the occlusal plane This should be placed so that 1–2 mm (↓ with age) of tooth are visible below the patient's upper lip at rest. The occlusal plane should lie midway between the ridges parallel to the inter-pupillary and the ala-tragus lines. At rest the tongue should rise just above the lower occlusal plane.

Horizontal jaw relationship Record the more reproducible centric relation position. In the natural dentition, MIP is ~1 mm forward of centric relation position, ∴ some prosthodontists advise adjusting the finished dentures to allow the patient to slide comfortably between the two positions.

Position of the anterior and posterior teeth Ideally, the artificial teeth should lie in the space occupied by the natural dentition. The extent to which it is possible to compensate for a Class II or III malocclusion depends on the retention afforded by the ridges. In the natural dentition the upper incisors lie ~10 mm anterior to the incisive papilla. With resorption this comes to lie on the ridge crest, ∴ the artificial teeth should be placed labial and buccal to the ridge, to give adequate lip support and a nasolabial angle of ~90°.

Mold and shade of artificial teeth Low cusped teeth are preferred with increasing residual ridge resorption, but cuspless teeth are useful for patients with poor natural retention or a "wandering" occlusal relationship. When considering the color, mold, and arrangement of the anterior teeth, the patient's age, facial appearance, and, most importantly, their opinion, must be taken into account. If you disagree about the suitability of their choice, document it.

Type of articulator to be used for setting-up the teeth Most textbooks advocate adjustable or average value articulators for F/F dentures. Dentures are made on simple hinge articulators to the satisfaction of the some patients, probably because they are able to adapt to the occlusion that results. An average value type will give some degree of balanced articulation that can then be refined in the mouth and will avoid the introduction of occlusal interferences, and is the preferred method.

Practical procedures

The occlusion is recorded using occlusal wax rims mounted on rigid acrylic or shellac bases. A heated wax trimmer, or a plaster knife and a bunsen burner, are required to adjust the rims. As head posture can affect interocclusal rest space, position the patient so that the Frankfort plane is horizontal.

- Check fit of bases. If it is poor, you can either repeat final impressions or take a ZOE or low-viscosity elastomer impression with the base and proceed.
- Adjust upper wax rim to give adequate lip support.
- Trim occlusal plane of upper rim.
- Trim lower wax rim to obtain correct lip support and buccolingual position of posterior teeth.
- Adjust lower rim so that it meets upper evenly in centric relation, with 2–4 mm of interocclusal rest space.
- Mark center lines.
- Locate rims in centric relation, e.g., with bite-recording paste.
- Prescribe mold and shade of artificial teeth for try-in.
- Consider using a facebow to mount the maxillary cast on the articulator

Common pitfalls

- Inaccuracies caused by poorly fitting bases
- Rims contacting prematurely posteriorly and flipping up anteriorly, or vice versa
- Failure to provide adequate interocclusal rest space
- Attempting to correct too much when replacing old, worn dentures and exceeding the adaptive capacity of the patient

Wax try-in of complete dentures

This is constructed by setting up the prescribed teeth in wax on acrylic or shellac bases. Both the dentist and patient must be satisfied before the dentures are processed in acrylic.

Clinical procedures

Check the trial dentures

On and off the articulator Comparison with the patient's existing dentures is helpful to see if the features to be copied or modified have been successfully incorporated.

- Singly in the mouth. To check extension, stability, and the position of the teeth relative to the soft tissues
- Together in mouth. Examine vertical dimension, occlusion, aesthetics, and phonetics ("S" sound will be affected by an ↑ or ↓ interocclusal space).

Seek the patient's opinion Confirm with the patient that they are satisfied with the appearance of the tooth set-up.

Prepare post-dam This should be placed just anterior to the vibrating line on the palate, which can be assessed by asking the patient to say "Aah." The degree of compressibility of the tissues is assessed and the depth of the post-dam cut accordingly (usually ~1 mm). The post-dam is prepared on the upper cast with a wax knife in the shape of a cupid's bow.

Complete prescription to the technician should include the following:

- Any changes in posterior tooth position or anterior tooth arrangement
- For fibrous undercuts >4 mm and bony undercuts >2 mm, decide whether they are to be plastered out or the flange thickened for adjustment at the time of insertion.
- Tin-foiling for relief of hard or nodular areas, if required
- Gingival color and contour
- Denture base material. This is usually heat-cure acrylic; however, metal bases are indicated for patients with a history of fractured dentures.
- Identification marker, which is preferably legible

Common problems and possible solutions

- Overextension of flanges. Reduce.
- Underextension of flanges. Try a temporary wax addition to flange first, to check effect of extending it. If this is satisfactory a new impression is required.
- Teeth outside the neutral zone. Remove offending teeth and replace with wax, which can be trimmed until correct.
- Incorrect VDO. If too small, it can be increased by adding wax to the occlusal surfaces of teeth, but if too large, you will need to replace lower teeth with wax and re-record VDO.
- Occlusal discrepancy or anterior open bite or posterior open bite. Replace lower posterior teeth with wax and re-record VDO.
- Too little of upper anterior teeth visible. Reset anterior teeth to correct position and adjust occlusal plane accordingly.

- Too much of upper anterior teeth showing. The effect of reducing the length of the incisors can be judged by coloring the incisal region with a black wax pencil and then indicating desired change in position to lab.
- Inadequate lip support. An increase in support can be assessed by adding wax to the labial aspect of the upper try-in.

A new try-in will be required if large errors are being corrected or if any doubt still exists about the occlusion.

Complete denture delivery

Some adjustment of completed dentures is inevitable following processing. On average, a 0.5 mm increase in height occurs, with a slight shift in tooth contact posteriorly. The main steps are described below.

Adjustment of fitting surface First, smooth any roughness and, if necessary, gradually reduce the bulk of the flanges in areas of undercut until the denture can be easily inserted without compromising retention.

Check occlusion The vertical dimension of the dentures is maintained by contact between the upper palatal and lower buccal cusps, ∴ adjustment of these should be avoided if possible. Get patient to occlude and check contact with articulating paper. If contact is uneven, or heavy contacts are seen, make necessary adjustments.

- For cusped teeth only, place articulating paper between occlusal surfaces and ask patient to make small lateral movements and adjust Buccal Upper and Lower Lingual (BULL rule) cusps only to remove any interferences.
- Remove any interferences to protrusive movements.
- Balancing contacts are desirable but not essential, unless they can be established easily by minor adjustments to working side contacts.

Advice to the patient Verbal and written instructions should be given.
- Most patients take some time to adapt to their new dentures. During this time a softer diet is advisable.
- If pain is experienced the patient should try to continue wearing their dentures and return for adjustment as soon as possible so that affected areas can be easily seen.
- Patients should be encouraged not to wear their dentures at night.
- When the dentures are not being worn they should be stored in water to prevent them from drying out and warping. Plastic denture boxes are cheap and safer than a glass of water at the bedside.
- Cleaning, see p. 328.

Review The patient should be seen 1–2 weeks after fitting to ease the dentures and adjust the occlusion. Localization of the cause of any irritation due to a flaw on the fitting surface can be helped by
- Pressure-indicating paste, which is painted onto the tissue surface of the denture revealing areas of excessive pressure
- Indelible pencil, (marking stick) or denture fixative powder mixed with zinc oxide, which is applied carefully to the area thought to be responsible and the denture inserted. On removal the mark will have been transferred to the adjacent mucosa and should correspond with the damaged area.

If there is no obvious cause relating to the fitting surface remember that occlusal faults can cause displacement and mucosal trauma, and an excessive VDO is a common cause of generalized soreness under -/F (p. 330).

Stress the importance of regular examination of all patients with dentures.

Denture maintenance

▶ Examine patients with F/F annually and perform routine oral cancer screening. Regular maintenance will help prevent damage from ill-fitting dentures and will ↑ the likelihood of early detection of oral pathology.

Problems caused by lack of aftercare of F/F As a result of resorption, all dentures become progressively ill-fitting, leading to loss of retention and stability. Movement of dentures in function may result in

- Resorption
- Predisposition to candidal infection
- Denture irritation hyperplasia, p. 388.
- Inflammatory papillary hyperplasia of the palate

All of these are exacerbated by wear of the occlusal surfaces.

Rebasing

The terms *rebasing* and *relining* are commonly used interchangeably. Strictly speaking, relining is replacement of the tissue surface (e.g., with a temporary material) and rebasing is replacement of all of the denture base.

Rebasing is indicated where the only feature of F/F that requires improvement is the fitting surface; otherwise consider replacement F/F using the duplication method. For rebasing the material of choice is heat-cure acrylic (p. 622), but this necessitates the patient being without their dentures while the addition is being made. Self-cure acrylic applied at the chairside appears attractive, but its properties are inferior. For a heat-cure rebase, a wash impression (ZOE or low-viscosity elastomer) must be recorded inside the denture.

Technique To avoid an ↑ in VDO, record the impression for one denture at a time while in occlusion.

- Check occlusion and adjust if required. Note VDO.
- Remove undercuts from tissue surface.
- Correct extension and place post-dam in compound.
- Apply impression material and insert in mouth. Get patient to close into contact with opposing denture. Check VDO and occlusion.
- Remove and examine impression; if unsatisfactory (or if in doubt), repeat.

An alternative method for inflamed tissues is to record a functional impression (p. 319) over several days with a tissue conditioner, in which case the resulting impression needs to be poured immediately.

Tissue conditioners

These are resilient materials that give a more even distribution of loading and thus promote tissue recovery. They are particularly useful where ill-fitting dentures have caused trauma, as it is important to allow the tissues to recover before impressions for replacement dentures or a rebase are taken.

Technique Relieve any areas of pressure on the fitting surface and reduce any overextension. A minimum thickness of 2 mm is required and the material should not be left for >1 week. Repeated applications may be necessary. If candidal infection is present it should be treated prior to impressions.

Soft linings are indicated for
- Older patients with a thin atrophic mucosa, usually for -/F
- Following prosthetic surgery
- Use of soft tissue undercuts for ↑ retention, e.g., following hemimaxillectomy, clefts

It is wise to make a new denture first in acrylic and adjust the occlusion, before placing soft lining. A minimum thickness of 2 mm is required, which may significantly weaken a lower denture, necessitating placement of a metal strengthener on the lingual aspect. No material is ideal and soft linings are best avoided (p. 624).

Cleaning dentures

When new dentures are fitted the importance of regular, thorough cleaning with soap, water, and a brush to prevent the buildup of plaque, stain, and calculus should be emphasized. Unfortunately, few patients are sufficiently diligent, in part from being conditioned by advertising, to expect to use a denture cleaner.

Advise patients to clean their dentures over a basin of water to act as a safety net.

Formulation	Active ingredients	Problems
Powder	Abrasives, e.g., calcium carbonate	Abrasion
Paste	Abrasives + eugenol	Abrasion + crazing
(Dentu-creme)	Abrasive + phenol oil	Abrasion + sensitivity
Hypochlorite	Sodium hypochlorite	Can corrode metal
Effervescent	Dissolves to give alkaline peroxide solution	Doubts about effectiveness
Enzymatic	Proteolytic enzymes	Not widely available

Practical tips

Hypochlorite solutions are effective for acrylic dentures when used overnight, but if used with hot water they are liable to cause bleaching, ∴ warn patient.[1] The peroxide cleaners are popular but are ineffective if used for only 15–30 min as the manufacturers advise.

	Avoid	Use
Viscogel	Acids, alkaline peroxide	Hypochlorite
Molloplast	Acids, alkaline peroxide	Hypochlorite
Coe-comfort	Hypochlorite, alkaline peroxide	Soap + water
Metal denture	Hypochlorite	Alkaline peroxide
Any denture	Household bleach	

1 C. A. Crawford 1986 *J Dent* **14** 258.

Denture problems and complaints

The most common complaints are of pain and/or looseness, which can be due to denture errors or patient factors. The latter should be foreseen and the patient warned in advance of the limitations of dentures. The wise prosthodontist will tend to overestimate the difficulty of providing successful dentures. Unless the cause is immediately obvious, e.g., a flaw on the fitting surface, a systematic examination of the tissue and polished and occlusal surfaces (including the jaw relationship) should be carried out.

Pain This can be due to a variety of causes, including roughness of the tissue surface, errors in the occlusion, lack of FWS, a bruxing habit, a retained root, or other pathology. Forward or lateral displacement of a denture due to a premature contact can lead to inflammation of the ridge on the lingual or lateral aspect, respectively. With continued resorption bony ridges become prominent and the mental foramina exposed, which can lead to localized areas of specific pain.

Pain from an individual tooth on P/P
• Excessive load and/or traumatic occlusion
• Leverage due to unstable denture
• Clasp arm too tight
• Inadequate lining under amalgam restoration failing to insulate against a galvanic couple with metal denture

Looseness This more commonly affects the lower than the upper denture.

Denture faults	Patient factors
Incorrect peripheral extension	Inadequate volume or amount of saliva
Teeth not in neutral zone	Poor ridge form
Unbalanced articulation	↓ adaptive skills, e.g., elderly patient
Polished surfaces unsatisfactory	

Burning mouth This can be due to **1** local causes: e.g., ↑ VDO or sensitivity to acrylic monomer, or be unrelated to the denture (e.g., irritant mouthwashes); **2** systemic causes: e.g., menopause, deficiency states, cancerphobia, xerostomia.

Speech

Patient's complaint	Possible cause
Difficulty with *f, v*	Incisors too far palatally
Difficulty with *d, s, t*	Alteration of palatal contour
	Incorrect overjet and overbite
s becomes *th*	Incisors too far palatally
	Palate too thick
Whistling	Palate vault too high behind incisors
Clicking teeth	↑ VDO
	Lack of retention

Cheek biting Check first that teeth are in neutral zone. If satisfactory, ↓ buccal "overjet," i.e., reduce buccal surface of lower molars (provided normal buccolingual relationship).

Nausea, gagging, and vomiting
- Map out extent of sensitive area on palate using a ball-ended instrument and firm pressure, and check extension of denture.
- Palateless dentures may be a solution, but their retention is poor.
- Training dentures. These can take the form of a simple palate to which teeth are added incrementally, starting with the incisors.
- Implants (p. 390) and a fixed prosthesis

The grossly resorbed lower ridge Resorption is progressive with time, which is a good argument for avoiding rendering young patients edentulous. The mandible resorbs more quickly than the maxilla, which exacerbates the problem of retention for -/F. Management is dependent on the severity of the problem and the patient's biological age.
- Minimizing destabilizing forces on the lower denture, e.g., **1** maximum extension of denture base; **2** ↓ number and width of teeth; **3** ↑ interocclusal rest space; **4** lowering occlusal plane
- Neutral zone impression technique (p. 318)
- Surgery (p. 388)
- Implants (p. 390)

Recurrent fracture Apart from carelessness, this is usually caused by occlusal faults or fatigue of the acrylic due to continual stressing by small forces. Flexing of the denture can occur with flabby ridges, palatal tori, and following resorption. Notching of a denture, e.g., relief for a prominent frenum, can also predispose to #. Treatment depends on the etiology, but in some cases provision of a metal plate or a cast-metal strengthener may be necessary.

Candida and dentures

Candida is a common oral pathogen. It becomes pathogenic if the environment favors its proliferation (e.g., dentures, antibiotic alteration of the bacterial flora) or the host's defenses are compromised.

Denture stomatitis

This is also known as denture sore mouth, a misnomer because the condition is usually symptomless. Classically, it is seen as redness of the palate under a F/- denture, with petechial and whitish areas. In 90% of cases it is due to *Candida albicans*, 9% to other candida, and <1% to other organisms, e.g., *Klebsiella* spp.

Incidence A common condition, it has been reported in 30–60% of patients wearing F/F. It affects women more commonly than men, in a ratio of 4:1, and usually affects the upper denture-bearing area only.

Etiology is still not completely understood.
- Infection with *Candida* species
- Poor denture hygiene
- Night-time wear of dentures
- Trauma is often cited as a contributing factor to denture stomatitis, BUT
  - it occurs more commonly under F/- than -/F;
  - it can affect patients wearing F/- only;
  - it is also found under well-fitting orthodontic appliances.
- Systemic factors can predispose to candida infection, e.g., iron and vitamin deficiency, steroids, drugs which cause xerostomia, and endocrine abnormalities.
- A high sugar intake provides substrate for candida to multiply. It has been postulated that the upper denture-bearing area is more commonly affected because it is related to the more serous nature of saliva from the submandibular glands and the poorer fit of -/F, which allows saliva to reach the underlying mucosa more easily.

Management
- Leave dentures out. Though not a realistic solution to most patients, they should be encouraged to remove their dentures at night.
- Improved denture hygiene, e.g., brushing fitting surface and soaking in hypochlorite cleanser.
- Reduce sugar intake.
- Antifungals (p. 560). Nystatin suspension 100,000 units/ml, 1 ml qid or amphotericin suspension 100 mg/ml, 1 ml qid, are the first choice. 2% Miconazole gel is more expensive and should ∴ be reserved for patients with candida that is unresponsive to other agents or associated with angular cheilitis.
- If you suspect systemic factors exacerbating this condition, refer patient to primary care physician.
- Coexisting papillary hyperplasia of palate may need surgical reduction.

Angular cheilitis See p. 432.

Denture duplication

Successful function with complete dentures depends to a marked degree on the patient's ability to control them. This ability is learned during a period of denture use. When replacement dentures become necessary, it is helpful if the new appliances require as little adaptation as possible to the existing skills. This is generally considered to be particularly important for the older patient. Not only may skills have been developed over a long period, but also the ability to relearn may be diminished. So-called denture-copying techniques provide a more reliable method for provision of replacements.

Treatment planning

Before undertaking treatment it is essential to decide which features of the previous dentures are satisfactory, and which require modification, and by how much. Consider the following:

- Tissue surface—if this is the only feature that requires improvement, then rebasing is a possibility.
- Polished surface shapes
- Occlusal surface, jaw relationship, VDO. The effect of an increase in VDO can be assessed by self-cure addition to the existing dentures, but remember that this irreversibly alters them.
- Anterior tooth size, arrangement, relation to lips
- Posterior tooth mold and arch width (relation to tongue and cheeks)

Duplicating complete dentures

A number of techniques have been described. They vary in the materials used, and these in turn affect the acceptability of laboratory work and the clinical freedom to incorporate "corrections." In general, copies of the old appliances are used as substitutes for occlusal rims and as custom trays.

A typical method involves the following stages:[1]

1. Clinic
- Correct underextension with stick compound.
- Record impressions with silicone putty of polished surface and teeth, using large disposable tray. Complete mold with second mix of putty to record tissue surface (use a separating medium—Vaseline or, better, emulsion hand cream).
- Open mold, clean dentures, and return to patient.
- Send putty molds to laboratory.

2. Laboratory
- Fabricate self-cure acrylic baseplates on the silicone model of the tissue surface.
- Pour wax into remaining space.
- After cooling remove completed copy, cut off sprues, and polish.

1 R. Yemm 1991 *Int Dent J* **41** 233.

3. Clinic
- Employ the copies ("replica record blocks") to record required changes in denture shapes (see Treatment Planning), by adding or removing wax.
- Record working impressions in low-viscosity silicone *with adhesive* to aid retention on base.
- Record jaw relationship with "bite recording paste."
- Select shade/molds for new teeth.

4. Laboratory
- Pour impressions and articulate.
- Set up, cutting away modified replica rims to substitute new teeth (rather like setting up an immediate denture!).
- Wax up, including borders defined by working impressions.

5. Clinic
- Try-in stage

6. Laboratory
- Finishing stages as normal

7. Clinic
- Normal delivery (insertion) stage (and subsequent follow-up)

Other methods use alternative materials (e.g., alginate for impressions of existing dentures, wax, and shellac to form the copy dentures). Choice will depend on acceptability to both clinic and laboratory. In no instance, however, is an all-wax copy regarded as acceptable, since rigidity is inadequate for use as an impression tray.

Duplicating partial dentures for immediate dentures[1]
In patients with successful P/P, for whom extraction of the remaining teeth is planned, the transition to complete dentures can be facilitated by using a copy technique.

Clinic 1 Correct underextended flanges with compound and then take impressions of the dentures with putty in stock trays (see F/F technique). Record an alginate impression of the opposing arch, if no denture is planned for that arch.

Lab 1 Wax/shellac or acrylic replica of partial denture is constructed.

Clinic 2 Use the replica denture to develop the prescription and then record a wash impression inside the base with a light-bodied silicone. Record the occlusion using bite registration paste. Finally, take a pick-up impression in a stock tray with the modified replica denture in situ.

Lab 2 The impression is cast and used as a base for articulating the wax replica with the cast of the opposing arch. The teeth prescribed are then set up, and the wash impression retained in the replica, for the try-in.

Try-in and finish as for complete immediate dentures (p. 314).

1 J. R. Drummond 1983 *BDJ* **155** 297.

Overdentures

An overdenture (OD) derives support from one or more abutment teeth by completely enclosing them beneath the tissue surface. It can be a partial or complete denture.

Advantages

- Alveolar bone preservation around the retained tooth
- Improved retention, stability, and support
- Preservation of proprioception via PDL
- Improved crown-to-root ratio, which ↓ damaging lateral forces
- ↑ masticatory force
- Additional retention possible using attachments
- Aids transition from P/P to F/F

Disadvantages

- RCT probably required
- To avoid excessive bulk in region of retained tooth, denture base may need to be thinned, which ↑ likelihood of #
- ↑ maintenance for both patient and dentist
- Caries of retained overdenture abutments

Indications

- Motivated patient with good oral hygiene.
- Because of ↓ retention and stability of -/F and ↑ rate of mandibular resorption, ODs are particularly useful for -/F
- Cleft lip and palate
- Hypodontia
- Severe toothwear

Choosing abutment teeth

- Ideally: bilateral, symmetrical with a minimum of one tooth space between them
- Order of preference: canines, premolars, incisors, molars
- Healthy attached gingiva, adequate periodontal support (>1/2 root in bone), and no or limited mobility
- Is RCT required and if so is it feasible?

Preparation of abutment teeth

Alternatives include
- Removal of undercuts only
- Preparation of crown for thimble/telescopic gold coping
- RCT, tooth cut to dome shape, and access cavity restored with amalgam or an adhesive restoration
- RCT and gold coping over root face
- RCT and precision attachment

Precision attachments[1] are useful for ↑ retention of dentures or bridges, especially in cases with tissue loss (e.g., trauma or CLP), but they ↑ loading on abutment teeth, and are expensive and difficult to rebase and repair. They are usually of two parts, which are matched to fit together. One part is attached to the abutment tooth and the other to the denture. A variety of attachments are available, including stud/anchor (e.g., Rother-man eccentric clip), bar (e.g., Dolder), and magnets.

Since precision attachments require the highest technical skill and are highly dependent on patient and professional maintenance, it is wise to first use a basic OD and then reassess the need for additional retention. Hybrid dentures are partial dentures that use precision attachments (either intra- or extracoronal) on the abutment teeth for retention. Implants inserted in edentulous areas can be used with a precision attachment to increase retention.

Clinical procedures
- Assessment (clinical examination, study models, radiographs, etc.)
- RCT if required

If abutment preparation is limited to crown reduction:
- The steps involved are as for immediate dentures, with the abutment teeth reduced less on cast than is planned clinically. At the visit during which the final dentures are to be delivered, the abutment teeth are prepared and the dentures relined with self-cure acrylic to improve their adaptation.

If precision attachments or copings to be used:
- The teeth are prepared and an impression of the abutments, including post holes, taken. In the lab, dies are prepared and transfer copings (usually metal) made. The transfer copings are tried on the abutments, and if satisfactory an overall impression is recorded to accurately locate the copings to the remainder of the denture-bearing area. Alternatively, a two-stage technique using a special tray with windows cut out over abutments can be employed.
- Regular examinations (6-monthly) and maintenance is necessary for success.

Problems
The most important problems are
- Caries of abutment teeth, ∴ need good oral and denture hygiene and topical fluoride, e.g., toothpaste, applied to the tissue surface of the denture. Patients should be encouraged to remove their denture at night.
- Periodontal breakdown

---

1 H. W. Preiskel 1984 *Precision Attachments in Prosthodontics*, Quintessence.

Geriatric Dentistry

(or Geriatrics or Gerontology)

Definition Dentistry for the elderly. For those who have not reached retirement age, the elderly is anyone over 65. Others suggest that it is >75 years of age. Rather than arbitrary cutoffs, biological age should be considered.

Epidemiology Two factors are mainly responsible for the increasing relevance of dentistry for the elderly: an increase in the proportion of the elderly in the population and the improvements in dental health that have resulted in more people keeping their natural teeth for a longer period of time. By 2005 the proportion of the U.S. population over 65 was over 12%.[1] It is estimated that in 2002, 7.7% of adults were edentulous, compared with 11% in 1988.

Problems

The major overall problems are
- Age changes, both physiological and pathological
- Disease and drug therapy (Chapter 10)
- Delivery of care

Restorative problems include the following:
- Root caries, which can occur following exposure of root surfaces by gingival recession, in association with changes in diet, ↓ self-care, and ↓ salivary flow. Details of management are given on p. 25. Prevention of root caries in susceptible patients is possible using either a topical fluoride mouth rinse or fluoride-containing artificial saliva.
- Toothwear (p. 276) is especially prevalent when partial tooth loss has occurred.
- Pulpal changes, including sclerosis (p. 298) and ↓ repair capacity.

Periodontal problems include
- Reduced manual dexterity, making OH procedures difficult. Epidemiological studies of the periodontal needs of the elderly population are sparse and some trends may be masked by edentulism. The available evidence suggests that, although older patients develop plaque more quickly, the need for periodontal treatment ↑ up to middle age, and thereafter most patients can be maintained by regular nonsurgical management.

Prosthetic problems include the following:
- Reduced adaptive capacity; ∴ if teeth are unlikely to last a lifetime, the transition to at least partial dentures should be made while the patient is able to learn the new skills necessary.
- Age changes in the denture-bearing areas, including bone resorption and mucosal atrophy.

1 http://www.census.gov

Age-related changes

Age changes are defined as an alteration in the form or function of a tissue or organ as a result of biological activity associated with a minor disturbance of normal cellular turnover.

In general

↓ microcirculation, ↓ cellular reproduction, ↓ tissue repair, ↓ metabolic rate, ↑ fibrosis. Degeneration of elastic and nervous tissue. These result in reduced function of several body systems.

Dental

Oral soft tissues ↓ in the thickness of the epithelium, mucosa, and sub-mucosa is seen. Taste bud function ↓. With age, an ↑ occurs in the number and size of Fordyce's spots (sebaceous glands), lingual varices, and foliate papillae. Recent evidence suggests that stimulated salivary flow rate does not fall purely as a result of age. However, medications or systemic disease can affect salivary output.

Dental hard tissues Enamel becomes less permeable with age. Clinically, older teeth appear more brittle, but there is no significant difference between the elastic modulus of dentine in old or young teeth. The rate of secondary dentine formation reduces with age, but still continues. Occlusion of the dentine tubules with calcified material spreads crownward with age.

Toothwear is an age-related phenomenon and can be regarded as physiological in many cases. However, excessive and pathological wear can be caused by parafunction, abrasion, erosion (dietary, gastric, or environmental), or a combination of these factors.

Dental pulp ↑ fibrosis and ↓ vascularity mean that the defensive capacities of the pulp ↓ with ↑ age, ∴ pulp capping is less likely to succeed. Also ↑ secondary dentine and ↑ pulp calcification.

Periodontium ↑ fibrosis, ↓ cellularity, ↓ vascularity, and ↓ cell turnover are found with ↑ age. Whether gingival recession is pathological or physiological (developmental) is still hotly debated.

Systemic

Immune system A ↓ in cell-mediated response and ↓ in number of circulating lymphocytes leads to an ↑ incidence of autoimmune disease as well as a ↓ in the older patient's defense against infection. Also, an ↑ in neoplasia is seen. Steroid treatment for autoimmune disease may complicate dental treatment.

Nervous system Aging involves both a physiological decline in function and dysfunction associated with age-related disease (e.g., strokes, parkinsonism). A ↓ in acuity compounds the problem.

Cardiovascular Hypertension and ischemic heart disease worsen with age. Anemia is more common in the elderly. In general, the greatest problems arise when a GA is required, or the practice is located on the second floor.

Pulmonary system Lung capacity ↓ with age and chronic obstructive airways disease ↑ in prevalence.

Endocrine system Diabetes is more common.

Muscles ↓ bulk, slower contractions, and less precision of control occur.

Nutrition Poverty, impaired mobility, ↓ taste acuity, and ↓ masticatory function can result in nutritional deficiencies in the elderly. These can manifest as changes in the oral mucosa.

Mucosal disease is more common with increasing age.
- Oral cancer, p. 444.
- Lichen planus, p. 456.
- Herpes zoster is more common with ↑ age due to a ↓ in T-cell function. Neuralgia occurs more frequently after an attack in the elderly.
- Benign mucous membrane pemphigoid, p. 436.
- Pemphigus, p. 435.
- Candida is seen more frequently in the older age groups because of an ↑ proportion of denture wearers and ↑ immune deficiencies.

This list is obviously not exhaustive.

Dental care for the elderly

The basis for delivery of care to the older patient has been, and is likely to continue to be, via the general dentist.

General management problems

Medical and drug history (Chapter 10) It is wise to check any complicated medical problems with the patient's primary care physician. Unfortunately, many doctors are only familiar with the dental treatment they have personally received, therefore it is important to give details of the proposed treatment.

Communication with the elderly requires patience and understanding. Often older patients will try to cover up deafness, poor eyesight, and lack of comprehension, so it is better to err on the side of overstressing an important point or instruction, but avoid sounding patronizing. It is often helpful to enlist the assistance of a relative or friend of the older patient. Dental and medical appointments are often social encounters for many of the elderly.

Oral hygiene may be compromised by arthritis, stroke, or any illness that may affect motor function. Advise an electric toothbrush or modifying the handle of an ordinary toothbrush to make it easier to grip, e.g., with bicycle handlebar grips. Alternatively, self-cure acrylic can be used to make a custom grip for a toothbrush.

Delivery of care

Dental practice

Consideration should be given to the following:

- Access for a wheelchair or Zimmer frame. This is easy to arrange when a purpose-designed practice is being built, but can pose considerable problems for the established practice. In surgery it is important to allow sufficient space around the dental chair.
- Timing of appointments; e.g., for a diabetic patient these need to be arranged around meals and drug regimens, and early morning visits are probably C/I for arthritic patients, as it may take them a couple of hours to "get going."
- Positioning of the patient. Many elderly patients are unhappy to be recumbent in the dental chair. In addition, this position is C/I for those with cardiovascular or pulmonary disease. Adjust dental chair gradually as rapid movement from a flat to upright position can result in postural hypotension.

Home care

An estimated >10% of the elderly population are bedridden or housebound to such a degree that they cannot visit their PCP or general dentist. Unfortunately, although the dental needs of this group are high, the uptake of dental care is low, from the low priority placed on such care and the difficulty experienced in obtaining it. In some communities, dentists are available who have the equipment to provide home care with portable dental units, or mobile dental offices. Check with the local dental association to determine if these services are available in your community.

- *Site* The kitchen is probably the most suitable room, with access to water and heat. However, it is wise to defer to the patient should they prefer another location for the improvised surgery. Care must be taken to protect the floor and work surfaces from any spills.
- *Seating* Where possible the patient should be seated in their wheelchair, or a straight-backed chair placed against a wall with a cushion for additional head support. When a patient is bedridden there is no choice, but the dentist(s) should take frequent rests from bending over, to prevent back strain.
- *Equipment* The expenditure on this will be determined by the volume of such work undertaken. Portable dental units are available, but costly. However, the outlay could be shared by several practices. A wheeled suitcase or fishing-tackle box is useful for transport of equipment.
- *Aftercare* This is particularly important. It is the dentist's responsibility to ensure that the relatives or caregivers appreciate the need for good oral and denture care and how to carry it out. In the homebound, chlorhexidine can be applied to the teeth by cotton swabs.

▶ Take a dental assistant along with you.

Key points

- Can treatment be provided successfully?
- Consider maintenance required by any proposed treatment. Failure of elaborate procedures may leave the patient worse off.
- The objective is to maintain optimum oral function. Sometimes retention of a few teeth can be a disadvantage.
- Medical crises (e.g., a period in hospital) can result in a very rapid change in a previously stable oral state, e.g., rapid caries, loss of denture-wearing skill through lack of use.
- Avoid sudden changes in occlusion. During restorative work refrain from introducing significant occlusal change. When extractions are necessary, it may be prudent to do so a few at a time, with additions to existing partial dentures.

Some clinical techniques of particular value in elderly

- Adhesive restorations, e.g., GI for root caries.
- Adhesive bridgework is less destructive to abutments and is ∴ more fail-safe.
- Gradual tooth loss, with additions to existing P/Ps, is less demanding of a ↓ adaptive capacity.
- Replacement dentures should be made with careful regard to existing appliances. Use of copying techniques again ↓ amount of adaptation required.
- If recording the occlusion proves difficult, use monoplane teeth.
- Mark dentures with the patient's name.

Oral and maxillofacial surgery

In general, maxillofacial surgery is a postgraduate subject that has evolved from oral surgery, with foundations in medicine, dentistry, and surgery. It is included here as an introduction to students, an *aide-mémoire* for junior hospital staff, and a guide for those who will be referring patients.

Principal sources: L. Peterson *et al.* 2003 *Contemporay Oral and Maxillofacial Surgery* 4th ed., Mosby. G. Dimitroulis 1997 A Synopsis of Minor Oral Surgery, Wright. K. Riden 1998 Key Topics in Oral and Maxillofacial Surgery, Bios. D. Mitchell 2006 An Introduction to Oral and Maxillofacial Surgery, OUP. J. Pedlar and J. Frame 2001 Oral and Maxillofacial Surgery: An Objective Based Textbook, Churchill Livingstone. J. Watkinson 2000 Head and Neck Surgery, Butterworth-Heinemann. ACS 1997 ATLS Core Course Manual. M. Yaremchuk 1992 Rigid Fixation of the Craniomaxillo-facial Skeleton, Butterworth-Heinemann. J. Shah 2003 Oral Cancer, Dunitz. R. Cawson 1997 Pathology and Surgery of the Salivary Glands, Isis Medical Media. Personal experience.

Additional background: Pathology: J. V. Soames and J. C. Southam 1999 Oral Pathology, 3rd ed., OUP. *Third molars:* NICE 2000 Guidance on Removal of Wisdom Teeth. A. J. MacGregor 1985 The Impacted Lower Wisdom Tooth, OUP. P. H. Kwon and D. M. Laskin 1997 Clinicians' Manual of Oral and Maxillofacial Surgery, 2nd ed., Quintessence.

Principles of surgery of the mouth

The mouth is a remarkably forgiving environment in which to operate, because of its excellent blood supply and the properties of saliva. It is compromised less than could be expected by its teeming hordes of commensal organisms. This does not, however, constitute *carte blanche* for ignoring the basic principles of surgery, although these can and should be modified to suit the nature and the site of the surgery.

Asepsis and antisepsis See p. 350.

Analgesia All patients should expect and receive painless surgery, both perioperatively and postoperatively. For analgesia and anesthesia, see Chapter 12.

Anatomy and pathology are the interdependent building blocks of surgery. Know the anatomy and you can understand or even devise the operation. Know the pathology and you know why you are doing it, what can be sacrificed, and what must be preserved.

Access For all minor and certain major oral surgical procedures, access is through the mouth via intraoral incisions. For extraoral surgery, see Chapter 8.

Incisions for dentoalveolar surgery are full thickness, i.e., mucoperiosteal flaps; for mucosal and periodontal surgery split-thickness flaps are raised (pp. 204 and 212). For mucoperiosteal flaps, although the base does not have to be longer than its length, this design improves the blood supply to the flap and should be used where this is a concern. Improved access via a large flap, allowing minimally traumatic surgery, virtually always outweighs the trauma of additional periosteal stripping.

Always plan the incision mindful of local structures. *One cut*, at right angles, through mucoperiosteum to bone, is the aim. Do not split interdental papillae. Try to cut in the depth of the gingival sulcus. Raise the flap cleanly, working subperiosteally with a blunt instrument, moving from easily elevated areas to the more difficult ones (p. 352).

Retraction of the raised flap should be gentle and precise. It is the assistant's duty to prevent trauma to the tissues by sharp edges and overheated drills.

Bone removal by drills must be accompanied by sterile irrigation to prevent heat necrosis of bone, damage to soft tissues, and clogging of the bur. When using chisels to remove bone remember the natural lines of cleavage of the jaws and make stop cuts (chisel technique, p. 364).

Removal of the tooth or root is carried out using controlled force.

Debridement is removal from the wound of debris generated by both the pathology and the operation. It is as important as any other part of the operation. Subperiosteal bone dust is a common cause of pain and delayed wound healing.

Hemostasis and wound closure are covered on p. 356.

Postoperative edema is, to some degree, inevitable; it is minimized by gentle, efficient surgery, which is more important than such measures as ice packs and peri- or postoperative steroids, although these can help.

Asepsis and antisepsis

Asepsis is the avoidance of pathogenic microorganisms. In practical terms, *aseptic technique* is one that aims to exclude all microorganisms. Surgical technique is aseptic in the use of sterile instruments, clothing, and the "no-touch" technique.

Antisepsis is an agent or the application of an agent that inhibits the growth of microorganisms while in contact with them. Scrubbing up and preparation of operative sites are examples of antisepsis.

Disinfection is the inhibition or destruction of pathogens, whereas *sterilization* is the destruction or removal of *all* forms of life. Prepackaged sterile supplies and the use of an autoclave (121°C for 15 min or 134°C for 3 min) for sterilizable equipment are the only really acceptable techniques in dentistry. Disinfection with gluteraldehyde or hypochlorite are second choices, for use where true sterilization is not feasible. There are strict restrictions on the use of gluteraldehyde that limit its usefulness outside hospitals. It is not possible to render the mouth aseptic and it is fruitless to try; there are, however, three basic techniques of value:

Avoid introducing infection This is achieved by **always** using *sterilized* instruments, and wearing gloves.

Avoid being infected yourself by the operative site Wear gloves, masks, and eye protection.

Reduce the contaminating load to the site by pre-extraction cleaning of teeth, use of chlorhexidine mouth rinse, and prophylactic antimicrobials, when appropriate.

Cross-infection and its control

Much attention has been focused on this problem in recent years, first with hepatitis B and its related agents, then with HIV, and now with prions. Although screening is possible in some instances, this is of little real value, since most individuals with communicable viral particles *are asymptomatic* and hence not identifiable. Therefore, safe practice mandates the use of sound infection control procedures as part of everyday practice on *all* patients.

Aerosols are easily created and are a potential source of cross-infection. Minimize wherever possible by high-vacuum suction. Wear glasses and a mask if exposure to an aerosol cannot be avoided. Masks are routine in the operating theater, although they are of unproven value in preventing wound infection.

Cleaning and sterilizing Use disposable equipment when possible and **never** reuse. Clean instruments prior to sterilization. Use disposable or easily disinfected work surfaces. This book cover can be wiped down!

Gloves should be worn routinely, and sterile gloves for surgery.

Immunization against hepatitis B is available. Get it and get all staff with clinical contact to do likewise.

Waste disposal It is everyone's responsibility to ensure that sharps are carefully placed in rigid, well-marked containers and disposed of by an appropriate service. For dealing with potentially contaminated impressions and appliances, see p. 614. For treatment of the known high-risk patient.

Needlestick injuries If this happens to you, rinse wound under running water and record date and patient details. In the hospital and dental school or institutional setting, follow the institutional policy; in practice, you should have a hazard communication plan in place. Universal source testing for hepatitis B and C and for HIV is recommended.

Forceps, elevators, and other instruments

Extraction forceps come in numerous shapes and sizes. The choice of forcep comes largely down to individual preference or, more frequently, availability. "Universal" forceps are straight-bladed upper or lower forceps used to grip the roots of teeth to allow a controlled extracting force. "Eagle beak" forceps are upper and lower molar forceps that engage the bifurcation of molar teeth, allowing a buccally directed extraction force. "Cowhorns" are designed to penetrate the molar bifurcation either to be used in a figure-eight loosening pattern or to split the roots. Most forceps come with a deciduous tooth equivalent.

Elevators are used to dilate sockets to facilitate extraction or to remove dental hard tissue by themselves. These are the instruments that should **always** be used to remove impacted teeth. They should be used with gentle (finger pressure) forces. The commonly used patterns are Couplands No. 1, 2, and 3, Cryers right and left, and Warwick–James right, left, and straight.

Scalpel A Bard–Parker handle with a No. 15 blade is most common.

Periosteal elevators A number of these are available.

Retractors Tongue, cheek, and flap retractors are needed and are legion in number; Dyson's tongue retractor, Kilner's cheek retractor, Bowdler–Henry's rake retractor, and the Minnesota flap retractor are favorites. Lack's is an all-purpose retractor (really a bent bit of metal)!

Chisels versus burs The choice depends on your training. Generally, burs (No. 8 round T-C for bone removal, medium-taper fissure T-C for tooth division) are kinder on the conscious patient and the best bet for the inexperienced. Chisels are more appropriate in the operating theater and are particularly useful (3 mm and 5 mm T-C tipped) for distoangular third molars and upper third molars.

Curettes The Mitchells trimmer is probably one of the most valuable instruments in this category.

Needle holders and sutures vary more than any of the above, depending on your location. The usual suture size for intraoral work is 4/0; the material may be nonresorbable (silk) or resorbable (Dexon®, Vicryl®). It is difficult to justify the continued use of any nonresorbable intraoral suture for routine use.

Scissors Remember to keep dissecting scissors, separate from suture-cutting scissors, and keep both sets sharp.

Dissecting forceps are designed to hold soft tissue without damaging it; Gillies dissectors are popular. College pliers are *not* dissecting forceps and are used to lift up sutures prior to removing them.

Aspirator Use a sterile and disposable suction tip small enough to get into the defect.

Extraction of teeth

The extraction of teeth must be viewed as a minor surgical procedure, ∴ the medical history will be pertinent, e.g., bleeding diathesis, at risk for bacteremia, etc. More common and specific considerations are the gender, age, and build of the patient. Extractions in children are technically simple; it is the child who is most likely to be a problem, whereas stoical old men who may not bat an eye at the procedure often have teeth aptly described as "glass in concrete." Malpositioned teeth present problems of access and isolated teeth, especially upper second molars, tend to be ankylosed. Heavily restored and root-filled teeth tend to be very brittle. In all these cases a pre-extraction X-ray can help.

Extraction of teeth begins with *positioning* After LA has taken effect, the patient is positioned supine at the height of the operator's elbow for upper teeth, and sitting with the operator behind for (right-handed dentists) lower extractions on the right and in front for lower extractions on the left. The position is reversed for left-handers, although unfortunately the world seems biased against this group, as many dental chair systems seem to preclude comfortable positioning for them.

Common technique The socket is dilated either using an elevator between the bone of the socket wall and the tooth or by driving the forceps blades into the socket. The blades of the forceps are applied to the buccal and palatal/lingual aspects of the tooth and pushed either along the root of the tooth or, in certain molar extractions, into the bifurcation. The tooth is then gripped in the forceps and, maintaining a consistent and quite substantial vertical force, the tooth is moved depending on its anatomy:

Mandibular incisors and canines have conical roots—rotate, then pull.

Mandibular premolars have either two fine roots or a flattened root—move buccopalatally until you feel them "give," then pull down and buccally.

Mandibular molars have three large divergent roots—these are moved buccally while maintaining upward pressure, but frequently need a variety of rocking movements before they are sufficiently disengaged to complete extraction.

Maxillary incisors and canines can usually be removed with a simple buccal movement, but sometimes need to be rocked or even rotated.

Maxillary premolars are rotated and lifted out.

Maxillary molars are two-rooted and can usually be removed by a controlled buccal movement. Remember to support the patient's jaw.

Deciduous teeth are extracted using the same principles, but while permanent molars can be removed with forceps that engage the bifurcation, these should not be used on deciduous teeth.

Third molars (p. 362)

As with all operative techniques in dentistry, the doing is worth a thousand words. To become competent there are three golden rules: practice, practice, and practice.

Complications of extracting teeth

Access Small mouths present an obvious but usually manageable problem. Crowded or malpositioned teeth may need transalveolar approach. Trismus, if due to infection, e.g., submasseteric abscess, should be managed in a hospital where facilities for external drainage and airway protection are available.

Pain Has the LA worked? Try further LA as regional block, infiltration, or intraligamentary injection. Is it pain or pressure? If pressure, reassure the patient and proceed. If it is pain, and other signs of adequate LA are present, then acute infection is the most likely culprit. Can the extraction wait by using delaying tactics such as draining an abscess? The vast majority can, and very few adult extractions really justify a GA.

Inability to move the tooth Don't worry; it happens to all of us. Do you have an X-ray? If not, get one and look for bulbous or diverging roots, very long roots, ankylosis, or sclerotic bone. Do not press on regardless; it will work sometimes, but shows lack of consideration and will cost you in time and goodwill in the long run. Most "solid" teeth have an easily identifiable cause, e.g., diverging roots, and raising a flap and using a transalveolar procedure (p. 358) will quickly and easily remedy this.

Breaking the tooth is a common occurrence and may even assist extraction if, e.g., the roots of a molar are separated. More often, unfortunately, the crown #, leaving a portion of root(s) in situ. It is quite acceptable to leave small (<3 mm) pieces of deeply buried apex, but provide antibiotics, tell the patient, and review. Larger pieces of root must be removed as they have a high incidence of infective sequela (p. 372).

# of alveolar and/or basal bone Breaking the alveolar bone is relatively common. If # only involves the alveolus containing the extracted tooth, remove any pieces of bone not attached to periosteum and close the wound. Rarely, the alveolus carrying other teeth will be involved, in which case remove tooth by a transalveolar procedure and splint remaining teeth (p. 109). Basal bone # is rare; ensure analgesia (LA and/or systemic analgesics) and arrange reduction and fixation (p. 406).

Loss of the tooth Stop and look; in the mouth, is it under the mucoperiosteum or in a tissue space: these can usually be milked out. Look in the suction apparatus. Is it in the antrum (p. 384) or even the inferior alveolar nerve (IFA) canal? Has it been swallowed or inhaled? Chest X-ray is mandatory if not found (see plate 4).

Damage to other teeth or tissues and extraction of the wrong tooth Prevent by confirming with the patient the teeth to be removed and making careful notes. Plan the operation; do not use inappropriate instruments or ones you don't know how to use. If the wrong tooth is extracted, replant if feasible and proceed to remove the correct tooth. Tell the patient and make careful notes.

Dislocated jaw Reduce (p. 410); bleeding (p. 355); pain, swelling, and trismus are common sequela and are discussed on p. 364.

Postoperative bleeding

Bleeding disorders are covered on p. 476.

Principles of management of postoperative bleeding

- Support the patient. If hypotensive and tachycardic, establish IV access and replace lost blood volume.
- Diagnose each cause, nature, and site of blood loss.
- Control the bleeding point.

Classically, postoperative bleeding is described as immediate (primary), reactionary, and secondary.

Immediate postoperative bleeding occurs when true hemostasis has not been achieved at completion of surgery.

Reactionary bleeding occurs within 48 h of surgery and is due to both general and local rise in BP, opening up small divided vessels that were not bleeding at completion of surgery.

Secondary bleeding occurs ~7 days postoperatively and is usually due to infection destroying the clot or ulcerating local vessels. In practice, bleeding following removal of teeth is common and usually simple to diagnose. Patients are seldom shocked or hypotensive but are often very anxious and nauseated by the taste, smell, and sight of blood and by blood in the stomach, which is irritant. Bleeding usually comes from one or all of three sources: **1** gingival capillaries, **2** vessels in the bone of the socket, and **3** a large vessel under a flap or in bone, such as the inferior alveolar artery. The first two are by far the more common sources.

Management

Reassure the patient that they won't bleed to death. Remove accompanying entourage and get the patient to an area with reasonable facilities. Take a drug history (anticoagulants?). *Wear gloves and gown*: patients often vomit. (If patient has to wait to be seen they should bite firmly on a clean gauze, rolled to fit the area the bleeding seems to be coming from.) In good light, with suction, clean the patient's face and mouth, remove any lumps of clot, and identify the source of bleeding. Is it from under a flap? If from a socket, squeeze the gingiva to the outer walls of the socket between finger and thumb; if bleeding stops it is from a gingival vessel. In these cases, LA and suturing are needed. If bleeding continues it is from vessels in bone, which need some form of pack.

Technique

Give LA if needed, and have assistance with suction. If a flap is involved remove old sutures, evacuate clot, identify bleeding point, and place a tight suture around it. Bleeding should be significantly reduced; if not, repeat until it is, then close wound and have the patient bite on gauze for at least 15 min. If it is a gingival bleed a tight interrupted or mattress suture will compress the capillaries, followed again by gauze to bite on. If bleeding is from the depths of the socket, the clot may need to be removed and replaced by a pack or supported by a resorbable mesh. If removing clot and packing the socket, remember this will delay healing and predispose to infection, so use iodoform paste. If all else fails, all the above measures plus a pressure pack, analgesia, a sedative antiemetic, and a night in a hospital bed will do the trick. Patients requiring this degree of treatment should be investigated hematologically and for liver disease.

Suturing

Every dentist should master the basic skills of suturing.

Materials Most sutures are suture material fused to a needle, although threaded reusable needles are used in some countries. Needles may be round bodied, cutting or reverse cutting, straight, curved, or J-shaped. Almost all intraoral work is done with a 16–22 mm curved cutting or reverse-cutting needle held in a needle holder. Suture material may be resorbable (Dexon®, Vicryl®, or Monocryl®) or nonresorbable (silk, nylon, or prolene). Monofilament suture (e.g., nylon) causes less tissue response than braided (e.g., silk).

Skin is best closed with nylon, prolene, or Novafil®. *Mucosa* and *deep tissues* are best closed with resorbable material. *Vessels* are tied off using resorbables, except major veins and arteries, which are transfixed and tied with silk. Black silk suture (BSS) can be used for skin but must be removed *early*. Suture strength is described as 0 (thickest) to 4/0 (most common in intraoral use) to 11/0 (thinnest for microvascular work).
Types of stitch are shown in the diagram.

Suture technique Closure of a wound or incision should, whenever possible, be without tension, by closing deep layers and over supporting tissue. Hold the needle in the needle holder ~2/3 of the way from its tip. Suture from free to fixed tissue taking a bite of 2–3 mm on both sides. Leave the sutured wound edges slightly everted in apposition. Except when swaging tissue to bone, e.g., when arresting hemorrhage or when tying vessels, do not overtighten the suture as wound margins become swollen, and you need to allow for this.

Knot tying The two most useful are the square (reef) knot and the surgeon's knot (see diagram).

Instrument tying is easy to learn from a book but needs considerable practice to perfect. The knot is started by passing the suture once (square knot) or twice (surgeon's knot) around the tip of the needle holders; the knot is tightened and then locked by passing the suture around the needle holder in the opposite direction once. It is possible to control the suture tension by completing the knot in three loops instead of two.

Hand tying is invaluable for those wishing to develop surgical expertise or be involved in major maxillofacial surgery. It takes a substantial amount of time and practice and is impossible to learn from a book. Get a sympathetic senior to demonstrate.

Suture removal is not someone else's job to be casually forgotten about. Do the stitches need to be removed? In inaccessible sites, difficult patients, or areas in which scar quality is less important, a resorbable suture should be used. An alternative is a tissue glue. Facial skin sutures should be removed at 3–5 days. When removing sutures use sharp scissors (avoid "stitch cutters" if you can), lifting up and cutting a bit of suture that has been in the tissue, thus avoiding dragging bacteria through the incision on removal.

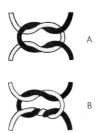

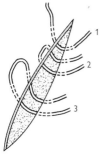

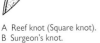

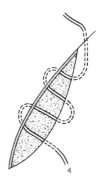

A Reef knot (Square knot).
B Surgeon's knot.

1 Simple interrupted suture.
2 Horizontal mattress suture.
3 Vertical mattress suture.
4 Continuous subcuticular suture.

Dentoalveolar surgery: removal of roots

Does the root need to be removed? If it is large, being extracted for pulpal or apical pathology, symptomatic, an impediment to denture construction, or in a patient in whom risk of minor local infection is not tolerable (e.g., immunocompromised or at risk from infective endocarditis [IE]), then the answer is yes.

Nonsurgical methods The use of root forceps or elevators may allow simple removal of roots close to the alveolar margin. When using root forceps ensure the root can be seen to be engaged by the blades. Elevators can be used to direct a root along its path of withdrawal providing (a) one exists and (b) an elevator can be introduced between bone and root. Do not waste time persisting with nonsurgical methods if your initial attempt is unsuccessful.

Surgical methods Plan your operation. Do you know why the root cannot be delivered, exactly where it is, and about any adjacent structures? If not, get an X-ray.

- The flap: if endentulous incise along the crest of the ridge; if dentate, in the gingival margin. Flaps may be envelope, two sided, or three sided. Relieving incisions make reflection of the flap easier but must be avoided in the region of the mental nerve ($\overline{45}$) and are better avoided around the buccal branch of the facial artery (mesial root $\overline{7}$). Include an interdental papilla at either side of the flap and start vertical cuts 2/3 of the way distal to the included papilla. Big flaps heal as well as small ones; the important consideration is access.
- Identify obstructions to the path of withdrawal of the root; these are either removed or the root is sectioned to create another path of withdrawal, depending on which approach is the least traumatic.
- Remove the minimum amount of buccal bone compatible with exposing the maximum diameter of the root and a point of application for an elevator (No. 8 round T-C surgical bur).
- Elevate by placing an elevator between bone and tooth (remember to apply to the convex surface of curved roots) and direct the root along its natural path of withdrawal.
- Finally, debride and close the wound.

Special cases

- Small apical fragments: use an apicoectomy approach.
- Multirooted teeth: always divide the roots, as this makes life much easier.
- Cannot find the root: re-X-ray and look in the soft tissues. The root may have been displaced into another cavity or even be in the aspirator; look carefully, but remember discretion is the better part of valor. Tell the patient.
- Patient refuses operation: it's their body; record your advice and their decision.

Under GA Mallet and chisel can replace bur and the "broken-instrument" technique can be used. This involves using a straight instrument or elevator guided through the bone with the mallet, and either then being used as an elevator or being placed in contact with the tooth or fragment, which is delivered by a sharp blow. Use with care.

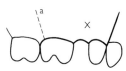

Outline of two-sided flap in heavy shade.
X Retained root or similar.
a Line of additional incision to convert to three-sided flap.

Dentoalveolar surgery: removal of unerupted teeth

The teeth most commonly requiring removal, other than third molars, are maxillary canines and premolars, supernumaries, and mandibular canines and premolars. Rarely, permanent or deciduous molars may be impacted or submerged.

Maxillary canines (pp. 143, 144) The canine may lie within or across the arch, buccally, or, most frequently, palatally. Assessment requires a careful examination, palpation, and X-rays (either two films at 90° or the parallax technique, p. 144).

Techniques Buccal impactions are approached via a buccal flap, palatal ones via a palatal flap, and cross- or within-arch impactions need a combination of the two. Buccal flaps are as previously described. Palatal flaps involve the reflection of the full thickness of the mucoperiosteum of the anterior hard palate, the incision running in the gingival crevice from 6 to 6 for bilateral canines or to the contralateral canine region for single impactions. The neurovascular bundle emerging from the incisive foramen is often sacrificed, with no noticeable morbidity. **Never** incise the palate at 90° to the gingival crevice and **always** use an envelope flap, otherwise you will section the palatine artery. Remove bone over the bulge of the crown of the tooth until the maximum bulbosity of the crown and the incisal tip are exposed. If the root curvature and path of withdrawal are favorable, the entire tooth can be elevated out. If not, section at the cervical margin with a tapered fissure bur and winkle the pieces out separately. Debride the socket and close with vertical mattress sutures to minimize hematoma formation.

Mandibular canines Most lie buccally, and can be elevated or removed with root forceps. Unerupted, deeply impacted buccal or lingual canines rarely need to be removed. If necessary, a degloving incision provides good access.

Maxillary premolars Most lie palatally. If partially erupted and conically rooted, they are simply elevated. Otherwise, a similar approach to that used for palatal canines is used. Premolars within the arch are approached buccally, sectioned, and removed piecemeal.

Mandibular premolars are often angled lingually. The "broken-instrument" technique can be invaluable. Otherwise, an extended buccal flap is raised to visualize and protect the mental nerve, buccal bone is removed, and the tooth sectioned at its cervical margin. The crown is then displaced downward into the space created and the root elevated upward.

Submerged deciduous molars If must be removed, they are approached buccally and sectioned vertically, then elevated along the individual root's path of withdrawal.

Supernumeraries (p. 66) These are removed with the approach used for the tooth they impede or replace. This can be a surprisingly difficult operation, usually because of difficulty in finding and identifying the supernumary.

Dentoalveolar surgery: removal of third molars

Not all wisdom teeth need to be removed.[1] Those that have space to erupt into functional occlusion should be left to do so, and those that are deeply impacted and asymptomatic are best left alone. Decisions about surgery vary widely.[2]

Etiology As the last tooth to erupt, the third molar is most liable to be prevented from doing so in a crowded mouth. *Causes*: soft Western diet not creating space by contact point abrasion, inherited tooth–jaw size incompatibility, and possibly an evolutionary tendency toward decreased jaw size.

Symptoms Pain, swelling, pericoronitis (p. 372), and sometimes a foul taste. These are mostly due to localized infection, less commonly to caries or resorption of second molar or cyst associated with third molar. Third molars covered by bone are very unlikely to become infected, whereas those where the crown has breached mucosa will almost inevitably do so. Infections in older, less vascular bone are more difficult to treat.

Indications for removal Recurrent pericoronitis, unrestorable caries in second or third molar, external or internal resorption, cystic change, periodontal disease distally in second molar. The prevention of lower labial segment (LLS) crowding on its own is **not** an indication, nor is vague TMJ pain.

Timing Symptoms are most common in the late teens and twenties; bone is soft, spongy, and elastic in this age group, so this is the usual and most favorable time to operate. Prophylactic removal of symptomless third molars is currently hard to justify.[3]

Choice of anesthetic Bilateral impacted third molars are more kindly treated under GA, as are those where surgery may be technically more difficult, e.g., distoangular third molars. LA and/or sedation is appropriate for most unilateral impactions not presenting particular difficulty. Consider the patient's medical history.

Assessment Look first: unerupted or partially erupted? Take a preoperative X-ray (DPT is ideal).

Assess angulation (vertical, mesioangular, distoangular, horizontal, or transverse); depth of impaction from the alveolar crest to the maximum diameter of the crown; degree of impaction (and against what); root shape; bone density; the relationship to the IFA canal; and the presence of any other pathology or complicating factors.

Plan the path of withdrawal. What impedes it? How much bone needs to be removed to provide a point of application for an elevator? How much to clear the path of withdrawal? Can this be done less traumatically by sectioning the tooth? In what direction?

---

1 NICE 2000 www.nice.org.uk
2 M. Brickley 1993 *BDJ* **175** 102.
3 University of York 1998 *Effectiveness Matters* **3**(2).

Warn the patient about pain, trismus, swelling, and the possibility of damage to the IFA and lingual nerves.

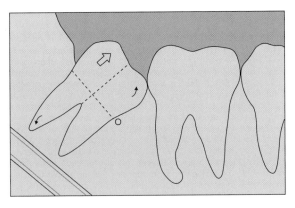

Diagram showing a schematic of planning for third molar removal.

Dentoalveolar surgery: third-molar technique

Technique

Mandible A buccal flap is incised along the external oblique ridge (lies well lateral to the arch) over the crest of the ridge if unerupted, or in the gingival margin if partially erupted. Extend to the distal aspect of the second molar and down into the buccal sulcus. Cut onto bone to create a full thickness flap. If there is a mesioangular or horizontal impaction, extend the incision around the lower second molar to the mesial border, but beware the buccal branch of the facial artery. Reflect and retract flap. There is now good evidence to suggest that manipulation from the lingual aspect results in unnecessary lingual nerve morbidity. Bone and tooth removal should be from a buccal approach. An attached mucosa distolingual flap for visibility that does not encroach on the lingual nerve is reasonable. Wide exposure and subperiosteal protection of the lingual nerve should be undertaken by those using the lingual split technique. Remove bone to provide a point of application for an elevator and clear obstruction to the path of withdrawal. This can be done with chisels or a bur. With a bur this is done by creating a distobuccal gutter, exposing the height of contour of the tooth. If needed, the bur can then be used to section the lower third molar to provide an unimpeded path of withdrawal.

With chisels, place mesial and distal stop cuts around the tooth and split off a collar of buccal and distal bone to expose the height of contour of the crown. This can then be extended into a lingual split, taking off a piece of lingual plate and allowing the tooth to be elevated lingually. Whichever technique is used, it is important to remember that if it is done properly, a minimum of directed force via an elevator will deliver the tooth or fragment out along its path of withdrawal. If this cannot be done, look carefully for another obstruction. Once the tooth is removed, debride the socket, remove the follicle, and close the wound with loose sutures to allow for swelling. Achieve hemostasis with pressure.

Maxilla A flap similar to that in the mandible can be used for inaccessible wisdom teeth but many can be approached using a "slash" incision (from distopalatally on the tuberosity to distobuccally at the second molar and into the buccal sulcus). Reflect and retract the flap. Bone removal can usually be effected by a hand-held chisel. The much softer bone rarely causes any problem with elevation, but care has to be taken to prevent displacement into the pterygoid space.

Postoperatively

Pain can be quite severe and responds best to nonsteroidal anti-inflammatory drugs (NSAIDs). Perioperative LA works well and leaves patients pain-free but numb for the duration. Trismus is due to pain and muscle spasm and can be ↓ by adequate analgesia (p. 526). It has obvious but often forgotten connotations for meals postoperatively. Swelling can also be ↓ by high-dose perioperative steroids. There is no evidence that ice-packs help, although they are often used. Hemorrhage can usually be controlled by biting on pressure packs. Rarely, it may be necessary to re-explore the wound. Antibiotic prophylaxis is probably beneficial.[1]

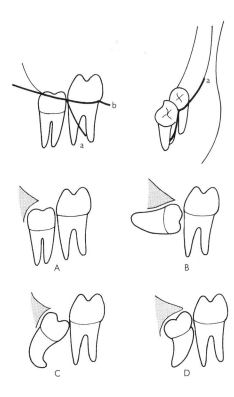

a Outline of incision for raising a third-molar buccal flap.
b Modification to create an envelope flap.
A Vertically impacted third molar.
B Horizontally impacted third molar.
C Mesioangular impaction of a third molar.
D Distoangular impaction of a third molar.
(Source: after Moore 1976.)

Dentoalveolar surgery: apicoectomy

There are three surgical aids to endodontics: apicoectomy, root hemisection, and removal of extruded endodontic paste.

Apicoectomy

This is by far the most common. It is a *second-line* treatment after failure of, or as a supplement to, orthograde endodontics (which has an 86–96% success rate in expert hands).[1]

Indications
- Impossible to prepare and fill apicial 1/3 of tooth, e.g., pulpal calcification, curved apex, open apex
- Irretrievable broken instrument in canal
- Post crown on tooth with apical pathology (only if post crown has sealed the coronal root and crown margin)
- Root perforation
- Fractured and infected apical 1/3
- Persistent infection due to apical cyst or other lesion requiring biopsy

Assessment Intraoral X-ray, best possible root filling in situ, free from acute infection, crown sealed with good-quality restoration.

Remember Nonsurgical retreatment: 72% success; apicoectomy and retrograde root filling (RRF): 60%, apicoectomy with no RRF: 51%.[1]

Technique This operation is best performed under LA. Ensure that an area of two tooth widths either side of the tooth being treated is anesthetized, and give palatal infiltration. In the mandible, give a block plus infiltration to aid hemostasis. If associated with infection, consider antibiotic prescription to begin preoperatively.

Flaps may be two or three sided, semilunar, or sublabial; the latter two avoid postoperative recession but give inferior access. Reflect and retract well above the apex (there is often a bulge or perforation of the cortical plate to aid location of the apex). A bony window is created to visualize the apex, which is often found sitting in a mass of granulation tissue. Excise the apical 1–2 mm and currette out the cystic and granulation tissue. Pack the cavity with bone wax or epinephrine-soaked ribbon gauze, identify the canal, and prepare it with a 1/2-round bur or ultrasonics (depending on availability). Seal with super-EBA (ethoxy benzoic acid), IRM, or MTA and debride. Close, using interrupted or vertical mattress sutures.

Surgical microscope Today the surgical microscope is supplanting the traditional surgical apicoectomy. The surgical microscopic technique minimizes the loss of tooth structure and allows visualization of accessory canals that may have been missed. It also allows precision fill of the root apex at the time of surgery.

---

1 N. P. Chandler *J R Coll Surg Edin* **47** 660.

Special points in apicoectomy

Warn patients about postoperative swelling. Lower incisors present an access problem eased but not erased by a degloving incision and experience. Think twice about the mental nerve in lower premolar apicectomies. Think hard about alternatives to apicoectomy of mandibular molars. Don't think at all about second or third molars. Remember the buccal and palatal roots in a mandibular first premolar; section the buccal root low to see the palatal. Apicoectomy of a mandibular molar is fine provided the palatal root can be treated by an orthograde approach and is hemisected, or you are happy to deal with breaching the antrum.

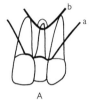 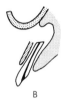

A An approach to apicoectomy.
   a Outline of incision for three-sided flap, with good access—best flap for the novice.
   b Outline of semilunar .flap incision.
B An approach to apicoectomy: a window is created in the buccal cortex to expose the apex, which is resected, leaving a smooth, raw, bony cavity.

Dentoalveolar surgery: other aids to endodontics

Root perforations are approached as for apicoectomy; however, multirooted tooth perforations, unrootfillable roots, or untreatable periodontal pockets may be dealt with using the aids described below.

Root hemisection This simply involves raising a flap around the tooth, identifying and horizontally sectioning the root, and atraumatically elevating it out. The wound is closed and a cleanable undersurface sealed with super-EBA, IRM, or MTA is left.

Endodontic implants have not received widespread acceptance. A sterile alloy implant passes through the prepared root canal into periapical bone, transfixing the tooth. Such implants have been superseded by single-tooth osseintegrated implants (p. 390).

Removal of extruded paste Usually, all that is required is an apicoectomy approach. However, careless use of "paste-only" techniques can result in paste in the floor of the nose, the antrum, or the IFA canal. The nasal floor can be approached sublabially or intranasally, the antrum by standard methods (p. 384), and the IFA canal by sagittally splitting the buccal cortex of the mandible.

Prognosis Single-rooted tooth apicoectomies should succeed 58–96% of the time. The range is due to an ill-defined definition of "success" and operator technique. Multirooted teeth, revision apicoectomy, and perforation repair have much lower success rates. The use of the surgical microscope may lead to an improved prognosis.

Dentoalveolar surgery: helping the orthodontist

Many minor oral surgical procedures, e.g., extraction of first premolars or removal of third molars, are carried out at the request of an orthodontist. Here we discuss the specific procedures of frenectomy, periodontal fiberectomy, tooth exposure, and tooth repositioning.

Frenectomy This is of value in closing a median diastema only if gentle traction on the upper lip and frenum produces blanching in a palatal insertion around the incisive papilla. It follows that the excision of the frenum must include those fibrous insertions, which leaves a raw area of alveolus after excision—this can be dressed with Surgicel, bismuth iodoform paraffin paste (BIPP), or a periodontal pack. It is a different operation from preprosthetic frenectomy and is performed for a different reason.

Periodontal fiberectomy is simply incising supra-alveolar periodontal fibers to prevent relapse when derotating teeth.

Tooth exposure Orthodontic traction is the treatment of choice for malpositioned, unerupted canines and incisors if the apices are in good position for eruption. The essential aspect of the operation is to remove any sacrificable impediments to tooth movement. Bonding an eyelet and gold chain or other bracket technique has a lower incidence of reoperation, but requires an orthodontist at the surgery.

Technique Palatal teeth are exposed by a palatal flap. Remove bone carefully with chisels, expose the greatest diameter of the crown and the tip. (Moving the tooth is counterproductive, ∴ don't do it.) Excise palatal mucoperiosteum generously, it grows back; bond a bracket if you're going to. Firmly pack the wound with, e.g., ribbon gauze, and secure, or use an acrylic dressing plate with periodontal paste, e.g., Coe-Pak. Close the remainder of the flap with vertical mattress sutures. Buccally located teeth are approached by a buccal flap, to preserve attached gingiva, and bonding should be done at operation. The flap can be repositioned coronally with the elastics or chain tunneling subgingivally. Teeth within the arch are approached buccally, removing crestal bone as needed.

Tooth repositioning (transplantation) Although there are claims of success rates as high as 93%, few people match this and most would transplant only when exposure and orthodontic movement were rejected. The most commonly transplanted tooth is the maxillary canine. It is essential to measure the available space and compare this with the erupted contralateral tooth or a good X-ray estimation, as it is not acceptable to grind down healthy teeth at operation to accommodate the retrieved tooth. If the tooth appears to be too big for the available space, then orthodontic Rx is required to create space. As this is often the reason the patient rejected exposure, an impasse is sometimes reached. This procedure has a poor long-term prognosis.

Technique The tooth is exposed by buccal or palatal flap, and once it is certain that it can be removed atraumatically, the deciduous tooth, if present, is extracted and a new socket surgically prepared with a bur. The tooth is reimplanted without force, the flaps sutured, and a close-fitting but **not** cemented splint placed. Functional splinting is continued for 7–10 days and the tooth root-filled as soon as possible after surgery. Regular follow-up is essential to allow early detection of root resorption, which is a common outcome.

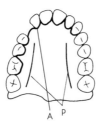

A Outline (heavy black line) of the incision for a palatal flap raised to expose a buried right maxillary canine.
P Position of the palatine arteries. Do not attempt a palatal "relieving" incision; exposure is achieved by the length of the envelope flap.
(Source: after Moore 1976.)

Dentofacial infections

▶ Infection associated with teeth is rarely, if ever, treated *definitively* by antibiotics and analgesics.

The vast majority of infections in this area requiring surgical treatment are bacterial, usually arising from necrotic pulps, periodontal pockets, or pericoronitis. They can be life threatening if allowed to progress, e.g., to the fascial spaces of the neck or the cavernous sinus, or as a focus for infective endocarditis (p. 477).

Microbiology Culture of dentofacial infections usually produces several commensal organisms, of which anaerobes are the most important. The predominant species *Bacteroides* (anaerobe) and streptococci (aerobe and anaerobe) are usually sensitive to the penicillins. Resistance is reported rarely. *Bacteroides* is nearly always sensitive to metronidazole. Remember the aerobic pathogens in established infection (don't just rely on metronidazole), and *Hemophilus* and staphylococci near the antrum (p. 384).

Diagnosis is usually simple and clinical, based on pain, swelling, temperature, and discharge.

Apical abscess Teeth with an apical abscess are TTP and non-vital. They may be discolored or crowned and have a history of trauma or RCT. Pain and TTP are often diminished when the intrabony pus tracks through the soft tissues and discharges, usually in the buccal sulcus (exceptions are maxillary lateral incisors and palatal roots of maxillary molars, which discharge palatally, and mandibular first premolars, which often discharge on the chin). Apical abscess may be associated periostitis with severe thickening.

Rx Drainage of pus either via the root canal, by incision of any fluctuant abscess, or by extraction under LA or GA. Palatal or buccal abscesses can be drained quite simply under LA by infiltrating a small amount of LA *between* the abscess cavity and the overlying mucosa, then incising the abscess. Explore using blunt closed forceps and keep patent either by excising an elipse of tissue or inserting and suturing a small rubber drain; this is particularly important in the palate. Cover the procedure with "best-guess" antibiotics such as amoxicillin 500 mg tid PO for 5–7 days, or metronidazole 400 mg tid PO for 5–7 days, or both.

Periodontal abscesses arise in a preexisting periodontal pocket (p. 190). Initial treatment involves incision and drainage, followed by elimination of the pocket, unless extraction is considered the only option.

Pericoronitis is inflammation and infection of a gum flap (operculum) overlying a partially erupted tooth, usually a mandibular third molar often traumatized by an overerupted third molar. Rx involves removal of the opposing maxillary third molar, irrigation under the operculum with saline or chlorhexidine, and antibiotics (see above) if necessary. Nearly all third molars associated with pericoronitis need removal.

Dry socket is osteitis of a socket following tooth removal. It is most common in the mandible after removal of molars, especially mandibular third molars. Predispo-sing factors are smoking, surgical trauma, LA, history, bone disease, oral contraceptives, or immunodeficiency.

Diagnosis Pain onset after (usually 2–4 days) extraction, similar in nature but worse than the preceding toothache. The socket looks inflamed and exposed bone is usually visible. Rx is to gently clean the socket by irrigation and dress the exposed bone with iodoform paste or gauze. Topical metronidazole is an alternative.[1] Chlorhexidine and/or warm salt mouthwashes may help. NSAIDs are the systemic analgesic of choice (p. 550). Prophylactic anaerobicidals such as metronidazole reduce the incidence of this condition.[2]

Actinomycosis (p. 176) Persistent low-grade infection, multiple sinuses. Rx: drainage and up to 6 weeks amoxicillin 500 mg tid. Doxycycline 100 mg od is an alternative.

Staphylococcal lymphadenitis is seen especially in children; small, occult skin or mucosal breach allows ingress. It may mimic a "slapped face" due to exotoxin. Drain and give flucloxacillin 125–500 mg qid (depending on age, p. 546).

Atypical mycobacteria Lymphadenitis with no obvious cause. Cold nodes, non-febrile patient. Drain or excise. Culture for up to 12 weeks. Do **not** start antituberculous therapy, as many atypical mycobacteria are resistant and side effects are common and significant. Clarithromycin is the most useful conventional antibiotic. Excision of nodes is definitive Rx.

1 L. Mitchell 1984 *BDJ* **156** 132.
2 J. Rood 1979 *Br J Oral Surg* **17** 62.

Biopsy

A *biopsy* is a sample of tissue taken from a patient for histopathological examination.

Types of biopsy Biopsies may be incisional or excisional. Examples of incisional biopsies are fine-needle aspirate (really cytology), punch biopsy, trephines, and "true-cut'" needle biopsy. The most common technique by far, however, is to excise an ellipse of tissue that includes a portion of the lesion and surrounding normal tissue. Excisional biopsy provides after-the-fact information on excised samples (reserve for lesions <0.5 mm).

What should be biopsied? Nearly everything that is worth excising is worth histological review, and so all excised specimens should be examined histopathologically. Any soft tissue lesion not amenable to accurate clinical Δ (by a reasonably trained eye) should be biopsied. All red lesions of oral mucosa and most white patches should be biopsied. If you think "should I biopsy this?" then do it; you will always get some unpleasant surprises.

Special considerations Frozen sections are biopsy specimens taken during major surgery, either when the extent of the procedure will depend on the histological Δ of the lesion or to verify clearance of excision. It is essential to contact the pathology lab before the patient goes to surgery to warn them. Advance warning is also necessary for certain special tests, e.g., immunohistochemistry.

How it is done Tell the patient you need a piece of tissue to help make the Δ. LA or GA. For simple incisional biopsy, stabilize the tissue to be sampled. Transfixing with a 3/0 BSS helps avoid crush artefact, and orientates the specimen. Cut an ellipse of tissue, including lesion and normal surrounding tissue, lift up and dissect out, then close primarily with sutures.

Biopsy and oral cancer Incisional biopsy carries a (theoretical) risk of shedding malignant cells into the circulation. The alternative is to subject a patient to mutilating surgery before definitive Δ. If you suspect an oral malignancy, refer before biopsy because most consultants have a preferred approach. This also allows integrated Δ and counseling.

Specimens are best laid out on paper. This allows orientation and decreases shrinkage artifact, which can be considerable. Usual preservative is 10% formalin; ask if you are not sure, as some specimens are needed fresh. Consider a specimen for culture as well (e.g., lymph node biopsy). Make a diagram of the specimen on the pathology form to accompany the clinical details. A photograph of the operative site can help.

▶ Tell the pathologist what you are thinking!

Cryosurgery

Cryosurgery is the therapeutic use of extreme cold.

Equipment The coolants (usually nitrous oxide or liquid nitrogen) act via a cryoprobe, a tubing system in which the coolant is not in direct contact with the tissues. The probe tip is applied to the lesion with an intervening layer of lubricant jelly; this gives rise to an "iceball," which is essential for success. Liquid nitrogen can also be directly sprayed onto lesions and, rarely, bone can be immersed into liquid nitrogen prior to reuse as a framework for grafting.

Mechanism Cell death and subsequent tissue necrosis by cellular disruption, dehydration, enzyme inhibition, and protein denaturation follow application of extreme cold. Indirect effects include vascular stasis and an immune response.[1] There is a curious lack of infection and scarring following cryosurgery.

Indications Some vascular malformations and hemangioma (not the same thing) respond very well. Areas of leukoplakia unsuitable for excision, and provided they have not already undergone malignant change, may respond. Occasionally, malignant change following cryosurgery of leukoplakia is reported, so some controversy surrounds the technique. Extensive hyperplastic lesions, e.g., palatal hyperplasisa under F/-, may respond. Viral warts respond in most instances and some advocate its use for mucoceles. Superficial basal cell carcinoma is frequently treated with cryosurgery, usually liquid nitrogen spray, although its use in more aggressive malignancy is controversial, as is its use following enucleation of keratocysts. Intractable facial pain is one of the more accepted uses, the freezing of peripheral nerves being followed by a period of analgesia that extends beyond the original postoperative numbness.

Technique
- Warn the patient about the procedure, postoperative edema (which can be severe), and a slough which forms over frozen sites. There is sometimes depigmentation of skin lesions.
- Use LA for larger lesions or if biopsy needed (LA may ↑ effectiveness of iceball).
- Select a probe tip suitable for the lesion; overlap ice zones if the lesion is large.
- Use KY jelly to improve contact between probe and tissues.
- Usual freeze–thaw cycles are ~1 min, repeated at least twice.
- Do not remove probe until defrosting has occurred.
- Do careful follow-up and check the histology of the lesion, except when using cryoanalgesia.

Simple analgesics and chlorhexidine mouthwash postop often help.

The treatment of frank malignancy by cryosurgery remains controversial, but freeze–thaw cycles used must be in excess of the usual (up to 3 min) and tissue temperatures monitored.

1 V.Popescu 1980 *J Maxiofac Surg* **8** 8.

Non-tumor soft tissue lumps in the mouth

Abscess (p. 372). Generalized gingival swelling and gingivitis (p. 182).

Brown "tumor" Not a tumor but a giant-cell lesion sometimes found in soft tissue but more commonly within bone (p. 378). It occurs 2° to hyperparathyroidism, although this is usually suggested after enucleation on finding giant cells in a fibrous stroma histologically. Check bone biochemistry (Ca^{2+}, $PO_4^{4+}\downarrow$, alkaline phosphatase $\uparrow$, PTH $\uparrow$). If hyperparathyroidism is confirmed and treated, these lesions regress.

Dermoid cyst A developmental cyst is most common at the lateral canthus of the eye, but is found next most often in the midline of the neck above mylohyoid, where it causes elevation of the tongue. Rx is complete but conservative excision.

Congenital epulis By definition present at birth; usually presents as a pedunculated nodule. Histology reveals large granular cells. Rx is complete but conservative excision.

Peripheral giant-cell granuloma (giant-cell epulis) Deep red gingival swelling, probably caused by chronic irritation. Histology reveals a vascular lesion with multinuclear giant cells. Rx is excision with stripping of periosteum and curettage of underlying bone.

Pregnancy epulis An $\uparrow$ inflammatory response to plaque during pregnancy causes a lesion indistinguishable from a pyogenic granuloma. Onset is usually in the 3rd month. Rx: none (other than OHI) if possible,, as it regresses after delivery. If very troublesome, do simple excision, but it may recur.

Pyogenic granuloma Red, fleshy swelling, often nodular, occurring as a response to recurrent trauma and nonspecific infection. Histology shows proliferation of vascular connective tissue, ∴ bleeds easily. Rx is excision, debride area, good OH.

Fibroepithelial polyp An overvigorous response to low-grade recurrent trauma. It may be cessile or pedunculated and range from small lumps to lesions covering the entire palate. Excise with base. Histology shows dense, collagenous, fibrous tissue lined by keratinized, stratified squamous epithelium.

Irritation (denture) hyperplasia A very common hyperplastic response to repeated trauma, e.g., following denture-induced ulceration. Classically, seen as rolls of tissue in the sulcus related to a denture flange. Histology is similar to fibroepithelial polyp. Rx: complete excision with temporary removal of dentures allows healing. Consider simple preprosthetic measures and replace F/F.

Mucoceles Usually mucous extravasation cysts, where saliva leaks from a traumatized duct and pools, creating a compressed connective tissue capsule. Rarely, they are mucous retention cysts. They mostly affect the lower lip—similar swellings in the upper lip are often minor salivary gland tumors (p. 418). Rx: excision with associated damaged glands and duct.

Ranula Mucoceles of the floor of the mouth, arising from the sublingual gland. They tend to recur if marsupialized. A plunging ranula crosses deep to mylohyoid and appears as a neck and floor of mouth swelling. Rx is excision of cyst and associated sublingual gland; submandibular gland may have to be excised if the duct is damaged.

Granulomata Lumps characterized by the histological finding of granulomata may be caused by Crohn's disease (p. 458) or its localized variant, orofacial granulomatosis, sarcoidosis (p. 447), or implanted foreign bodies such as amalgam.

Hemangioma Developmental lesion of blood vessels. Present at birth, they can grow with the child, remain static, or regress. Blanch on pressure. Do **not** biopsy, as 80% spontaneously regress. Rx for those that don't is laser or cryotherapy.

Lymphangioma Rarer developmental lesion, this time of lymphatics. May present as an enlarged tongue or lip. Rx is difficult; some can be beneficially excised.

Vascular malformations Developmental lesions of blood vessels that *do not* regress but grow with the patient. Characterized by rate of blood flow in lesion. Rx is interventional radiology and surgery.

Warts/squamous papillomata The main etiological factor is human papilloma virus (HPV). True warts are rare in the mouth and usually transmitted from skin warts. They are found in patients with sexually transmitted disease (STD) or AIDS, but most have no such link.

Papillomas are common in the mouth; they appear as multiply papillated pink or white asymptomatic lumps. Rx is excision biopsy (if on a stalk—ligate or diathermy base, as they contain a prominent vessel).

Non-tumor hard tissue lumps

Cysts (p. 380); benign tumors (p. 382); malignant tumors (p. 420).

Tori are bony exostoses found in both jaws. *Torus palatinus* is found in the center of the hard palate; *torus mandibularis* is on the lingual premolar/molar region of the mandible. Rx: reassurance that these developmental anomalies cause no harm (they are *not* part of the Gardener syndrome, p. 682). Rarely, excision for denture construction is indicated.

Giant cell granuloma (p. 377) This can present as an intrabony swelling or symptomless radiolucency. Carefully enucleate.

Brown "tumor" (p. 376) Again, this imitates the giant-cell granuloma; the difference lies in bone biochemistry.

Paget's disease of bone This is relatively common over the age of 55 and affects the skull, pelvis, and long bones, as well as the jaws. Although etiology is uncertain, both measles and respiratory syncytial virus have been implicated. The maxilla is more frequently affected than the mandible. Hypercementosis of roots makes extractions difficult in this group. There is a replacement of normal bone remodeling by a chaotic alternation of resorption and deposition, with resorption dominating in the early stages. Bone pain and cranial neuropathies can occur. X-rays show a "cotton wool" appearance. Biochemistry shows an ↑ alkaline phosphatase and urinary hydroxyproline. Avoid GA; use prophylactic antibiotics and plan extractions surgically. Diphosphonates and calcitonin are used in treatment.

Fibrous dysplasia Areas of bone are replaced by fibrous tissue. Onset is in childhood; the dysplasia ossifies and stabilizes with age. Jaw involvement usually presents as a painless hard swelling. Characteristic X-ray appearance is of "ground-glass" bone. Histology shows fibrous replacement of bone with osseous trabeculae that look like irregular Chinese characters. Rx is skeletal resculpting after stabilization of growth and/or orthognathic surgery/orthodontics.

Cherubism is hereditary, and presents at 2–4 yr. It is a bilateral variant of fibrous dysplasia. In addition to the histological pattern for fibrous dysplasia, there are also multinucleated giant cells. The natural history is not well understood; it may burn out or regress. Skeletal resculpting after cessation may be necessary.

Cysts of the jaws

Cysts are abnormal epithelium-lined cavities that often contain fluid but only contain pus if they become infected. Jaw cysts predominantly arise from odontogenic epithelium and grow by a means not fully understood but involving epithelial proliferation, bone resorption by prostaglandins, and variations in intracystic osmotic pressure.

Diagnosis

Many are detected as asymptomatic radiolucencies on X-ray; others present as painless swellings, almost always of the buccal cortex. Infected cysts present with pain, swelling, and discharge. Vitality test associated teeth. Take a DPT and a periapical film when possible to screen for size and coexisting pathology. Transillumination rarely helps, but aspiration is sometimes useful and can help distinguish some lesions. Rarely, cysts may present with a pathological #, especially of the mandible.

Treatment

- Enucleation with 1° closure is most common and generally the Rx of choice. It consists of removing the cyst lining from the bony walls of the cavity and repositioning the access flap. Any relevant dental pathology is treated at the same time, e.g., by apicoectomy.
- Enucleation with packing and delayed closure is used when badly infected cysts, particularly very large ones, are unsuitable for 1° closure. Pack with Whitehead's varnish or BIPP.
- Enucleation with 1° bone grafting is rarely useful.
- Marsupialization. This is the opening of the cyst to allow continuity with the oral mucosa; healing is slower than with enucleation and a cavity persists for some time. It is useful to allow tooth eruption through the cyst or where enucleation is C/I.

▶ Always submit cyst lining for histopathology.

Types of cysts

Many classifications exist, few are helpful.

Inflammatory dental cysts are very common and described as apical or lateral, depending on position in relation to tooth root, or residual if left behind after tooth extraction. Necrotic pulp is the stimulus, and the epithelium comes from cell rests of Malassez. Rx is enucleation plus endodontics or extraction.

Eruption cysts See p. 65.

Dentigerous cysts form around the crown of an unerupted permanent tooth and arise from reduced enamel epithelium. They may delay eruption. Rx is marsupialization or enucleation, depending on position.

Keratocysts are lined by parakeratinized epithelium derived from the remnants of the dental lamina and are thought to replace a missing tooth. They have a fluid filling with a protein content <4 g/dl. Aspiration of samples for biochemistry and cytology for parakeratinized squames can be helpful. It is important to identify these cysts, as outpouching walls and "daughter" or "satellite" cysts make them more liable to recur. Their multiloculated appearance on X-ray may confuse them with an ameloblastoma (p. 382). Rx is careful enucleation, and/or cryotherapy and/or Carnoy's solution, or aggressive curettage of the cavity. Rarely, excision is needed if recurrent.

Calcifying epithelial odontogenic cysts are rare and distinguished by areas of calcification and "ghost cells" on histology. Rx: enucleate.

Solitary bone cysts are usually an incidental finding on X-ray and devoid of a lining, but may contain straw-colored fluid. They probably arise following breakdown of an intraosseous hematoma, and are distinguished by a scalloped upper border on X-ray where the cyst pushes into cancellous bone between teeth but spares the lamina dura. Opening the cyst, gentle curettage, and closure heals these "cysts"; associated teeth need no Rx.

Aneurysmal bone cysts are expansile lesions full of vascular spongy bone. They present as a symptomless swelling, unless traumatized, when bleeding causes pain and rapid expansion. Small ones can be carefully enucleated, but larger aneurysmal bone cysts need excision and possible reconstruction since they will recur if incompletely excised.

Fissural cysts are not associated with dental epithelium but arise from embryonic junctional epithelium. They are rare and include incisive canal cysts, incisive papilla cysts, and nasolabial cysts. Rx is enucleation.

Benign tumors of the mouth

Nonodontogenic tumors

Epithelial

Squamous cell papilloma (p. 377) Resembles a white or pink cauliflower and is caused by HPV. Usually presents on the palate. Does not undergo malignant change. Excise.

Connective tissue

Fibroma Very rare. Benign fibrous tumor, usually pink and pedunculated. Excise with a narrow margin.

Lipoma Soft, smooth, slow-growing yellowish lump composed of fat cells. Enucleate or excise with narrow margin.

Osteoma Smooth, hard, benign neoplasm of bone. Usually unilateral and covered by normal oral mucosa. Not situated in the classical position of tori (p. 378). Associated with Gardener syndrome (p. 682).

Neurofibroma Rare tumor of the fibroblasts of a peripheral nerve. Usually affects the tongue; may be part of von Recklinghausen disease (p. 686). Can undergo sarcomatous change. Excise with a small margin.

Neurolemmoma (schwanomma) Tumor composed of Schwann cells (cells of the axonal sheath). Rx is excision; nerve fibers can sometimes be preserved due to eccentric tumor growth.

Granular cell myoblastoma Rare tumor of histiocyte origin, usually arising as a nodule on the tongue. Excise with a margin.

Ossifying fibroma May be neoplasm or developmental anomaly. It is a well-demarcated fibro-osseous lesion of the jaws. It presents as a painless, slow-growing swelling, expanding both buccal and lingual cortices. X-ray shows a radiolucent area, circumscribed by a radiopaque margin. Histology is similar to that of fibrous dysplasia. Enucleation or conservative excision is curative. A faster-growing but equally benign version occurs in children.

Odontogenic tumors

Many of these are (to some) fascinating rarities. Only the more important ones are discussed here.

Ameloblastoma One of the more common odontogenic tumors. Most common in men and Africans, and in the posterior mandible. There are three basic types: unicystic, polycystic, and peripheral. The unicystic type is the least aggressive; the polycystic and peripheral types show a tendency to invade surrounding tissue, whereas the unicystic type expands it. Metastases are very rare. Histologically, two types are seen: plexiform and follicular. Rx: the unicystic type can be enucleated provided a rim of enclosing bone is removed as well; the other types require excision with a margin.

Adenoameloblastoma Tends to occur in the anterior maxilla in females. Rx is conservative excision, as recurrence is not a problem.

Calcifying epithelial odontogenic tumor (Pindborg tumor) Characteristically, a radiolucency on X-ray with scattered radiopacities. Needs excision with a margin.

Myxoma Occurs in both hard and soft tissues. Those arising in the jaws are tumors of odontogenic mesenchyme. This is a tumor of young adults arising within bone and can invade the surrounding tissue extensively. Characteristically, it has a "soap bubble" appearance on X-ray. Histology reveals spindle cells in a mucoid stroma. These tumors need excision with a margin of surrounding normal bone.

Ameloblastic fibroma Rare; affects young adults and appears as a unilocular radiolucency on X-ray, causing painless expansion of the jaws. Enucleation is usually curative.

Odontomes Not true neoplasms, but malformations of dental hard tissues. Classically, they are classified as *compound* when they are multiple small "teeth" in a fibrous sac, and *complex* when they are a congealed, irregular mass of dental hard tissue. These are best regarded and treated as unerupted, malpositioned, or impacted teeth, and removed using standard dentoalveolar techniques when required (p. 360).

Disturbances in tooth formation can lead to isolated abnormalities of enamel, dentine, and cementum. Cementomas are worthy of mention bec-ause they create extreme difficulty in tooth removal. Dens in dente, p. 70.

The maxillary antrum

These are the largest of the four paired paranasal air sinuses, lying in each half of the maxilla between the alveolus inferiorly, nasal cavity medially, and orbits superiorly.

Antral pathology often mimics symptoms attributable to maxillary teeth. Δ is by exclusion of dental pathology, nasal discharge or stuffiness, tenderness over the cheeks, and pain worse on moving the head. Occipitomental X-rays (15° and 30°) may reveal antral opacity, fluid level, or # (p. 404). To define fluid level, repeat film with head tilted. Other X-rays: DPT for cysts and roots and CT scans for tumors, pansinusitis, and blow out #.

Extractions and the antrum The proximity of maxillary cheek teeth to the antral floor makes it easy for roots and even teeth to be displaced into the antrum. It also predisposes to # of the alveolar process during 6,7,8 extraction. Displaced roots can be retrieved either by an extended transalveolar approach similar to that for removing roots (useful when the roots are lying under the antral lining) or via a *Caldwell–Luc* approach.

Maxillary sinusitis

Acute sinusitis usually follows a viral upper respiratory tract infection (URTI), which has ↓ cilia activity, and is due to bacterial superinfection (usually mixed—anaerobes, haemophilus, staphylococci, and streptococci). Less commonly, it is due to a foreign body, e.g., roots, water. Poor drainage via the osteum exacerbates the situation. Δ is as above and confirmed by proof puncture if necessary. Rx: erythromycin 500 mg PO qid or doxycycline 100 mg PO od. Decongestants.

Chronic sinusitis may then develop, particularly if a foreign body or poor drainage is present. Mucosal lining hypertrophies and may form polyps. A postnasal discharge (drip) is often present. Rx is aimed at ventilation of the sinus. Foreign bodies, if present, should be removed via an incision in the canine fossa (above the premolars) and creation of a bony window into the antrum (Caldwell–Luc). Ventilation is provided by either intra-nasal antrostomy or (ideally) endoscopic enlargement of the osteum and/or drainage of anterior ethmoids, depending on cause (functional endoscopic sinus surgery [FESS], p. 393).

Oro-antral fistula

This is the creation of a pathological epithelium-lined tract between the mouth and maxillary sinus. It most often occurs following the extraction of isolated molar teeth when the fistula tends to persist. Post-extraction reflux of fluids into the nose or minor nosebleeds are a diagnostic pointer. Confirm by getting patient to attempt to blow out against a closed nose; there will be air bubbles through the fistula. Occasionally, there are antral mucosa prolapses through the socket. Rx: many small fistulae are asymptomatic and close spontaneously. Closure if Δ is made at time of extraction: close the socket by suture or buccal advancement flap, give antibiotics and decongestants as above, and advise not to blow nose. Closure if Δ is made >2 days after extraction: place on antibiotics, etc., for 2 weeks and review after 6 weeks. Many will have closed. If not, repair using one of the following methods.

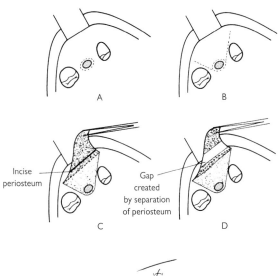

The buccal advancement flap (after Rehrmann).

Steps:

A Excise the fistulous tract; this is easiest with a No.11 blade.

B Outline (dashed line) incision for a full-thickness mucoperiosteal buccal flap.

C Reflect full-thickness mucoperiosteal flap and incise the periosteal layer ONLY.
 This makes it possible to mobilize the flap.

D "Stretch" the flap to assess the degree of elasticity once the restraining effect of
 the periosteum is lost.

E The flap is advanced across the fistula and sutured to palatal mucosa over bone.

- *Buccal advancement flap* Excise fistula to prepare a line of closure over bone and raise a broad-based buccal flap. Incise periosteum to allow mucosa to stretch over the socket and close, *over bone*, with vertical mattress sutures. Use antibiotics, etc., remove sutures at 10 days. Disadvantages: thin tissue may break down; reduces sulcus depth.
- *Palatal rotation flap* Excise fistula as above. Dissect a palatal mucoperiosteal flap based on palatine artery, rotate over socket, and suture in similar fashion. Disadvantages: bare bone is left to granulate; this is a difficult flap to rotate without distortion.
- *Buccal fat pad flap* If after raising the buccal advancement flap the periosteal incision is opened with artery forceps, the buccal fat pad is exposed. This can be easily mobilized as a pedicled flap to suture into and obtund the defect.

Sinus lift operation (p. 412).

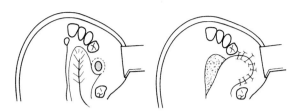

The palatal rotation flap (after Ashley).
A Excise fistula; outline palatal flap based on greater palatine artery.
B Mobilize and rotate palatal flap, suturing its leading edge to buccal mucosa
   over bone. Leave donor site to granulate under surgical dressing or pack.

Minor preprosthetic surgery

When teeth are extracted alveolar bone resorbs, ∴ you should aim to preserve alveolar bone whenever possible, by either not extracting teeth (overdentures, p. 336) or using a minimally traumatic technique.

At time of extraction of remaining teeth Extract carefully, compress the sockets, remove only small unattached pieces of bone, cover any exposed areas of bone with gingival flaps, and surgically remove roots *only* when necessary (infected, loose, >1/3 root length). Consider interseptal alveoloplasty if ridge is prominent and heavily undercut (e.g., Class II). This consists of creating a labial osteomucosal flap by dividing the septa and extending bone cut at the maxillary canine region through the buccal plate and collapsing-in the bone flap. Prominent frena should simply be excised. Attempts at decreasing the rate of ridge resorption have been made by leaving roots under mucosal flaps and by implanting hydroxyapatite or biocoral cones into extraction sockets.

Problems in denture wearers

▶ Only use surgery when denture faults and psychogenic disorders have been excluded. Screen jaws with PAN.

Retained roots and bone sequestra are removed using standard transalveolar technique, except in the maxilla, where buried canines may be removed using an osteoplastic flap (where bone is raised on a mucoperiosteal hinge).

Small bony irregularities can be smoothed with a bur but consider ridge augmentation if extensive.

Fibrous (flabby) ridges ↓ by raising a flap of attached gingiva to repair the defect, excise remaining soft tissue ridge, and repair with flap raised first. Fibrous tuberosities can be dealt with similarly.

Fibrous bands and irritation hyperplasia should be excised. Results are improved if palatal mucosal grafts are used to repair the defects and minimize scarring.

Tori can be reduced with a bur under a local flap, or resected with a combination of bur and chisel.

Muscle attachments to the mylohyoid ridge or genial tubercles can be displaced by resecting the bone from the mandible with a chisel and dissecting away the muscles. Genioglossus and geniohyoid should be reattached to the labial sulcus.

Ridge augmentation (p. 412) The use of subperiosteal injected porous hydroxyapatite as an outpatient procedure under LA is useful in a very limited number of cases, mainly because of ridge type. In this technique, a subperiosteal tunnel is raised along the crest of the ridge and filled with a hydroxyapatite/saline sludge. It is dependent on the shape of the ridge, and works best with concave ridges, not the more often seen feather-edge ridge. Problems include migration of particles after periosteal elevation.

Sulcus deepening (p. 412) When adequate vertical and horizontal basal bone exists but there is a shortage of ridge and/or attached gingiva, these procedures can help. Successful use depends on (a) dissecting away non-attached mucosa to leave a raw "new" sulcus; (b) lining this new sulcus with skin or mucosa; (c) *securing the new depth with a "surgical stent"*—a denture or base lined with tissue conditioner or impression compound, which is held in place by nylon sutures for 10–14 days, then replaced immediately by a new denture with a soft lining extended to the new sulcus and worn continually for the first 3 months.

Implantology

Dental implants are beginning to supplant the use of a fixed partial denture to replace a single tooth. They allow the replacement of teeth using available bone without having to treat adjacent teeth. This makes implants an attractive alternative to fixed partial dentures for patients who have few restorations or are adverse to connecting teeth to one another to replace missing teeth.

History Numerous procedures for dental implants have been described, including subperiosteal, endosseous, transosseous and submucosal. All have been strongly advocated by groups of enthusiasts. Genuine advances in the discipline have come about, thanks to a major contribution by Bränemark "osseointegration." All current implants are based on this now well-accepted concept.

Osseointegration is the direct aposition of bone to implant surface such that osteoblasts can be seen on electron micrographs to be growing on the implant surface. In addition, a tight fibrous/epithelial attachment above the crestal bone between gingiva and implant is essential. Finally, the implant must be designed to resist displacement and evenly dissipate occlusal loads.

Types of implant There is a large range. Materials are primarily titanium alloys with variations of surface treatment to increase surface area and improve initial integration of the implant. Bioceramic is less common. An implant may be inserted transmucosally or in two stages (see below). Attached mucoperiosteum is the "best" perimplant tissue.

Indications Edentulous patients unable to retain dentures, partially dentate for bridge abutments, single anterior tooth replacement, and maxillofacial prostheses after cancer surgery or trauma. If implants survive the first 2 yr there is a 98% success rate with dramatic improvement in all functional parameters.[1] Success for mandible > maxilla (bone quality). Irradiated bone may benefit from hyperbaric O_2 preoperatively.

Techniques A "team approach" requires joint planning between the dentist placing the implant and the restorative dentist for success. In the United States, it is common for an individual dentist to be trained in both the surgical and restorative aspects of implant placement. Excellent OH is mandatory. The surgical procedure is highly equipment dependent, and the surgeon needs to be trained in the particular technique used. Most commonly, this involves the following:

- Fixture installation. A gingival–mucosal flap is raised, and an osteotomy is prepared, using drills matched to the implant size and type. The fixture, depending on the type of implant, is either pressed or screwed into place. In two-stage procedures, the implant is covered by the flap at the end of the procedure. When placing multiple implants a direction indicator is helpful for achieving parallelism. Bone overheating must be avoided by constant irrigation.

1 R. Adell 1983 *J Prosthetic Dent* **49** 251.

In two-stage procedures, healing periods as short as 1.5 months in the mandible and 2 months in the maxilla are recommended. In one-stage procedures the implant heals partially exposed to the oral cavity for the same healing period.

- In two-stage procedures, abutment connection is then carried out by punch excision of mucosa overlying the implants, removal of cover screws, and insertion of the abutment. Prosthetic procedures start at abutment connection.
- Computer-aided design and computer-aided manufacturing (CAD/CAM) systems are now being used for implant placement and restoration on the same day, e.g., Nobelguide teeth-in-an-hour, Materialise SimPlant.
- *Craniofacial implants* (p. 425)
- *Transmandibular implants* (p. 412)

Lasers

Definition Light amplification by the stimulated emission of radiation. Light consists of packets of photons transmitted in electromagnetic waves (visible light 400–700 nm). Laser energy is produced by light stimulation of active media to generate collimated light energy at a specific frequency. The active media determines the characteristics of the laser.

Clinical lasers

These consist of two main groups, *hard* and *soft* lasers.

Hard lasers work principally by thermal effect, although certain benefits such as decreased scarring and pain are thought to be due to the photochemical effects of the laser beam.

Carbon dioxide laser A hard laser in common use in the hospital service. Its main role is as a cutting beam that seals small vessels as it cuts. It is also used to evaporate benign white patches of oral mucosa. Used as continuous wave or pulsed beam at 10–20 watts of energy.

KTP laser Similar to carbon dioxide laser, giving initially painless wounds. It becomes painful after 48–72 h, however.

Argon laser Produces a light beam that is selectively absorbed by hemoglobin and melanin, ∴ particularly useful for pigmented and vascular lesions.

Neodymium–yttrium aluminum garnet (Nd–Yag) laser Originally marketed as a hard laser with a relatively low-power output, it is now available as a soft dental laser.

Tuneable dye laser Expensive variable-frequency laser.

Soft lasers Thought to work by stabilizing cell membranes by a nonthermal photochemical process, increasing cellular metabolism by a minor thermal change, and possibly by inducing endorphin release.

Helium–neon The red-aiming beam on hard lasers, classroom pointers, and the "Terminator's" weaponry. Part of the soft laser group, it has no cutting effect but seems to act photochemically on cells.

Neodymium–Yag A system using this active media is now marketed for use in dentistry and is purported to ↑ cell turnover, ↓ inflammatory response, inhibit edema, ↑ rate of cell regeneration, e.g., peripheral neurons, and ↓ wound scarring. All this without any recognized side effects. Many of these claims have yet to be widely validated.

Summary

Lasers are available for a range of uses in dentistry; they are expensive and require special safety precautions. Some benefits can be achieved in other ways and some have yet to be proven. They are a tool, not a magic wand.

Minimally invasive surgery

While some specialties such as orthopedics and gynecology have been using endoscopic technology for many years, a recent surge in fiber-optic technology coupled with the "discovery" of the laparoscope by general surgeons made minimally invasive (minimal access) surgery one of the hot topics of the late 1990s.

One of the spin-offs of the sudden uncontrolled ↑ in the number of laparoscopic operations was bad publicity about some of the adverse outcomes following this type of surgery, and questions about surgeons' training. One very positive result of this has been the development of surgical skills laboratories, structured courses, and a real interest in training and education.

In the field of oral and maxillofacial surgery minimally invasive surgery has yet to make a significant impact. Current examples are described below.

Temporomandibular joint arthroscopy uses specialized small, rigid endoscopes with a fiber-optic light source that can be placed in the TMJ space (usually upper joint space) through a tiny incision in the preauricular skin. The joint is distended by a flow of sterile irrigant that exits via a needle placed about 1 cm anterior to the arthroscope. Reasonable visualization is possible but significant surgery is fairly limited.

Functional endoscopic sinus surgery (FESS) Rigid endoscopes with angled viewing ports allow visualization and a certain amount of surgery of the paranasal sinuses. Biopsy and sampling of a wide range of paranasal tissues are possible and may prove to be an ideal tool in the treatment for chronic sinusitis. This technique has been rapidly developed by many ENT specialists but indications for its use will take a few more years to become stabilized.

Endoscopically assisted internal fixation Internal fixation of facial # is now widely accepted and standard practice; however, some areas, particularly of the mandible, are very difficult to access safely. Condylar neck # and some angle # may be more easily treated using a modified trocar system and light source.

Endoscopically assisted face and brow lifting Aesthetic facial surgery by its very nature requires distant and minimalist scars. Endoscopic brow lifting from the anterior scalp is reasonably straightforward and popular in France and the United States. Long-term stability is awaited. Endoscopic facelifting makes a tedious operation more so.

Note: While flexible fiber-optic scopes play quite an extensive role in examination of the upper respiratory tract, the extent to which significant head and neck surgery can be performed is currently limited.

Advanced trauma life support (ATLS)

ATLS is a system providing one safe way of resuscitating a trauma victim. It was first conceived in Nebraska, subsequently developed by the American College of Surgeons (ACS), and has now reached international acceptance. It is not the only approach, but it is one that works. It is highly recommended.

Trauma deaths have a trimodal distribution. The first peak is within seconds to minutes of injury. The second is within the first hour, the "golden hour," and is the area of main concern. The third is days to weeks later but may reflect management within the golden hour.

The core concept behind ATLS is the *primary survey* with simultaneous resuscitation, followed by a *secondary survey* leading to definitive care.

Primary survey

This uses the mnemonic **ABCDE** on the basis of identifying and treating the most lethal injury first.

- *Airway with cervical spine control* Establish a patent airway and protect the cervical spine from further injury. Chin lift, jaw thrust, oral airway, nasopharyngeal airway, intubation, and surgical airway as needed, coupled with immobilization of cervical spine.
- *Breathing and ventilation* Inspect, palpate, and auscultate the chest. Count respiratory rate. Give 100% O_2. Perform chest decompression by needle puncture in 2nd intercostal space mid-clavicular line if indicated for tension pneumothorax. Use chest drain as indicated.
- *Circulation with hemorrhage control* Assess level of consciousness, skin color, pulse, and BP, manual pressure control of extreme hemorrhage. Establish two large venous cannula, take blood for X-match and baseline studies. Give 2 l of prewarmed Hartmann's solution. Establish electrocardiogram (ECG), seek help for operative control of bleeding if needed. Establish urinary catheter unless urethral transection is suspected, and oro- or nasogastric tube.
- *Disability* (neuro-evaluation) Glasgow coma score. Pupillary response to light, visual acuity. Prevent hypotension and hypoxia.
- *Exposure* Remove all clothing to allow full assessment of injuries. Ensure monitoring: respiratory rate, BP, pulse, arterial blood gases, pulse oximetry, and ECG. Prevent hypothermia.

If all these can be established and monitored parameters are normalized, the patient's chances of living are optimized.

X-rays At this stage obtain a chest and pelvis film in the resuscitation room. Cervical spine film may help but cervical spine should remain immobilized until fully assessed if mechanism of injury suggests spinal trauma.

Reassess the ABCs

If all is stable, move to the *secondary survey*, which is a head-to-toe examination of the patient. It is at this stage *only* that specific non-immediately life-threatening conditions should be identified and dealt with in turn.

Maxillofacial injuries other than those with a direct effect on the airway or cervical spine, or causing exsanguinating hemorrhage, should not be dealt with until the **ABCs** have been completed, and this question should be asked of all referring doctors prior to accepting responsibility for a patient. Remember to exclude intracranial, visceral, and major orthopedic injuries.

ATLS is designed primarily for front-line physicians, and recommended to anyone caring for trauma patients.

Basic life support (BLS)

BLS is a specific level of prehospital medical care provided by trained responders in the absence of advanced medical care. In the dental office trained responders include dentist, dental hygienists, and dental assistants. It is prudent to have other office staff trained in BLS/ardiopulmonary resuscitation (CPR) as well. Most state licensing agencies require dentists, hygienists, and assistants to be certified in BLS.

Heart disease is the leading cause of death in the United States. Annually 685,000 deaths are attributed to heart diseases.[1] Sudden cardiac arrest is one of the leading causes of death in the United States and Canada.[2,3] The CDC estimates approximately 330,000 people die each year from coronary heart diseases before reaching a hospital. The elapsed time from cardiac arrest to defibrillation is one of the most important determinants of survival. Automated external defibrillators (AEDs) are reliable and simple to operate, allowing dentists and their office staff to safely provide defibrillation.

Steps

Survey the area and make sure it is safe. Check the patient for a response. If no response, call the emergency response system—**911** and get **AED.** Have a second person do this if someone is available. Place the patient in a supine position on a firm surface (floor or dental chair).

Then begin CPR adult algorithm.

CPR has four main parts: **ABCD**.
- **A**irway Open the patient's **A**irway.
- **B**reathing Check for breathing. If no breathing give **2** breaths that make the chest rise.
- **C**irculation Check pulse. If there is no pulse give cycles of **30** compressions and **2** breaths until **AED** arrives, an advanced life support ALS provider arrives, or the patient starts to move.
- **D**efibrillation Connect AED and follow directions. If there is shockable rhythm give one shock and resume CPR for 5 cycles. If no pulse or breathing repeat until ALS provider/emergency response team arrives, checking patient every 5 cycles. If not shockable continue CPR for 5 cycles and check rhythm every 5 cycles until ALS provider/emergency response team arrives.

1 Centers for Disease Control and Prevention. Web-based Injury statistics query and reporting system (WISQARS)[online]. http://cdc.gov./ncipc/wisqars.
2 Z. Zheng 2001 *Circulation* **104** 2158.
3 S. Chugh 2004 *J Am Coll Cardiol* **44** 1268.

Primary management of maxillofacial trauma

The first consideration is whether the patient has suffered polytrauma, which may have multiple and life-threatening ramifications, or, as is more commonly the case, trauma confined to the face. In the former the prime concern is keeping the patient alive, and the maxillofacial injuries can await Rx (p. 394). Remember that isolated facial injuries rarely cause sufficient bleeding to induce hypovolemic shock. Ask yourself: Can they see?

Airway The brain can tolerate hypoxia for 3 min. Most conscious patients can maintain a patent airway if the oropharynx is cleared. Give all traumatized patients maximal O_2 initially. Oral airways are not tolerated unless the patient is unconscious. Nasopharyngeal airways are only of value if they can be inserted safely and kept patent. If the patient is unconscious and the airway is obstructed they should be intubated. If this is not possible, an emergency airway can be maintained by cricothyroid puncture with a wide-bore cannula. Long-term security of the airway can be achieved by surgical cricothyroidotomy as an emergency, or tracheostomy as a planned operation. Conscious patients with severe isolated facial trauma maintain their airway by sitting leaning forward.

Cervical spine injuries Until these are excluded, the patient should be immobilized.

Bleeding Same as above. Gunshot wounds and lacerated major vessels are exceptions that can cause extensive bleeding. Specific techniques to control naso- and oropharyngeal bleeding are bilateral rubber mouth props to immobilize the maxilla; bilateral balloon catheters passed into the postnasal space, inflated then pulled forward; and bilateral anterior nasal packs.

Scalp wounds can exsanguinate children; control with pressure and heavy full-thickness sutures.

Head injuries The main cause of death and disability in patients with isolated maxillofacial trauma. Assessment: p. 398. Do no further harm.

CSF leaks Facial and skull # can create dural tears, leading to cerebrospinal fluid (CSF) rhinorrhea (from the nose) or otorrhea (from the ear).

Tetanus immunity If in doubt, give tetanus toxoid.

Analgesia May not be needed. Avoid opioids if possible, as they interfere with neuro-observations. If needed, give codeine phosphate 60 mg IM every 4 h.

Patients to admit Any question of danger to the airway, skull #, history of unconsciousness, retrograde amnesia, bleeding, middle 1/3 #, mandibular # (except when very simple), zygoma # if +ve eye signs, children, and those with domestic or social problems. If in doubt, *admit*. Place on, at least, initial hourly neurological observations (most will need 1/4 hourly observation initially). IV access and antibiotic. If not admitting, give the patient a head-injury card.

If teeth have been lost ensure they are not in the chest (CXR) or soft tissues.

X-rays See pp. 400, 402, 406, plate 4.

Assessing head injury

▶ All patients with recent facial trauma warranting hospital admission need at least initial assessment for head injury.

A change in the level of consciousness is the earliest and most valuable sign of head injury.

A combination of the following is generally used.

Glasgow coma scale (GCS)

Eyes open
- spontaneously   4
- to speech   3
- to pain   2
- do not open   1

Best verbal response
- orientated   5
- confused   4
- inappropriate   3
- incomprehensible   2
- none   1

Best motor response
- obeys commands   6
- localizes pain   5
- normal flexion   4
- abnormal flexion   3
- extension   2
- none   1

Pulse and BP ↓ pulse and ↑ BP is a late sign of ↑ intracranial pressure.

Pupils Measure size (1–8 mm) and reaction to light in both pupils.

Respiration ↓ rate is a sign of raised intracranial pressure.

Limb movement

Indicate   normal
             mild weakness
             severe weakness
             extension
             no response

for arms and legs (record right and left separately if there is a difference).

CT scan The definitive investigation. However, patients must never be transferred before correcting hypoxia and hypovolemia.

Using GCS

Severe head injury and/or deterioration = call for help.

One accepted method of categorizing head injury patients by severity using GCS is[1]

Severe   <8
Moderate   9–12
Minor   13–15

In addition

A severe head injury is present if the following are seen:
- Unequal pupils (except traumatic mydriasis)
- Unequal limb movement (except orthopedic injury)
- Open head injury (i.e., compound to brain)

- Deterioration in measured parameters
- Depressed skull #

Subtle signs of deterioration include
- Severe and/or worsening headache
- Early unilateral pupillary dilatation
- Early unilateral limb weakness

A GCS of <6 in the absence of drugs has a dismal prognosis.

A change in GCS of 2 or more is significant. Beware changes in monitoring staff!

Optimizing outcome Preventing brain injury:
- Oxygenate.
- Moderate hyperventilation to control PCO_2.
- Control hemorrhage and optimize fluid balance.
- Contact neurosurgery and ask for advice.
- Only use mannitol under expert advice.
- Do not use steroids at all.[1]

---

1 R. Bullock 1996 *Eur J. Emerg Med* **3** 109.

Mandibular fractures

These are the most common # of the facial skeleton. Most are the result of fights and road traffic accidents (the former appear to be increasing whereas the latter are decreasing as a result of seat belts, etc.). Rarely, they may be comminuted with hard and soft tissue loss, e.g., gunshot wounds.

Classification The most useful is based on site of injury: dentoalveolar, condyle, coronoid, ramus, angle, body, symphyseal, or parasymphyseal. Further subclassification into unilateral, bilateral, multiple, or comminuted aids Rx planning. In common with all # they can be grouped into greenstick (incomplete # with flexible bone), simple (closed linear #), compound (open to mouth or skin), pathological (# through an area weakened by other pathology), or comminuted; again, this influences Rx.

Muscle pull Pull on # segments renders the # favorable or unfavorable, depending on whether or not the # line resists displacement. This is of less importance than recognizing the # and its associated injuries.

Common # Condylar neck # are the most common and range from easiest to most difficult. Often found with a # of the angle or canine region of the opposite side of the jaw. Rarely, bilateral condylar # is found with a symphyseal # "guardsman's #" from falling on the point of the chin. Angle # usually occurs through wisdom-tooth socket, and body # commonly through canine socket.

Anatomic distribution of fractures[1]	
Condylar	29.1%
Angle	24.5%
Symphysis	22%
Body	16%
Dentoalveolar	3.1%
Ramus	1.7%
Coronoid	1.3%

Diagnosis History of trauma. Ask if the patient can bite their teeth or dentures together in the manner that is normal to them. Inability to do this and a lingual mucosal hematoma is pathognomonic of a mandibular #. Look at the face; there is usually bruising and swelling over the # site and sometimes lacerations. If the # is displaced, there may be gagging on the posterior teeth and the mouth hangs open. The saliva is usually bloodstained. The patient may complain of paresthesia in the distribution of the inferior alveolar nerve.

Gentle palpation over the mandible will reveal step deformities, bony crepitus, and tenderness. All have trismus.

1 R. Olson 1982 *J Oral Max Surg* **40** 23.

Examination of the mouth may reveal broken teeth or dentures that should be removed. Suction the mouth to clean away blood clots prior to examining both the buccal and lingual sulcus. Look for step deformities in the occlusion, and examine the teeth. Palpate for steps in the lingual and buccal sulcus. If Δ is uncertain it is sometimes worth trying to elicit abnormal mobility across the suspected # site, using gentle pressure. In cases where you are very unsure, place one hand over each angle of the mandible and exert gentle pressure; this will produce pain if there is a #, even if it is only a crack #. Never perform this if you have proved otherwise that there is a #.

X-rays PAN and PA mandible are the essentials. Get right and left lateral obliques if PAN is unobtainable. Rotated PA (helpful for # between the symphysis and canine region), intraoral periapicals, occlusal, high PAN, open-mouth Townes view, and CT/3-D reconstruction are second-line investigations that may help.

Preliminary Rx (p. 397) Most patients will be admitted to the hospital. Keep NPO and maintain hydration by IV. Compound # need antibiotics. Assess need for analgesia; LA, temporary immobilization, parenteral NSAIDs, or opioids may be needed.

Mid-face fractures

The mid-facial skeleton is a complex composite of fine fragile bones, which rarely # in isolation. It forms a detachable framework that protects the brain from trauma. Severe trauma can move the entire mid-face downward and backward along the base of the skull, lengthening the face and obstructing the airway (clot and swelling exacerbate this). Most *conscious* patients, however, can compensate for this. # of the cribriform plate of the ethmoids can lead to dural tears and CSF leak (p. 397).

Orbit The globe and optic nerve are well-protected by the bony buttress of the orbit. Most # lines pass around the optic foramen; however, swelling can cause proptosis. Late changes can include tethering and enopthalmos.

Retrobulbar hemorrhage is an arterial bleed behind the globe following trauma. It presents as a painful, proptosed eye with decreasing visual acuity, and is a surgical emergency.

Bleeding Severe bleeding is rare, but severe mid-facial trauma may lacerate the third part of the maxillary artery, resulting in profuse bleeding into the nasopharynx that requires anterior and posterior nasal packs and possibly direct ligation.

Classification is mainly based on the experimental work of Rene Le Fort. In Le Fort I # the tooth-bearing portion of the jaw is detached via a # line from the anterior margin of the anterior nasal aperture running laterally and back to the lower 1/3 of the pterygoid plate. In Le Fort II the true mid-face is deatched in a pyramidal shape (see diagram). In Le Fort III the entire facial skeleton is detached from the cranial base, as in the diagram.

Diagnosis Le Fort I may occur singly or associated with other facial #. The tooth-bearing portion of the upper jaw is mobile, unless impacted superiorly. There is bruising in the buccal sulcus bilaterally, disturbed occlusion, and posterior "gagging" of the bite. Grasp the upper jaw between the thumb and forefinger anteriorly, place thumb and forefinger of other hand over the supraorbital ridges, and attempt to mobilize the upper jaw to assess mobility. Spring the maxillary teeth to detect a palatal split. Percussion of the upper teeth may produce a "cracked cup" sound. Le Fort II and III # produce similar clinical appearances, namely, gross edema of soft tissues, bilateral black eyes (panda facies), subconjunctival hemorrhage, mobile mid-face, dish-face appearance, and extensive bruising of the soft palate. Look for a CSF leak and assess visual acuity. Le Fort II # may also show infraorbital nerve paresthesia and step deformity in the orbital rim. Peculiar to Le Fort III # are tenderness and separation of the frontozygomatic suture, deformity of zygomatic arches bilaterally, and mobility of entire facial skeleton.

X-rays Occipitomental 10° and 30°, submentovertex, lateral skull, posternterior skull **only** if C-spine is confirmed to be intact. Otherwise, secure C-spine and await CT scan as the definitive imaging technique.

Preliminary Rx as on pp. 394, 397; definitive Rx, p. 406.

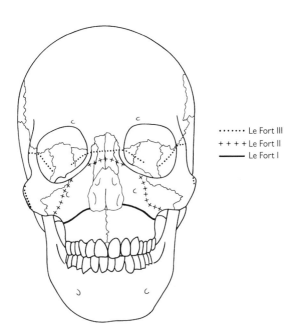

•••••• Le Fort III
+ + + + Le Fort II
———— Le Fort I

Nasal and zygomatic fractures

Zygomatic (or malar) # A common and easily missed injury, usually the result of a blow with a blunt object (e.g., fist). The zygoma forms the cheekbone and resembles a four-pointed star on occipitomental X-ray. The "star" points to the maxilla (orbital margin and lateral wall of antrum), frontal bone, and temporal bone. # can involve the arch alone or the whole zygoma, which may or may not be displaced. The nature of the displacement is of value in planning the Rx.

Diagnosis is from history, examination, and X-ray. Bruising around eye with subconjunctival hemorrhage (unilateral). Diplopia, a step deformity of the orbital rim, sometimes paresthesia of the infraorbital nerve, limitation of lateral excursion of the mandible on mouth opening, and unilateral epistaxis. There is often tenderness on palpation of the zygomatic buttress IO and usually some flattening of the cheek prominence.

Orbital floor # Main signs are those of the zygoma # (or middle 1/3 # if that is the presenting injury). Late signs are enopthalmos and tethering of inferior rectus, causing diplopia in upward gaze. Also known as orbital blowout #; fat and muscle herniates through the thin orbital floor (a similar injury can occur to the medial wall). Classically, seen on X-ray as "hanging drop sign" (radiolucent fat hanging into antrum). Confirm with coronal CT scan. Lateral wall and/or roof # are much less common.

Nasal # Simple nasal trauma is seen by a number of different specialities and considered rather trivial. This is unfair to the patients, as long-term results of nasal # leave a lot to be desired. Nasal # are frequently associated with deviation or crumpling of the septum, obvious nasal deformity, epistaxis, and a degree of nasal obstruction. Rx often consists of simply manipulating the nasal bones with the thumb and splinting. This leaves the septum untreated and contributes to poor long-term results, many needing rhinoplasty later.

Nasoethmoid # Consists of nasal bones, frontal process of maxilla, lacrimal bones, orbital plate of ethmoid, and displacement of the medial canthus of the eye. These # require accurate reduction, stabilization, and fixation of the medial canthus. Δ: bilateral black eyes, obvious nasal deformity (particularly depression of the nasal bridge), septal deviation, epistaxis, and obstruction. Look for CSF leak.

Septal hematoma A comparatively uncommon complication of nasal trauma requiring immediate evacuation. If ignored, it can lead to septal necrosis.

Treatment of facial fractures

Treatment essentially involves reduction, fixation, and immobilization of the # segments. In mandibular and maxillary #, this was traditionally achieved by intermaxillary fixation (IMF), i.e., immobilizing the jaws in occlusion. Today, elastic traction is sometimes used to supplement internal fixation. Third molar teeth and grossly broken down or periodontally infected teeth in the # line should be removed. Otherwise, provide antibiotics and adequate reduction and immobilizatiion with good follow-up.

Open reduction and internal fixation (ORIF) of facial bone # has revolutionized Rx. # sites are exposed, usually via mucosal incisions, and reduced under direct vision; the teeth are placed in temporary IMF and/or a wire around the tooth on either side of the # and rigid plate fixation to immobilize the reduction. IMF can then be released for recovery and elastics placed instead on the ward if needed. Very rarely interosseous wires replace plates, or IMF alone may be used. Resorbable systems are now on the market that use plates fabricated from polylactic acid and polyglycolic acid, but they have yet to match titanium's reliability.

Edentulous mandible The absence of teeth in occlusion creates problems when relying on IMF, and modified dentures can be used. The denture is wired to the mandible and the maxillary denture wired or screwed into the maxilla. The fixed dentures are then wired to one another to create IMF. This technique has been superseded by the use of bone plates in most cases. Pencil-thin edentulous mandibles can be managed by thick (2.4 mm) plates with bicortical screws.

Condylar # Management depends on age and type of injury. <12 yr: analgesia, soft diet, and intermaxillary elastic guidance (if needed) produces optimal results. >12 yr: pain-free, pre-injury occlusion should be established (by elastic traction if need be), and the patient reassessed at 7 days. If spontaneous pain-free occlusion not possible at this stage: ORIF.[1]

Mid-face # Use one of the following methods:

Internal fixation Interosseous wiring, plating, transfixation with wires. Plating to recreate the pyriform and zygomatic buttress system is used.

External fixation e.g., Halo, box frame, which fix the mid-face to the cranium.

Zygoma # Are elevated by a combination of intraoral, infraorbital and lateral eyebrow approach. An instrument is used to elevate and reduce the fracture. If the reduction is not stable it is supplemented by internal fixation with a range of plating techniques.

Nasal bones Are manipulated and splinted. There is some benefit from mini-submucous resection of the septum.

Nasoethmoidal # Are openly reduced and wired or microplated to reposition the medial canthi and restore anatomy.

---

1 Faculty of Dental Surgery 1997 National clinical guidelines. *RCS Eng.*

Fractures in children are considerably rarer. Plates and pins tend to be avoided because of risk to unerupted teeth. Patients <10 yr may require a form of acrylic splint taht fits over the mixed dentition. # are usually firmly united within 3 weeks.

Postop care Antibiotics and scrupulous OH are required. IMF requires a liquid diet of 2000–2500 calories and 3 l of fluid daily. Do not discharge until this can be maintained at home. ORIF requires a soft diet for up to 3 weeks.

Complications
Mandible Infection, paresthesia, damage to teeth, TMJ pain, malunion, delayed union, non-union, bony sequestration, plate and wire infection.

Maxilla Postoperative deformity, epiphora, diplopia, late enophthalmus, anosmia. Failure of union is very rare, although malunion is a problem with poor reduction or late referral.

Zygoma Diplopia, retrobulbar hemorrhage, enophthalmos, paresthesia.

Nasal Deformity, nasal obstruction.

Composite tissue loss Gunshot wounds have led to more facial # presenting as composite defects of hard and soft tissue with tissue loss. These patients need to be stabilized, often with surgical debridement and external fixation prior to free-tissue transfer as part of definitive Rx.

Facial soft tissue injuries

The face is highly visible and once cut no one can make the scar disappear. You can, however, give the patient the best possible scar by following certain principles. Soft tissue injuries are treated after hard tissues have been treated.

Assessment ABCs, mechanism of injury, allergies, and PMH, need for tetanus and rabies prophylaxis. Wounds should be closed within 24 h.

Examination Type of patient, type of wound (cut, burst, flap, tissue loss), special anatomy, eye, eyelid, lip, V/VII, parotid/lacrimal duct.

Investigation X-ray for foreign body (FB).

Plan treatment Clean simple wounds in a cooperative patient are best closed under LA. Otherwise, admit for treatment under GA in the operating room.

Clean wound Irrigate clean wounds with saline. Pulsed saline irrigation is more effective then a continuous stream. Bites or dirty wounds with ingrained FB need aggressive scrubbing with surgical soap. Minimal or no excision of tissue is needed for debridement. Explore all wounds for FB, #, nerve, duct, or vessel damage. Get hemostasis.

Wound closure In layers, mucosa, and muscle: resorbable 3/0–4/0; skin: monofilament 4/0–6/0 (suturing, p. 356.) Avoid tension on skin edge.

Types of wound

Simple lacerations Close in layers with accurate anatomical apposition. Approximate, don't strangulate. Use minimum number of sutures to achieve intact wound with slight eversion. Remove sutures in 7–10 days.

Crush lacerations Skin has burst: minimal edge excision, deep closure, and light skin approximation. Tends to swell. Remove sutures at 5–7 days.

Slicing/shelving lacerations Convert to simple where possible by excision, as these tend to "trap door" otherwise. If excision would be excessive, tack down carefully.

Avulsion If flap, and seems viable: reposition and avoid hematoma. If complete: skin graft or local flap.

Penetrating injuries especially through platysma should be explored and evaluated by a general surgeon.

Anatomical sites

Eye Exclude globe injury.

Ear Drain hematoma if present to avoid "cauliflower."

Septum Drain hematoma to prevent perforation/collapse.

Eyelid, ala of the nose, eyebrow, and vermilion border Require precise matching. Test preanesthetic for facial and trigeminal nerve function.

Special wounds

Abrasions heal spontaneously but must be cleaned thoroughly.

Bites are readily infected. Clean very carefully, and close. Infectious disease consultation required.

Burns need specialist referral.

Tissue loss Nasal tip, ala, and lip are most common. Skin graft or local flap repair is more likely to succeed than stitching severed part back on.

Gunshot wounds See p. 407.

Surgery and the temporomandibular joint

TMD See p. 470.

Ankylosis may be true or false.

True ankylosis is restriction of movement caused by a pathological joint condition, usually due to trauma (intracapsular # in childhood) or infection. Extreme limitation of movement and X-rays will confirm degree of bony union. In fibrous union, exercises are of value. In bony union, interpositional arthroplasty or condylectomy with reconstruction is needed. Postop exercise is crucial.

False ankylosis Restriction of movement imposed by extra-articular abnormalities is very rare. Rx depends on cause. Trismus (limitation of movement due to spasm of muscles of mastication) may be confused with ankylosis but does not affect the joint. It is much more common and complicates many oral surgical procedures; it may follow trauma or infection, or may be a manifestation of occult malignancy.

Trauma Condylar #, p. 400.

Intracapsular # is essentially a childhood injury (relatively shorter, thicker condylar neck). Keep in function to prevent ankylosis.

Dislocation can occur spontaneously as a result of wide opening or during dental procedures. It occurs in normal joints under exceptional circumstances, or in lax joints where dislocation is recurrent. It may be unilateral or bilateral. Condyle can be palpated anterior to articular eminence, X-rays can be used to confirm position, mouth is gagged open. Rx: immediate reduction; the vast majority can be performed with LA by placing thumbs over the molar teeth and exerting downward and backward pressure (if LA is used, less force is needed and thumbs can be placed in buccal sulcus, avoiding the risk of being bitten). Advise jaw support when yawning, etc.; this is usually enough, and avoids IMF. In chronically recurring dislocations, patients can be taught to self-reduce. Exercises are of limited benefit but may avoid surgery. Sclerosing injections are unpleasant and no longer used. Operations are legion: capsular plication, arthroscopic disckectomy, condylotomy, obliteration of upper joint space, eminectomy, high condylectomy. No one operation has gained pre-eminence.

Condylar hyperplasia Rare. Rx: high condylectomy if active (bone scan, but interpretation variable and condylar replacement, e.g., with costochondral cartilage, is unpredictable) or wait for it to "burn out," then perform definitive orthognathic surgery.

Tumors are rare. Rx: ablation, reconstruction, and radiotherapy if malignant.

Arthritic conditions Rheumatoid, degenerative, and gout all manifest in the TMJ but in <15% of patients with the systemic disease. The signs and symptoms are joint stiffness, pain, tenderness, and crepitus. Δ: knowledge of systemic disease and local signs. Rx: treat systemic condition. Symptomatic

Rx of joint is with appliances, physiotherapy, exercises, NSAIDs, and intra-articular steroids. The main long-term problem is limitation of function.

Osteoarthritis is a distinct entity of the TMJ, with a different clinical course from that seen in other joints. It appears to be a degenerative condition of articular cartilage. Δ: crepitus, limitation, and pain on movement, tenderness over condyle, often with X-ray evidence of condylar erosions. Most patients have symptoms for ~1 yr that gradually ↓ over the next 2 yr. X-rays show condylar remodeling to a flat smooth surface. Patients then enter a long period of remission. Rx is ∴ aimed at pain relief, using standard TMD measures (p. 470). Those remaining unresponsive may benefit from intra-articular steroids (p. 552), which probably accelerate natural remodeling. A small group will remain with pain 3–4 months after steroids, usually with X-ray abnormalities. They should be considered for high condylar shave or high condylectomy.

Surgery and TMD Approximately 20% of patients with TMD remain unresponsive to conservative Rx. They may benefit from arthrography or arthroscopy both as an investigation and a Rx (distension of the joint space-releasing adhesions). Surgery for pure TMD in patients unresponsive to the above may be of benefit (probably by cutting the nerve supply to the joint), although clicking can certainly be eliminated by meniscal plication and/or pterygoid myotomy, and irrevocably damaged menisci can be removed but require some form of interpositional reconstruction.

Major preprosthetic surgery

Minor procedures, p. 388; implantology, p. 390. The aim is to enable an edentulous patient to live comfortably with functioning dentures, ∴ surgery without liaison with an understanding and competent prosthodontist is pointless. All procedures for improving the denture-bearing area of the jaws are dependent on the use of a denture with a modified fitting surface (surgical stent), which is placed during surgery and must be worn for up to 8 weeks postoperatively, the tissue surface being modified at intervals with a soft acrylic lining material. There are many who would claim these procedures do not work, and indeed there is little scientific support for them.

► Warn all patients undergoing lower jaw procedures about postop mental nerve damage.

Vestibuloplasty Basically, this is a skin graft to the alveolar surface of the jaw, creating a deeper sulcus. Important points: excise all areas of scarred or hyperplastic tissue, dissect off any strands of mentalis in the lower jaw, ensure preservation of the alveolar periosteum, ensure that the surgical stent extends to the new sulcus depth, and ensure that the skin–mucosa junction lies on the labial surface.

Combination mucosal flap and vestibuloplasty usually suffices in the maxilla due to its ↑ potential for denture retention.

Mental nerve repositioning Mental nerve compression by a denture flange following alveolar resorption is a common problem, producing a sensation like an electric shock but with a background ache that ↑ during the day and ↓ overnight. Leaving the -/F out for several days ↓ the pain. The mental nerve is repositioned by creating a new foramen under its present position or laterally transposing the entire nerve into the soft tissues in grossly atrophic mandibles.

Alveolar augmentation Problems with osseous donor site morbidity and length of procedure have put these operations out of favor. The use of "sandwich" procedures (where the augmenting material is literally sandwiched between horizontally osteotomized jaw), coupled with effective bone substitutes and tunneling procedures (p. 388), has made augmentation a better proposition. Healthy patients with severe jaw atrophy or those with incipient or actual pathological # may still benefit from split rib grafting.

Distraction osteogenesis A preprosthetic component to this well-accepted technique for "growing" bone by osteotomizing and gradually moving bone apart using an appliance (1–2 mm/day) will probably replace all major augmentation procedures.

Sinus lift ↑ popular procedure combined with simultaneous or delayed implants. After raising subperiosteal buccal flaps a window is created to expose antral lining. Lining of the floor and walls is elevated intact and this space is filled with autogenous bone from the iliac crest, tibia, or chin to provide retention for implants.

Transmandibular implant (staple implant) A box frame construction is placed in the mandible from a submental incision. Transmandibular implant has been supplanted by osseointegrated implants.

Clefts and craniofacial anomalies

Orofacial clefts include cleft lip, cleft palate, and combined cleft lip and cleft palate and are estimated to occur in 1 in 700 births in the United States. Cleft lip is more common than cleft palate. Worldwide, orofacial clefts affect about 1 in 700 to 1000 babies.[1] Clefts occur with ↑ frequency in Asians and ↓ frequency in African Americans. Boys are affected more than girls by 3:2. Cleft lip and palate 2x ↑ in boys. Cleft palate alone is ↑ in girls. 3/4 clefts are unilateral.[2]

Cleft lip and palate (see also p. 172)

▶ The aim is to replace anatomical structures in their correct position; the price is scarring, which will restrict growth to some degree. It is important to recognize that the stigmata of surgery is due to growth of the patient. At least as much deformity has been caused in the past by poor surgery as has been caused by the cleft.

Lip closure There are two main philosophies:
- *"Plastic" approach* Performed neonatally or up to 3 months; flaps transgress skin boundaries and use supraperiosteal dissection. This gives good early aesthetic results (e.g., Millard).
- *"Functional" approach* All skin boundaries are respected; subperiosteal dissection is used. Immediate aesthetics are less good due to pout caused by muscle repair but there is ↑ function and growth potential.

Palatal closure Extensive surgery restricts maxillary growth, ∴ use minimal simple repair that recreates a functioning soft palate (e.g., Von Langenbeck technique).

Alveolus Vomer flap to close anterior hard palate cleft.

Ears Preschool audiology.

Nasal deformity Perhaps the greatest surgical challenge. 1° functional lip/nose repair may alter this.

Secondary surgery Lip revision (simple or complex). Sometimes required preschool or at time of alveolar bone graft.

Alveolar bone graft See p. 173.

Speech, nasendoscopy, and pharyngoplasty All cleft palate patients have impaired speech. Fiber-optic nasendoscopy allows visualization of the palate during speech and aids assessment. Pharyngoplasty narrows the velopharyngeal opening to ↓ hypernasal speech. Successful palate repair ↓ need for pharyngoplasty.

Orthognathic surgery See p. 416.

---

1 http://www.cdc.gov
2 C.Jones 2000 The genetics of cleft lip and palate: information for families, Cleft Lip and Palate Foundation.

Craniofacial anomalies

This includes a broad group of conditions involving the craniomaxillofacial region. A simple classification is as follows:

Congenital

- Orbital malformations (hypertelorism, orbital dystopia)
- Craniosynostoses (premature fusion of cranial sutures)
- Craniofacial synostoses (Apert syndromes, Crouzon, pp. 680, 681)
- Encephaloceles
- Others (Treacher–Collins, hemifacial microsomia, hemifacial hypertrophy and atrophy)

Acquired

- Tumors (benign or malignant)
- Dysplasias (fibro-osseous)
- Neurofibromatosis
- Post-trauma deformity

These patients need craniofacial surgical teams. Coronal flaps to deglove the face are the mainstay of access, followed by craniotomy and osteotomy as required. The main risks are cerebral edema, infection, damage to optic nerves and vessels, and, in neonates and children, pediatric fluid balance.

Orthognathic surgery

This is the surgery of facial skeletal deformity and merges with cleft and craniofacial surgery. Prime indications are functional: speech, eating. Secondary indications are aesthetic.

▶ Patients may not see these as quite such separate issues. Their reasons and motivation for seeking surgery must be understood and the limitations of surgery made absolutely clear before embarking on protracted and complex Rx.

Diagnosis and treatment planning See p. 170.

Mandibular procedures

These involve ramus, body, alveolus, or chin.

Intraoral vertical subsigmoid osteotomy is used to push back the mandible. EO approach used when suitable equipment for IO not available. The IO procedure is straightforward, performed via an extended third-molar type incision. Bone cuts are made with a right-angled oscillating saw from sigmoid notch to lower border. Technique is very instrument dependent.

Sagital split osteotomy(bilateral) can move mandible backward or forward. IO incision is similar to above. Bone cuts are made from above lingula, across retromolar region, down buccal aspect to lower border. Split sagitally with osteotome followed by spreaders. Main complication is paresthesia of IFAN.

Inverted L- and C-shaped osteotomy Usually EO approach. Rarely used; can lengthen ramus if used with bone graft.

Body ostectomy shortens body of mandible. Need to gain space ortho-dontically or remove tooth. Watch mental nerve.

Subapical osteotomy is used to move dentoalveolar segments. Technically it is more difficult than it looks. There is risk to tooth vitality.

Genioplasty The tip of the chin can be moved pretty much anywhere; the secret is to keep a sliding contact with bone and a muscle pedicle. Fixation should be kept away from areas of muscle activity as this leads to bone resorption.

Maxillary procedures

Segmental Can be single-tooth, or bone and tooth blocks that involve tunneling incisions in buccal sulcus and palate to move premaxilla. Problems are finding space for bone cuts and avoiding damaging teeth.

Le Fort I Primary maxillary procedure. Standard approach is the "down-fracture" with horseshoe buccal incision, bone cuts at Le Fort I level, and segment pedicle on the palate. The free maxilla can be moved up, down, or forward. In cleft palate cases, concern over the adequacy of the palatal blood supply has led to some surgeons using tunneled buccal incisions to make the bone cuts, thus preserving some of the buccal blood supply to the maxilla. Fixation can be a problem when using this technique.

Le Fort II Usually used for mid-face advancement. Bilateral canthal and vestibular incisions allow bone cuts at the Le Fort II level.

Le Fort III Really a subcranial craniofacial operation using a coronal flap plus vestibular and orbital incisions to move the entire mid-face and zygomatic complex.

Zygomatic osteotomy is used for post-traumatic defects. Approach via coronal incisions. There is risk to infraorbital nerve from maxillary bone cut.

Rhinoplasty The correction of isolated nasal deformity. Usually done intranasally, supplemented by tiny incisions over the nasal bones to allow bone cuts. "Open rhinoplasty," which involves degloving the nasal skeleton via a columella incision, is becoming popular.

Stability ↑ use of mini-plates in the fixation of the osteotomized segments has ↓ the reliance on bone grafts. Presurgical orthodontics (p. 170) makes a significant contribution to ↓ rate of relapse. IMF and/or elastic traction remains vital for long-term success. Good dental interdigitation and planning movements within the capacity of the soft tissues are probably the best measures to prevent relapse.[1]

1 D. Tuinzing 1993 *Surgical Orthodontics*, VU University Press.

Salivary gland tumors

Diseases (see also pp. 448, 450)

Classified by the World Health Organization (WHO) into epithelial tumors, non-epithelial tumors, and unclassified tumors.

Common benign tumors Pleomorphic adenoma, p. 450. Monomorphic adenoma papillary cystadenoma lymphoma (Warthin's tumor) affects M > F; rare <50 yr. Bilateral in 10%. Feels soft and cystic. Benign, very unlikely to recur despite being multifocal.

Carcinomas Rare.
  Adenoid cystic carcinoma Characteristic "Swiss cheese" appearance histologically. Spreads locally, particularly along perineural spaces. Can be compatible with long-term survival despite propensity for 2° in lungs, although rarely cured.
  Adenocarcinomas There is a wide range of these malignant tumors, from the highly aggressive to the relatively indolent, e.g., polymorphous low-grade adenocarcinoma. It is essential that an adequate histological diagnosis be made by an oral pathologist. Other carcinomas are rare but may arise in a preexisting pleomorphic adenoma or de novo. 5-yr survival 730%.

Other epithelial tumors include *acinic cell tumor* and *mucoepidermoid tumor*. Both have variable, unpredictable behavior, can recur locally, metastasize, and can occur at any age. On average, both are compatible with ~80% survival.

Nonepithelial tumors include hemangioma, lymphangioma, and neurofibroma. They account for 50% of salivary tumors in children.

Unclassified group This includes lymphomas, secondaries, lipomas, and chemodectomas.

Parotid History and examination are the prime diagnostic tools. Long history, no pain, and no facial nerve involvement suggest benign tumor. Facial palsy, pain, and rapid growth suggest malignancy. The feel of many tumors is characteristic. CT, fine-needle aspiration cytology (FNAC), ultrasound scanning (USS), MRI may help; however, Rx almost always involves parotidectomy and most investigations simply delay this.

Submandibular Less common tumors. Pleomorphic adenoma remains most common. Malignant tumors account for up to 30%. Rx of most is gland excision via a skin crease in the neck. Modified neck dissection required for malignant or recurrent tumors.

Sublingual and minor glands >50% of tumors are malignant (mostly adenoid cystic) and require extensive surgery and reconstruction similar to floor of mouth cancer.

Surgery of the salivary glands

Surgery of the major salivary glands is primarily for tumors, obstruction, and, less commonly, inflammatory conditions. The minor glands are most commonly removed for mucoceles (p. 376) and more rarely for tumors. With the exception of lymphomas *all* salivary gland tumors should have surgery initially, patient permitting.

Parotidectomy Principles are complete excision of tumor with margin of healthy tissue and preservation of facial nerve. Clinically benign tumors in superficial lobe have superficial parotidectomy, and in deep lobe, total conservative parotidectomy. Malignant tumors require radical excision and/or radiotherapy. Whether to sacrifice the facial nerve adjacent to malignant parotid tumor is a complex decision. Many would accept *nerve clinically affected*—preop, sacrifice, and reconstruct; *nerve clinically intact*—preop, preserve, and rely on postop radiotherapy.

Salivary duct calculi History is of recurrent pain and swelling in the obstructed gland, particularly before and during meals. Plain X-rays (lower occlusal for submandibular, cheek for parotid) reveal radio-opaque calculi, but do not exclude the radiolucent calculi and mucous plugs. Sialography reveals a stricture or obstruction. Most common in the submandibular duct. Rx: *submandibular duct* for calculi lying anterior in duct—remove by passing a suture behind the calculus to prevent it from slipping further down the duct, dissect the duct from an IO approach, and lift out stone; either marsupialize the duct or reconstruct. Posterior calculi—excise gland and duct. Rx: *parotid duct*—expose duct via IO approach for anterior stones or via a small skin flap onto a probe in the duct for more posterior calculi. Otherwise, selective superficial parotidectomy is the only safe approach.

Lithotripsy is available in some centers for proximal calculi in patients who want to avoid gland excision. It has been successful with stones <3 mm in size

Sialadenitis Severe infection of the parotid or submandibular glands leads to dilatation and ballooning of the ducts and alveoli called *sialectasis*. Sialography is the investigation of choice and often therapeutic, inducing long remissions between episodes of infection. *Conservative* Rx: culture and sensitivity with appropriate antibiotic Rx. Most likely is *Staphylococcus aureus*–treat with cephalosporin. When remission periods are short or intolerable, or the patient requires *definitive* Rx, use gland excision.

Surgery for drooling In severe cases it is possible to re-site the parotid ducts into the hypopharynx and/or perform bilateral submandibular gland excision to control drooling without impairing lubrication for swallowing and oral health (Wilkes procedure). A more physiological approach is to reposition submandibular ducts and excise sublingual glands, as these are a major source of pooled saliva at rest. Intraglandular botulinum toxin can help.

Mucoceles See p. 376.

Oral cancer

Etiology, epidemiology, Δ, and staging, p. 444; neck masses, p. 422; salivary tumors, p. 418.

Various parameters affect the choice of Rx for patients with oral cancer; not least among these, but often forgotten, are the patients themselves, their general health, understanding of their disease, geographical location, and social and domestic commitments. Classically, broad Rx principles are based on tumor staging, using TNM classification (p. 444), and the patient's fitness for surgery (this tends to imply that if they can't cope with surgery they can cope with traveling for radiotherapy, which is not always the case). In many instances of oral cancer, combined surgery and radiotherapy constitute optimal Rx.

Suggested management plan (this will vary according to the surgeon concerned)

- Establish provisional Δ. History, examination, and get to know patient. Check full blood count (FBC), erythrocyte sedimentation rate (ESR), urea and electrolytes (U&Es), liver function tests (LFTs) (including albumin), bone biochemistry, VDRL, blood group, CXR, ECG, PAN.
- Arrange tissue Δ. By biopsy—usually under LA. Flexible nasendoscopy, head, neck, thorax, imaging (CT/MRI). This is to exclude synchronous 1° tumor in upper aerodigestive tract (present in, at most, 15% of cases). Palpate the neck for nodes. Stage tumor (TNM).
  - T1–N0: Surgery or radiotherapy (often brachytherapy—radioactive implants) offers equal cure rate.
  - Tumor close to bone having radiotherapy: safest to remove associated teeth to prevent osteoradionecrosis.
  - T2 and T3: >50% of patients will have occult metastases; consider watch and wait; prophylactic radiotherapy (works for occult but not for obvious bulky nodes); or prophylactic selective neck dissection. Later is usually best.
  - For large tumors, close or +ve margins, and extracapsular spread, radiotherapy is given postoperatively.
  - Vastly ↑ access is obtained for resection by osteotomizing the mandible (position plate beforehand).
  - Anterior floor of mouth cancer may spread to bilateral lymph nodes; bilateral selective neck dissection can be simultaneous and is usual.
  - Presence or absence of extracapsular spread in cervical lymph nodes is strongest prognostic indicator.

Simultaneous chemotherapy and radiotherapy can have a dramatic effect on poorly differentiated squamous cell carcinomas (SCCs), especially those originating from postnasal space, tonsil, and tongue base.

5-yr survival 90% for T1–N0, but 30% for T2/3–N1 and worse for T4; however, this does *not* mean that extensive combination therapy and reconstruction is pointless in those with advanced oral cancers. Death comes in many ways, and a fungating uncontrolled cancer of the head and neck is one of the less pleasant. Attempted surgical "cure" that alleviates local disease and symptoms and allows the patient a few more years of life and a gradual demise from carcinomatosis or another disease is still worthwhile from all viewpoints (palliative surgery with curative intent).

Chemotherapy There is, as yet, no proven role for cytotoxics in oral cancer, other than in combination with radiotherapy or in palliation.

Neck masses

▶ Do not leave chronic cervical lymphadenopathy undiagnosed.
▶ A head and neck malignancy must be excluded before biopsy.

Children are an exception; inflammation is common and tumor is rare, so a watch-and-wait policy is reasonable.

Diagnosis History, look at the patient and mass. Palpate it. If needed, carry out a full head and neck examination. Most diagnoses will be made by then.

Investigation Ultrasound, aspiration cytology, biopsy.

Causes Think (a) anatomy, (b) pathology, (c) oddity.

Skin Lesions lie superficially.

Sebaceous cyst Look for punctum; it is within skin. Excise.

Lipoma Soft, often yellowish. Excise.

Sublingual dermoid cyst Lies in floor of mouth, often under mylohyoid. Arises from trapped epithelium during embryonic fusion; contains keratin. Rx: total excision.

Lymph nodes Deep to platysma. Try to diagnose before biopsy. Opening of malignant nodes ↓ survival (p. 421).

Infection (p. 466) Nodes are large and tender. Causes: viral (e.g., glandular fever, HIV), bacterial (e.g., mycobacterial, which can calcify, actinomycosis), or reactive to other head and neck infection.

Malignancy Either metastatic from head and neck 1° (hard, rock-like nodes) or lymphoma/leukemia (large rubbery), p. 466. FNAC unhelpful in lymphoma; biopsy is needed.

Glandular Think anatomically.

Salivary (p. 418) Submandibular/lower pole of parotid: abscess, sialadenitis, obstruction, sarcoidosis, Sjögren syndrome. Sublingual: ranula, tumor.

Thyroid Benign and malignant tumors, goiter, thyroglossal cyst (may lie anywhere between foramen cecum of tongue and thyroid, tract goes behind, around, or through hyoid bone, moves with swallowing).

Arterial Don't biopsy!

Carotid aneurysm (pulsatile).

Carotid body tumor Found around carotid bifurcation. Usually firm, not hormonally active, 5% malignant. Rx: excise if symptomatic.

Schwannoma/neurofibroma All major nerves in neck can develop painless masses. Rx: excision, preserving healthy fibers if possible.

Pharynx

Diverticulum (or pharyngeal pouch) Fills on swallowing. Evert endoscopically or excise.

Larynx

   Laryngocele Rare. Mainly M >60. 80% unilateral. Excise.

Sternomastoid

   'Sternomastoid tumor' (congenital ischemic fibrosis causing torticollis).

   True muscle tumors Rare.

Bone Cervical rib, prominent hyoid bone.

Infections (see also p. 372) Ludwig's angina, submasseteric abscess, retropharyngeal abscess, parapharyngeal cellulitis, tuberculosis (TB), infected cysts or pouches.

Oddities

Branchial cyst Either a remnant from 2nd and 3rd branchial arches or degeneration of lymphoid tissue. This is an epithelial lined cyst that presents as a deep-seated swelling lying anterior to sternomastoid at or above the level of the hyoid. It is prone to infection. Rx: total excision.

Branchial fistula A fistula from the tonsillar fossa to the skin overlying anterior lower 1/3 of sternomastoid. It is present at birth; discharges intermittently. Rx: total excision of tract.

Cystic hygroma Presents in infancy and is a form of lymphangioma that appears as endothelium-lined multilocular cysts containing lymph. It may be found anywhere in head–neck but classically behind lower end of sternomastoid. May suddenly ↑ in size if bled into or ruptured. Rx: total excision (in practice, excise as much as possible) as soon as child is healthy enough for surgery.

Flaps and grafts

A *graft* is transferred tissue dependent on the recipient site capillaries for its survival. A *flap* is transferred tissue independent, at least initially, of the recipient site capillaries for survival.

The possibility of functional reconstruction of the head and neck in conjunction with the potential for cure justifies the mutilation of radical surgery for oral cancer; however, head and neck reconstruction is used in other aspects of maxillofacial surgery, particularly trauma.

Mucosal grafts, p. 213. Mucosal flaps, p. 206.

Skin grafts may be split thickness or full thickness. Split-thickness grafts (taken by knife or dermatome from thigh or inner arm) take quickly and become wettable in the mouth. They are "quilted" in place with sutures. Full-thickness grafts (supraclavicular, post-auricular, or abdominal) provide a mediocre color match when repairing skin defects of the face. Full-thickness donor sites are closed.

Free bone grafts are from rib, iliac crest, or calvarium. Rib, which is partially split at 1 cm intervals, can be bent to conform to the shape of the mandible. Iliac crest supplies cortical or cancellous bone and can be cut to a template, but ↑ risk of deep venous thrombosis (DVT). Various synthetic mesh containers as a mold for cancellous bone exist.

Nasolabial flap Random-pattern pedicle flap based above and lateral to the upper lip; a useful local flap. It requires division ~3 weeks later.

Tongue flaps Random-pattern pedicle flap for lip and palate repair. It requires division and inset 3 weeks later.

Forehead flap Based on anterior branch of superficial temporal artery; very safe flap, rarely used because of the poor donor site defect. It requires division later.

Masseter muscle flap Limited in size; can be used intraorally.

Temperoparietal fuscia flap Pedicle or free flap based on superficial temporal vessels. Long, flexible reconstruction. It is difficult to raise.

Temporalis flap Inferiorly based on deep temporal branches of maxillary artery. Its use is limited because of size and tendency to fibrose.

Deltopectoral flap Based on perforating internal mammary vessels. Thin skin suitable for skin or mucosa repair. It is usually divided and inset after 3 weeks.

Pectoralis major myocutaneous flap Also described with bone, but the bone is really a free rib graft. Based on acromiothoracic axis. Usually tunnelled after neck dissection. Very bulky flap; covers carotids after radical neck dissection. This is a workhorse head-and-neck pedicle flap.

Latissimus dorsi myocutaneous flap Very bulky flap based on thoracodorsal vessels. Needs to be tunneled through axilla if pedicled. it is more commonly used as a free flap.

Free tissue transfer by microvascular r-anastomosis has been the biggest advance in reconstruction. The following are useful and commonly used flaps.

Radial forearm flap A fasciocutaneous flap based on the radial artery. The skin available is thin and supple and can conform to the complex anatomy of the mouth (skin is often hairless, which is a big bonus). A thin segment of up to 10 cm of radius can also be transferred for bony reconstruction.

Deep circumflex iliac artery flap Based on the deep circumflex iliac artery. This flap has potential for sufficient bone transfer to reconstruct the entire mandible. Internal oblique muscle is usually transferred for soft tissue, which is good where nonmobile soft tissue repair needed. Skin transfer is possible but less useful.

Free fibula flap 25 cm of fibula can be excised within a muscle cuff supplied by the peroneal vessels. Excellent length and thickness of bone for mandibular reconstruction. Skin transfer for mobile soft tissue available.

Free rectus abdominus Bulky skin/muscle flap based on inferior epigastric vessels. Useful for massive facial defects but often limited by fat volume.

Anterolateral thigh free flap Recently popularized soft tissue flap from thigh (descending branch of lateral circumflex femoral artery). Skin thickness can limit usefulness infraorally.

Subscapular system flaps Several skin, fat, and bone flaps can be harvested from these vessels; the disadvantage is the need to turn patient perioperatively.

Craniofacial implants Prosthetic eyes, ears, and noses can be securely fixed to the facial skeleton with implants using techniques similar to those for oral implants. Probably the best available ear reconstruction.

Oral medicine

Principal sources   Much of the skill of oral medicine lies in the clinical recognition of lesions, therefore a color atlas of oral mucosal disease is invaluable.

C. Scully 1999 *Slide Interpretation in Oral Diseases*, OUP. J. Soames 1999 *Oral Pathology*, 3rd ed., OUP. J. A. Regezi 1999 *Oral Pathology*, 3rd ed., W.B. Saunders. R. Gray 1995 *Temporomandibular Disorders: A Clinical Approach*, BDJ.

Bacterial infections of the mouth

Caries (p. 24); periodontal disease (p. 179); dentofacial infections (p. 372).

This page refers primarily to mucosal infections.

Scarlet fever may be due to a delayed type hypersensitivity to streptococcal erythrogenic toxin produced by some strains of group A streptococci that cause capillary damage. It usually causes a urinary tract infection (UTI). The sore throat is accompanied by a skin rash, general malaise, and fever. The oral mucosa is reddened and the tongue undergoes pathognomonic changes; the dorsum develops a white coating through which white edematous fungiform papillae project—the "strawberry tongue" of scarlet fever. Later the white coating is shed and the dorsum becomes smooth and red with enlarged fungiform papillae—"raspberry tongue." Rx is directed toward the systemic condition with high-dose penicillin or erythromycin in patients allergic to penicillin. The oral manifestations resolve within 14 days.

Tuberculosis A re-emerging infectious disease caused by *Mycobacterium tuberculosis*. Spread of infection is through small airborne droplets, which carry the organisms to pulmonary air spaces. Histopathology shows necrotizing granuloma with giant and epithelioid cells, and a Ziehl–Neelsen stain reveals mycobacteria. TB is commonly seen in immuno-compromised patients, including elderly persons; although 1/3 of global population is affected by TB, oral involvement with it is rare. When it does occur, it is usually 2° to open pulmonary infection or coexisting HIV. The oral lesion presents as a deep painful ulcer, gradually increasing in size. Any part of the oral mucosa may be involved, although the posterior aspect of the dorsum of the tongue is the most common site. A positive inflammatory skin reaction (Mantoux test/PPD tuberculosis test) indicates a previous exposure and subclinical infection, but does not necessarily imply active disease. If the test is positive, the physician will order a chest X-ray and/or sputum culture. Tuberculosis can be successfully treated with specific antibiotics taken for at least 6 months. A person who does not have symptoms but has a positive TB test may need antibiotics to prevent an active infection from developing. If untreated, TB can be fatal. Multidrug-resistant (MDR-TB) strains of TB and extreme drug resistance (XDR-TB) in TB are emerging.

Syphilis is a sexually transmitted or congenital infection caused by the bacterium *Treponema pallidum*. The drug of choice for treating all stages of syphilis is penicillin. Syphilis has several stages.

1° stage A chancre (a firm ulcerated nodule) develops at the site of inoculation, usually the lips or tongue. This lesion is highly infectious and *T. pallidum* can easily be isolated. There is usually marked cervical lymphadenopathy, which resolves spontaneously in 1–2 months.

2° stage Develops 2–4 months (latent period) after the 1° with a cutaneous rash, condylomata, and ulceration of the oral mucosa. This oral involvement occurs regardless of the site of 1° infection, with superficial gray, sloughy ulcers known as mucous patches or snail-track ulcers.

These are also highly contagious, and *T. pallidum* can be easily isolated. Syphilis serology is positive at this stage. The ulcers generally clear up within a few weeks, although there may be recurrences.

3° stage Develops several years later and is marked by gumma formation. This is a necrotic granulomatous reaction usually affecting the palate or tongue, which enlarges and ulcerates and may lead to perforation of the palate. In the past, syphilis of the tongue was associated with malignant change, often presenting as a leukoplakia. It is not entirely clear whether it was the condition or its Rx that caused this. Lesions are noninfectious.

Congenital syphilis occurs during the latter half of pregnancy, when the *T. pallidum* crosses the placenta from the infected mother. This might cause numerous inflammatory and destructive lesions in various fetal organs, or it may cause abortion. Classical appearances include saddle nose, frontal bossing and Hutchinson's triad (an inflammatory reaction in the cornea, eighth nerve deafness, and dental abnormalities consisting of notched or screwdriver-shaped incisors and mulberry molars).

Gonorrhea is a sexually transmitted infection caused by bacteria called *Neisseria gonorrhea*. This is a result of orogenital contact with an infected partner and presents as a nonspecific stomatitis or pharyngitis with frequent persisting superficial ulcers. Swabs may reveal gram-negative intracellular diplococci. No specific clinical signs have been consistently associated with oral gonorrhea. Rx is with high-dose penicillin; this STD should be referred to a specialist.

Viral infections of the mouth

Herpes simplex virus (HSV) is responsible for common vesicular eruptions of the skin and mucosa. Although oral infection with HSV-1 and HSV-2 is described below, most oral-facial herpetic lesions are due to HSV-1. Antibodies indicating past infection are virtually ubiquitous in adults. There are two oral manifestations.

Primary herpetic gingivostomatitis varies widely in severity (↑ with age). In infancy is often mistakenly attributed to teething. Presents with a single episode of widespread stomatitis with vesicles, which break down to form shallow painful ulcers, enlarged, tender cervical lymph nodes, halitosis, coated tongue, fever, and a general malaise for 10–14 days. Thus, lesions may appear on any intraoral mucosal surface. Although generally self-limiting, rare complications include herpetic encephalitis. Diagnosis is based on the clinical features and history, although the virus can be grown in cell culture. Microscopically ballooning degeneration of epithelial cells with intranuclear viral inclusions "Lipschutz bodies" are seen. A fourfold ↑ in convalescent-phase antibodies is also diagnostic, but gives the diagnosis retrospectively. Rx: topical and systemic analgesia (Benzydamine, acetaminophen), a soft or liquid diet with extra fluid intake, and prevention of 2° infection (chlorhexidine mouthwash) are usually adequate in healthy patients. Severely ill or immuno-compromised patients should receive systemic acyclovir.

Secondary herpes (herpes labialis, cold sore) is a reactivation of the 1° infection, which is believed to lie dormant in the trigeminal ganglion. Precipitating factors include trauma, immunosuppression, and, less commonly, exposure to sunlight, stress, or other illness. It usually recurs on the skin of lip or nose supplied by one branch of trigeminal nerve, classically at the mucocutaneous junction, or rarely as an IO blister. The prodromal phase is over 24 h when there is a prickling sensation on the lips followed by vesiculation and pain. Lesions may respond to topical acyclovir 5% cream. Systemic acyclovir should be considered in the immunosuppressed. Recurrence appears to decline with age.

Herpes (varicella) zoster is a neurogenic DNA virus that causes chickenpox as a 1° infection and shingles as a reactivation.

Chickenpox is classically an itchy, vesicular, cutaneous rash that may rarely affect the oral mucosa. Fever, chills, malaise, and headache may accompany rash that involves primarily the trunk, head and neck. The infection is self-limited and lasts several weeks.

Shingles is confined to the distribution of a nerve, the virus staying either in the dorsal root ganglion of a peripheral nerve or the trigeminal ganglion. It always presents as a unilateral lesion never crossing the midline. Facial or oral lesions may arise in the area supplied by the branches of the trigeminal nerve. Diagnosis: pre-eruption pain, followed by development of painful vesicles on skin or oral mucosa, which rupture to give ulcers or crusting skin wounds in the distribution outlined above. These usually clear in 2–4 weeks, but apparent resolution is often followed by severe postherpetic neuralgia, which may continue for years. Rx: symptomatic relief for chickenpox. There is some evidence to suggest that early Rx of shingles with acyclovir ↓ the incidence and severity of postherpetic neuralgia in immuno-compromised patients. Refer to an ophthalmologist if the eye is involved.

Coxsackie virus is an RNA virus causing 2° oral mucosal conditions.

Herpangina Highly contagious viral infection caused by Coxsackie A virus (A1 + A6, A8, A10, A12, A16, or A22) is confined to children and presents with widespread small ulcers on the oral mucosa with fever and general upset. Clinically, it resembles herpetic stomatitis, but with no gingivitis and only moderate cervical lymphadenitis. It may be preceded by sore throat and conjunctivitis. Can also be mistaken as teething. It is self-limiting in 10–14 days, and is fairly rare.

Hand, foot, and mouth disease is caused by Coxsackie virus (usually A16) and is also confined to children. A papular, vesicular rash appears on the hands and feet in conjunction with nasal congestion and oral mucosal vesicles. These break down, leaving painful superficial ulcers, particularly on the palate. The gingiva is rarely involved. It is self-limiting in 10–14 days. Rx is as for herpetic stomatitis.

Human papilloma virus has been associated with squamous cell papilloma, condyloma acuminatum (multiple white/pink nodules), focal epithelial hyperplasia (multiple painless papules), and verruca vulgaris (white exophytic lumps). The last three are very rare. Rx: local surgery and interferon.

Measles (Rubeola) A highly contagious viral infection caused by a member of the pramyxovirus family of viruses. The prodromal phase of measles may be marked by small white spots with an erythematous margin on the buccal mucosa, known as Koplik's spots. A few days later the maculo-papular rash of measles appears, usually behind the ears, then spreading to the face and trunk. There is no specific treatment for measles.

Glandular fever (infectious mononucleosis) is seen mostly in children and young adults and spread by infected saliva. It varies widely in severity and presents with sore throat, generalized lymphadenopathy, fever, headaches, general malaise, and often a maculopapular rash. There may be hepatosplenomegaly. Oral manifestations may mimic 1° herpetic gingivostomatitis, with widespread oral ulceration, and in addition petechial hemorrhages, especially at the junction of hard and soft palate (pathognomonic), and bruising may be present. The cause is usually Epstein–Barr virus (EBV), and less commonly cytomegalovirus (CMV). Toxoplasmosis can give a similar picture. Diagnosis: initially monospot test, Paul–Bunnell test to exclude EBV, and acute and convalescent titres for CMV and toxoplasmosis. Be aware that early HIV infection can mimic this condition. Rx: symptomatic as for 1° herpes, except toxoplasmosis, which may respond to sulfa drugs; seek expert advice.

Note: Ampicillin should not be given to patients with a sore throat who may have glandular fever as it inevitably produces an unwanted response, ranging from a rash to anaphylaxis. Opportunistic infection on the tongue mucosa by EBV is thought to be the pathological mechanism behind "hairy leukoplakia."

Reiter's syndrome The causative agent is unknown but appears to be a postinfective response. The syndrome consists of urethritis, arthritis, conjunctivitis and/or oral ulcers, or erosions. It predominantly affects young males and is associated with HLA B27 in 80% of patients—leukocytosis and ↑ ESR are common. NSAIDs are generally used in the treatment of this disease.

Candidiasis

Although over 100 *Candida* species can be isolated, only a handful are clinically important. Candidiasis is caused by *C. albicans* and related but far less common species such as *C. parapsilosis, C. tropicalis, C. glabrata, C. krusei, C. pseudotropicalis,* and *C. guilliermondi. C. albicans* is a commensal organism residing in the oral cavity in a majority of healthy persons. Overt infection occurs when there are local or systemic predisposing factors. Therefore, the prime tenet of management is to look for and treat these factors.

Acute candidiasis

Acute pseudomembranous candidiasis (thrush) is most common in infancy, old age and the immunosuppressed or debilitated (e.g., those on radiotherapy, cytotoxics, or steroids, or with diabetes, cancer, HIV, or hematological malignancy), or those on broad-spectrum antibiotics. Clinically it appears as creamy, lightly adherent plaques on an erythematous oral mucosa, usually on the cheek, palate, or oropharynx. Occasionally they are symptomless, but more commonly cause discomfort on eating. These plaques can be gently stripped off, leaving an erythematous, eroded, or ulcerated surface that is often tender. Rx: nystatin (oral or topical) and chlorhexidine mouthwash as an effective adjunct to Rx. Amphotericin and miconazole are more expensive (and mutually antagonistic) alternatives. Fluconazole is the systemic drug of choice. *C. glabrata, C. tropicalis,* and *C. knusiei* are fluconazole resistant. Therefore, candida subtyping should be performed for resistant cases.

Acute atrophic (erythematous) candidiasis is an opportunistic infection following the use of broad-spectrum antibiotics and sometimes inhaled steroids, and in patients with HIV and those with xerostomia. It is painful and exacerbated by hot or spicy foods. The oral mucosa has a red, shiny, atrophic appearance and there may be coexisting areas of thrush. Rx: eliminate cause (if due to inhaled steroids, rinse mouth with water after inhaling).

Chronic candidiasis

Chronic atrophic candidiasis (denture stomatitis) The reported prevalence of denture stomatitis is 10–75%. Chronic low-grade trauma secondary to poor prosthesis fit, less than ideal occlusal relationships, and failure to remove the appliance at night all contribute to the development of this condition. The clinical appearance is that of a bright red, somewhat velvety to pebbly surface, with relatively little keratinization.

Angular cheilitis is a combined staphylococcal, streptococcal, and candidal infection involving the tissues at the angle of the mouth, often with an underlying precipitating factor, e.g., iron deficiency and B12 deficiency anemia. Therefore, hematological deficiency should be investigated with a FBC red cell folate, B12, and glucose. Anecdote suggests an inadequate occlusal vertical dimension (OVD) can also predispose, but correction of this alone will not resolve the condition. It is often associated with chronic atrophic candidiasis. Clinical findings are red, cracked, macerated skin at angles of the mouth, often with a gold crust. Infecting organisms can be identified on culture of swabs of the area. Rx: miconazole cream, which is active against all three infecting organisms. Rx needs to be prolonged, up to 10 days after resolution of clinical lesion, and carried out in conjunction with elimination of any underlying factors.

Median rhomboid glossitis is no longer considered an anatomical abnormality but a form of chronic atrophic candidiasis affecting the dorsum of the tongue. It is seen in patients using inhaled steroids and in smokers. Some patients have lesions in the center of the dorsum of tongue and palate (kissing lesions). Rx only if symptomatic, as discomfort can be improved with topical antifungals, but the appearance cannot.

Chronic hyperplastic candidiasis (candidal leukoplakia) More commonly seen in smokers. Typically presents as a white patch on the oral commissural buccal mucosa bilaterally. Although there is an ↑ risk of malignant change, the initial approach after ensuring the diagnosis (microbiologically and histopathologically) is to eradicate the candidal infection. Candidal hyphae can be seen in the superficial layers of the epidermis, which is one reason why eradication is so difficult. Rx: systemic antifungals such as fluconazole and itraconazole, while expensive, are indicated in an attempt to remove the infecting organism. This condition is often associated with iron, folate, and B12 deficiency and smoking, which should be corrected. Most lesions resolve after such Rx; if not, reassess degree of dysplasia.

Chronic mucocutaneous candidiasis A rare syndrome complex with several subgroups, including *candidal endocrinopathy*, where skin and mouth lesions occur in conjunction with endocrine abnormalities, *granulomatous skin candidiasis*, a *late-onset predominantly male-affecting group*, and an *AIDS-associated group*. Rx: fluconazole and itraconazole.

Histoplasmosis This and other rare fungal infections have occasional oral manifestations.

Recurrent aphthous stomatitis (ulcers)

This is the term given to a fairly well-defined group of conditions characterized by recurrent oral ulceration. There are three subgroups:

Minor aphthous ulcers A very common condition (~25% of population) affecting ~80% of RAS patients. Usually appears as a group of 1–6 ulcers at a time, of variable size (usually 2–5 mm diameter). Lesions mainly occur on non-keratinized mucosa and heal within 1–2 weeks without scarring. Prodromal discomfort may precede painful ulcers. Exacerbated by stress, local trauma, menstruation and may be an oral "marker" of iron, B12, or folate deficiencies. In some cases they could be a manifestation of Crohn's disease, ulcerative colitis, or gluten enteropathy. The etiology, although not fully understood, is almost certainly autoimmune. There is a familial history in 45% of cases. Rx: prevent superinfection with chlorhexidine mouthwash and relieve pain (simple analgesics, benzydamine mouth rinse). It is important to look for and treat any underlying deficiency or coexisting pathology.

Major aphthous ulcers are seen in 10% of RAS patients. This is a more severe variant with fewer but larger ulcers >10 mm that may last 5–10 weeks and most commonly affect keratinized mucosa. They are associated with tissue destruction and scarring, and any site in the mouth and oropharynx may be affected. There is an even higher association between major aphthae and gastrointestinal and hematological disorders. They are also seen in HIV-positive patients. Seldom is there a cyclical pattern. Rx: as for minor aphthae, plus topical or systemic steroids.

Herpetiform aphthous ulcers Least common. This is a descriptive term, as these ulcers have nothing whatsoever to do with infection with the herpes virus. They manifest as a crop of small but painful ulcers that usually last 1–2 weeks, the most common site being the floor of mouth, lateral margins, and tip of tongue. They heal without scarring and may occur on both keratinized and non-keratinized surfaces. They rarely merge to form a large ulcer, which heals with scarring. Rx: as for minor aphthous ulceration.

Behçet's syndrome A severe refractory, systemic vasculitis of unknown etiology, characteristically affecting venules. All organs of the body can be concurrently or consecutively affected. Recurrent oral aphthae are a consistent feature. It has a worldwide distribution, but is most prevalent in the Far East, along the Silk Route and in the Middle East. It is a disease of young adults, and rare before the age of 10 years and after 50 years. it is more common and severe in males. It is associated with HLA subtype, and is diagnosed clinically because of the absence of laboratory tests, and with the presence of recurrent oral ulcers and two of the following: recurrent genital ulceration, eye lesions (uveitis), or skin lesions (erythema nodosum, folliculitis). There is good evidence that prophylactic Rx with azathioprine can prevent blindness. Steroids are mainstay. Rx: ophthalmic referral if eye involved. Monoclonal anti-tumor necrosis factor (TNF) and similar agents may be of benefit. Thalidomide is effective, but neuropathy is a major side effect.

Oral ulcers See p. 468.

Vesiculobullous lesions—intraepithelial

Vesicle is a small blister a few millimeters in diameter.

Bulla is a larger blister.

Intraepithelial bullae are caused by loss of attachment between individual cells (acantholysis).

Subepithelial bullae separate the epithelium from the underlying corium.

Ulcer is a breach in the mucous membrane. Immunopathology: immunofluorescence is a prime diagnostic test. Direct immunofluorescence is performed on a fresh biopsy specimen. Indirect immunofluorescence is performed on a serum sample.

Erosions are shallower than ulcers.

Note: Because the vesiculobullous lesions constitute a defined group with examples from several different pathological processes, they are favorite examination topics. One method of classifying this group is into intraepithelial and subepithelial, according to where the blisters form.

Pemphigus is a chronic skin disease that is lethal if not treated. Oral mucosa is affected in 95% of patients with pemphigus vulgaris and may be the initial presentation of pemphigus in 50%. Autoimmune in etiology, there are circulating autoantibodies to epithelial intercellular substance. Acantholysis and intercellular IgG and/or C3 are typical (autoantibodies against desmoglein adhesion molecules of squamous epithelium) and cause separation of epithelium above the basal cell layer, and edema into this potential space produces a superficial, easily burst, fluid-filled bulla. Rupture leaves a large superficial, easily infected ulcer. The first identifiable lesions are quite often found in the mouth, especially on the palate, although these are usually seen as ulcers because the bullae break down rapidly. It is mainly a disease of middle age (F > M), with ↑ incidence in Semitic people. Rarely, it may be drug induced. Diagnosis: stroking the mucosa produces a bulla (Nikolsky's sign), but this is inducing pathology for the sake of diagnosis. Other methods are by direct or indirect immunofluorescent techniques (biopsy samples need to be fresh). Rx: systemic steroids and/or azathioprine, dapsone, mycophenolate mofetil, or cyclophosphamide (especially in refractory and severe cases).

Benign familial chronic pemphigus differs from the above by having a strong family history, with onset of disease in young adults.

Viral infections p. 430.

Epidermolysis bullosa Other variants are subepithelial. Due to genetic defect in basement membrane proteins. Skin blisters are due to mild trauma, leading to scarring and disfigurement. Caries and periodontal disease are common from inability to maintain good OH. Simplex type (most common form) is due to mutations in *K5* or *K14* gene, leading to disruption of basal cells and formation of bullae. Therapy includes avoidance of trauma, supportive measures, and chemotherapeutic agents.

Vesiculobullous lesions—subepithelial

Angina bullosa hemorrhagica This term is used to describe benign and generally subepithelial oral mucosal blisters filled with blood, which are not attributable to a systemic disorder or hemostatic defect. They are of unknown etiology, although steroid inhalers may predispose. Diagnosis: exclude other bullous conditions. Rx: puncture and/or reassure pateint (must differentiate from pemphigus/pemphigoid).

Benign mucous membrane pemphigoid is idiopathic and is also considered an autoimmune process with an unknown stimulus. It is most common in females >60. It presents as mucous membrane bullae, which rupture and heal with scar formation. It is rare to see skin bullae. Conjunctiva may be affected and if scarring occurs can lead to loss of vision, therefore regard oral signs as a warning to prevent ocular damage. The natural history is of a long-lasting disease that persists with periods of activity and inactivity alternating and may be quiescent for several years. Diagnosis: again, direct and indirect immunofluorescence is used, the antibodies being found at the level of the basement membrane. The bullae are blood filled and tense and may be found in conjunction with atrophic gingivitis. Positive Nikolsky's sign. Rx: topical steroids, systemic steroids, or dapsone. Refer patient to ophthalmologist.

Pemphigoid affects >60-yr age group. Subepithelial bullae form that are firm and less likely to break down than those in pemphigus because of autoantibodies to epithelial basement membrane. The oral mucosa is only affected in ~20% of patients. It may be an external "marker" of internal malignancy or a drug-related immune response.

Dermatitis herpetiformis is a rare, chronic condition of unknown etiology, but often associated with gluten sensitivity with autoantibodies against reticullin, gliadin, endomysium, and transglutaminase. Oral lesions are seen in 70% of patients with skin lesion. Common in middle-aged men, it affects both skin and mucous membranes; bullae in the mouth break down to leave large erosions. Rx: dapsone may be used for both diagnostic and therapeutic purposes. A gluten-free diet helps. Sulfapyridine is an alternative to dapsone.

Lichen planus is a relatively common, chronic mucocutaneous disease of unknown cause. It affects both skin and mucous membranes. In oral mucosa, it typically presents as bilateral white lesions, occasionally with associated ulcers. Among the many different types of lichen planus within the oral cavity, bullous lichen planus is a rare variant in which subepithelial bullae form and break down, leaving large erosions. Although lichen planus cannot be cured, some drugs can provide satisfactory control (e.g., corticosteroids).

Epidermolysis bullosa is a rare skin disease that exists in numerous different forms. The dystrophic autosomal recessive form is most likely to present with oral manifestations and appears shortly after birth. It is associated with bullae formation after minor trauma to skin or mucosa; these break down, leaving painful erosions. Healing is with scarring, resulting in difficulty in eating, speaking and swallowing, as scar tissue limits movement.

Skin involvement can lead to destruction of extremities and may be overtaken by carcinomatous change. Prognosis varies widely depending on type. Therapy includes avoidance of trauma, supportive measures and chemotherapeutic agents. Phenytoin and steroids may help some varieties.

Erythema multiforme This is a group of signs and symptoms of multifactorial etiology; the most severe form is known as Stevens–Johnson syndrome (p. 685). It affects skin and mucous membranes with an acute onset, usually in young adult males, and is probably due to deposition of immune complexes. It is associated with exposure to certain drugs (sulfas, barbiturates) or infecting organisms (herpes, mycoplasma) in a susceptible individual (hormonal changes). Diagnosis is from clinical features, which include "target lesions," concentric rings of erythema on the palms, legs, face, or neck. The oral mucosa is covered in bullae, which break down, the lips and gingiva becoming crusted with painful erosions. There is usually a fever. It is a self-limiting condition in 3–4 weeks, but can recur once or twice a year.

Management Hospitalization may be required in severe forms. Do biopsy; perform virological studies to exclude herpes; identify and avoid precipitating factors; acyclovir may be needed if it is related to herpes. Improve OH with chlorhexidine. Severe form: Rx with steroids. Minor form: Rx with topical steroids.

Linear IgA disease is a chronic autoimmune disease of skin that frequently affects mucous membranes, including gingiva. Oral lesions are ulcerative in nature. It may be a variation of dermatitis herpetiformis.

White patches

Numerous conditions manifest as white patches of the oral mucosa; some of these are transient, such as thrush or chemical burns (e.g., aspirin). More are persistent, and there is some confusion over the terminology applied to these white patches.

White sponge nevus This is an autosomal dominant condition that appears from keratin 4 and/or 13 point mutations. It appears as asymptomatic diffuse, soft, uneven thickening of the superficial layer of the epithelium, which characteristically has no definite boundary and may affect any part of the mouth. Histology shows hyperplastic epithelium with gross intra-epithelial edema. Rx: there is no specific treatment because it is asymptomatic, benign, and has no malignant potential.

Focal (frictional) hyperkeratosis This is a white patch due to hyperplastic hyperkeratotic epithelium induced by local trauma, e.g., sharp tooth and cheek biting. It is managed by removal of the source of the friction, which will generally allow complete resolution of the lesion. If this doesn't happen, biopsy is indicated. This condition can be seen as self-mutilation in psychiatric disorders or learning disability.

Smokers' keratosis Characteristically a white patch affecting buccal mucosa, tongue, or palate. It appears as discrete white patch and is due to a combination of low-grade burn and the chemical irritants of smoke; it is seen particularly in pipe smokers. There is little evidence that these patches are premalignant and they resolve with smoking cessation.

Nicotine stomatitis is most typically associated with pipe and cigar smoking, with a positive correlation between severity of the condition and intensity of smoking. It affects the palate, with numerous red papules on a white/gray base. These red papules represent inflammation of the salivary gland excretory ducts.

Syphilitic leukoplakia A white patch on the dorsum of the tongue is one of the classical appearances of tertiary syphilis (p. 429). Active disease must be treated; however, this will not resolve the area of leukoplakia, which has a propensity to undergo malignant change. Diagnosis is usually suggested by histology, serology, or dark-ground microscopy of smears.

Chronic hyperplastic candidiasis/candidal leukoplakia See p. 433.

Lichen planus See p. 456.

Lupus erythematosis See p. 457.

Leukoplakia See p . 442.

Hairy leukoplakia See p. 464.

Panoral leukoplakia is where the entire oral mucosa appears to be undergoing hyperplastic field change. There is risk of malignant change.

Oral carcinoma Occasionally, oral cancer may appear as a white patch, as distinct from a leukoplakia becoming malignant.

Skin grafts may appear as a white patch in the mouth and are a trap for the unwary in exams.

Renal failure can produce soft, oval white patches taht resolve on Rx of renal failure.

Darier's disease A rare skin condition whose oral lesions (present in ~50%) are coalescing white papules on gingiva and palate.

Pachyonychia congenita A rare genetic condition affecting nails, skin, and sweat glands. Oval, benign white patches on the tongue are common.

Pigmented lesions of the mouth

Oral melanin pigmentation ranges from brown to black to blue, depending on the amount of melanin produced and the depth or location of the pigment. Generally, superficial pigmentation is brown, whereas deeper pigmentation is black to blue. Diagnosis is aided by whether the pigmentation is localized or generalized throughout the mouth. Evaluation of a patient presenting with a pigmented lesion should include a full medical and dental history, extraoral and intraoral examinations, and, in some cases, biopsy and laboratory investigations.

Localized

Foreign body amalgam tattoo is the most common form of a localized dense blue/black area of mucosal pigmentation. It may result from implantation at the time of restoration or from a broken filling. It is radio-opaque, and may be palpable, but often is not. Amalgam tends to become granular and fragmented; if removal is planned, cut out as full-thickness wedge. If asymptomatic, diagnose and reassure. "Road rash" from grit after a traffic accident or graphite from pencils can cause similar pigmentation.

Local response to chronic trauma usually presents as an area of keratosis, but sometimes can appear pigmented.

Ephelis A freckle of the oral mucosa. Harmless.

Pigmented nevi Rare and benign, analogous to a mole. These are mostly harmless, and are most commonly seen on the vermilion border of lips and palate. If <1 cm, they do not change in size or color.

Peutz–Jegher syndrome Multiple small, perioral nevi.

Kaposi's sarcoma (p. 464) A radiosensitive tumor associated with AIDS.

Malignant melanoma Potentially lethal, relatively rare IO malignancy. It is very dark, has an irregular outline, and enlarges rapidly; it has a poor prognosis. A rare variant is nonpigmented.

Generalized

Racial pigmentation of the oral mucosa varies with skin type and is obviously not pathological.

Drugs Antimalarials, phenothiazines, cisplatin, zidovudine, busulfan and oral contraceptives can all cause mucosal pigmentation. The most common offender is chlorhexidine mouthwash, especially if "blended" with tea and tobacco.

Heavy metal salts These are now rare; they are classically deposited along the gingival margin in lead or mercury poisoning.

Endocrine associated Addison's disease, Adrenocorticotrophic hormone (ACTH)-secreting tumors, adenomatous pituitary dysfunction (Nelson syndrome), and ACTH Rx.

Hemochromatosis Hemosiderin deposits cause hyperpigmentation. Rare.

Black hairy tongue is caused by overgrowth of pigment-producing microorganisms combined with benign overgrowth of the filiform papillae of the dorsum of the tongue and a lack of normal desquamation. Rx: reassurance, improve OH, tongue scrape or tongue shave, depending on patient need and severity of condition.

Premalignant lesions

There is a group of conditions that have an ↑ risk of malignant transformation of the oropharyngeal mucosa. Although a great deal of attention has been paid to these premalignant conditions, it should be remembered that only a small number of oral cancers are preceded by them, and that the designation "premalignant" does not necessarily imply certain malignant transformation. Indeed, most patients with so-called premalignant lesions will not go on to develop oral cancer. The ↑ risk of progression to carcinoma necessitates accurate diagnosis, Rx if indicated, and long-term follow-up in an attempt to pre-empt life-threatening disease.

Leukoplakia is described as white patch or plaque that cannot be characterized clinically or pathologically as any other disease and is not associated with any physical or chemical agent except the use of tobacco (WHO).

The histopathology of these lesions varies widely from the essentially benign to carcinoma in situ. They are usually characterized by a thick surface layer of keratin with thickening of the prickle cell layer of the epithelium, acanthosis, and infiltration of the corium by plasma cells; however, the most important variable is cellular atypia among the epithelial cells. Pointers to look for are: nuclear hyperchromatism, an ↑ nuclear/cytoplasmic ratio, cellular and nuclear pleomorphism, ↑ and/or atypical mitoses, individual cell keratinization, and focal disturbance in cell arrangement and adhesion. The degree of cellular atypia is one of the most important factors to be considered in the management of a leukoplakia. However, histology of epithelial dysplasia is not reliable, and in one study pathologists in 20% of cases could not confirm or refute their own earlier diagnosis of dysplasia. Furthermore, there is no guarantee that the biopsy specimen is representative of the whole lesion. The second major consideration is the site, e.g., floor of mouth and ventral surface of tongue are more likely to undergo malignant change than most other sites. Third, relation to cause, e.g., buccal leukoplakia, in the preferred site for chewing tobacco and paan is at high risk if the habit is not discontinued.

On average, 5% of leukoplakias progress to carcinomas; however, in certain sites, e.g., floor of mouth, >25% may progress and certain variants, e.g., "candidal leukoplakia," have a claimed 10–40% incidence of malignant change. Diagnosis and treatment: referral to specialist is indicated—biopsy guided by toluidine blue to select the most appropriate area and Rx as appropriate. Malignant transformation is more common among nonsmokers (idiopathic leukoplakia): 2.4% are malignant in 10 yr, 5% are malignant in 20 yr, with a 50–100 times greater risk than for a normal mouth.

Erythroleukoplakia (speckled leukoplakia) This is basically leukoplakia with areas of erythroplakia. Exhibits an ↑ risk of malignant transformation.

Erythroplakia is generally a well-demarcated, red, velvety patch of the oral mucosa that histologically shows marked cellular atypia, no surface keratinization and a degree of atrophy of the surface layer. Most of these lesions are carcinoma *in situ* or frank carcinoma and are found at high-risk sites (>80%).

Erosive lichen planus is a comparatively rare variant of lichen planus, which some authorities believe to be premalignant. The common forms of lichen planus have no premalignant potential.

Submucous fibrosis is a condition found particularly in those of South Asian extraction, and is thought to be a tanning of the oral mucous membrane induced by betel chewing *without* the addition of tobacco (some cultures use betel leaf, areca nut, and slake lime; others add tobacco to this; the first seems to produce submucous fibrosis; the second, carcinoma). The mucosa is pale, with constraining fibrous bands, and fibrosis of the submucosa occurs, making the lips and cheeks immobile and resulting in trismus. Histology shows hyalinization and acellular dense fibrous tissue with narrowed blood vessels and a lymphocytic infiltrate. There is epithelial atrophy and cellular atypia. Pathogenesis is unclear; ↑ levels of copper due to areca nut chewing lead to cross-linking of collagen by up-regulation of lysyl oxidase, and thus ↑ fibrosis and DNA damage. Malignant transformation is seen in 10% in 10–15 yr. Rx: stop habit, intralesional steroids/exercise, or surgery with flap reconstruction.

Dyskeratosis congenita A rare autosomal dominant condition of pigmented skin, nail dystrophy, and leukoplakia evident in childhood. White plaques have premalignant potential (p. 456).

Patterson–Brown–Kelly syndrome (Plummer–Vinson syndrome) p. 684.

Management of premalignant lesions Record in detail, along with clinical pictures. Consider site, histology, age, and health of the patient, in conjunction with etiological factors, before deciding on long-term observation or active intervention. Convince patient to smoking and 60% of cases will disappear.[1] Observation may consist of clinical examination with repeated cytology (although cytology has generally been disappointing), or biopsy if change is seen. Guided biopsy with toluidine blue may ↑ diagnostic accuracy. Rx options: laser excision, cryotherapy, surgical excision, or topical bleomycin after removal of any identifiable etiological factors. Follow up at 3-month intervals.

Note: It is impossible to predict the behavior of a patch of leukoplakia with precision.

---

1 J Pindburg 1980 *Oral Cancer and Precancer*. Wright, Bristol.

Oral cancer

Cancer of the mouth accounts for ~2% of all malignant tumors in northern Europe and the United States, but ~30–40% in the Indian subcontinent. As much as >90% of these are squamous cell carcinomas. Globally it is the 6th most common cause of cancer-related death. Almost all gingival carcinomas are SCCs, and most are well differentiated.[1] In the United States, carcinoma of the gingiva constitutes 4–16% of all oral carcinomas and is predominantly a disease of the elderly, with persons <40 years of age accounting for about 2% of patients.[2] In other countries such as Japan, SCC of the gingiva is also the second most common carcinomas of the oral cavity, next to those of the tongue.[3] Even though oral cancer is mostly preventable, overall mortality rate is 50%.

Site The floor of the mouth is the most common single site, and when combined with lingual sulcus and ventral surface of tongue creates a horseshoe area, accounting for over 75% of carcinomas seen in European or American practice. Occurrence in M > F, although this difference is less marked than in the past, possibly because of changes in smoking habits between the sexes. It is an age-related disease, with 98% of patients >40 years of age.

Etiology The main etiological factor in cancer of the lip is exposure to sunlight, as with skin cancer. It is estimated that the risk of developing lip cancer doubles every 250 miles nearer the equator. Excessive alcohol and tobacco use are the important factors in the etiology of cancer of the mouth, showing a synergistic effect. Perhaps the most clear-cut etiological factor is the chewing of tobacco and paan. Late-stage syphilis is now an exceedingly rare risk factor. Immunosuppression, e.g., of renal transplant and HIV patients, ↑ risk of this and other tumors.

Clinical appearance Oral cancer is most often seen as a painless ulcer, although it may present as a swelling, an area of leukoplakia, erythroleukoplakia or erythroplakia, or as malignant change of long-standing benign tumors or rarely as cyst linings. Pain is usually a *late* feature when the lesion becomes superinfected or during eating of spicy foods. Referred otalgia is a common manifestation of pain from oral cancer. The ulcer is described as firm with raised edges, with an indurated, inflamed, granular base and is fixed to surrounding tissues.

Staging The **TNM** classification is most commonly used:

T	primary tumor		**N**	lymph nodes
T1	<2 cm diameter		**N0**	no nodes
T2	2–4 cm diameter		**N1**	single node <3 cm
T3	>4 cm diameter		**N2**	single 3–6 cm node (N2a), multiple
T4	massive, invading			nodes (N2b) or contralateral
	beyond mouth			node(s) (N2c)
			N3	node >6 cm
			M	distant metastases
			M0	absent
			M1	present

Survival is dependent on site, stage and comorbidity. The presence or absence of extracapsular spread of tumor in metastatic cervical nodes is the most important single prognostic factor.

Histopathology Almost always SCC. Characteristically shows invasion of deep tissues with cellular pleomorphism and ↑ nuclear staining. The presence of a lymphocytic response may have prognostic value, as does the manner of invasion (pushing or spreading). It can spread via local infiltration or lymphatic system (cervical nodes), and late spread occurs via the bloodstream. However, histologically similar tumors can show quite different biological behavior and this is a focus of current research.

Verrucous carcinoma A distinctive exophytic, wart-like lesion that grows slowly, is locally invasive, and is regarded as a lower-grade SCC, characterized by folded hyperplastic epithelium and a lower degree of cellular atypia. Surgical excision and/or radiotherapy is the Rx. Inadequate radiotherapy has been reported to induce more aggressive behavior.

Other tumors Malignant connective tissue tumors (sarcomas) are rare in the mouth, but fibrosarcoma and rhabdomyosarcoma are seen in children. Osteosarcoma of the jaws has a slightly better prognosis than when found in long bones.

Salivary gland tumors See p. 418.

Management of oral malignancy See p. 420.

1 K. D. McClatchy 1999 *Diagnostic Surgical Pathology*, p. 822, Lippincott Williams and Wilkins.
2 L. Barnes 2001 *Cancer of the Oral Cavity and Oropharynx*, p. 387, Marcel Dekker.
3 Y. Uchida 1988 *Jpn J Oral Biol* **7** 16.

Abnormalities of the lips and tongue

Although many diseases of the oral mucosa will involve the lips and tongue, there are a number of conditions specific to these structures, in part because of their highly specialized nature. The tongue is a peculiar muscular organ covered with specialized sensory epithelium, and the lips form the interface between skin and mucosa.

The tongue

Ankyloglossia (tongue tie) This is one of the most common developmental variation of the tongue and may be associated with microglossia. Rx: frenectomy.

Macroglossia is a disorder in which the tongue is larger than normal. Congenital; Down syndrome, Hurler syndrome, Beckwith–Weidemann syndrome. Benign tumors (e.g., lymphangioma) or acquired; acromegaly, amyloidosis. Most cases of macroglossia are treated surgically.

Fissured tongue Deep fissuring of the tongue is not pathological in itself (affects 3% of tongues), but may harbor pathogenic microorganisms. It is more common in Down syndrome patients than in the average population. Different fissure patterns are identified by various names such as scrotal tongue. The Melkersson–Rosenthal syndrome is a deeply fissured tongue in association with recurrent facial nerve palsy and swelling. Rx: no definitive therapy or medication is required. If symptomatic, patients are encouraged to brush the dorsum of the tongue to eliminate debris that may serve as an irritant. Additional consultation may be necessary if the patient exhibits manifestations of Melkersson-Rosenthal syndrome, particularly cranial nerve VII paralysis.

Hairy tongue A peculiar condition of unknown etiology, probably due to elongation of the filiform papillae, which may or may not be accompanied by abnormal pigmentation. Brushing the tongue and maintaining fastidious oral hygiene should be of some benefit (application of a 1% solution of podophyllum resin has also been described as a useful treatment).

Median rhomboid glossitis, See p. 433.

Geographic tongue (benign migratory glossitis, erythema migrans) This peculiar inflammatory condition of unknown etiology involves the rapid appearance and disappearance of atrophic areas with a white demarcated border on the dorsum and lateral surface of the tongue, giving it the appearance of moving around the tongue surface. It is due to temporary loss of the filiform papillae. Several clinical variants exist. A familial pattern is common; 4% have psoriasis. Rx: reassurance about benign self-limiting nature. However, when symptoms occur, topical steroids may be helpful.

Depapillation of the tongue also appears in a number of hematological and deficiency states, and in severe cases may also appear lobulated.

Sore tongue (glossodynia) may occur in the presence or absence of clinical changes; however, it should be remembered that even the presence of glossitis may not explain the symptoms of sore or burning tongue. The main causes of glossitis are iron deficiency anemia, pernicious anemia, candidiasis, vitamin B group deficiencies, and lichen planus. Sore but clinically normal tongue is a common problem and often psychogenic in origin; however, the first line of Rx is to exclude any possible causes, e.g., hematological deficiency states and unwanted reactions to self-administered or professionally administered medicines or mouthwashes.

The lips

Granulomatous cheilitis (orofacial granulomatosis) This is characterized by swelling of the lips and is histologically similar to Crohn's disease (non-caseating granuloma being found on biopsy, but no systemic features). Intralesional steroids, e.g., triamincinolone, 40 mg into affected lip, may help. Rx: clofazimine or metronidazole may produce resolution in granulomatous cheilitis. Intralesional corticosteroid (triamcinolone) injections may reduce swelling.

Persistent median fissure This may be found as a developmental abnormality but is usually secondarily infected, which is extremely difficult to eradicate. It may be associated with granulomatous cheilitis.

Sarcoidosis A chronic granulomatous condition that can affect any body system. Lip swelling, and gingival and palatal nodules occur. This may be associated with parotid gland swelling and fever, so-called uveoparotid fever or Heerfordt's syndrome. Although no specific cause has been identified, it has been suggested that this disease represents an infection or a hypersensitivity response to atypical mycobacteria. Biopsy reveals non-caseating granuloma with inclusion bodies. Chest X-ray shows hilar lymphadenopathy. Serum adenosine deaminase, angiotensin converting enzyme level is ↑. Ask an ophthalmologist to exclude uveal tract involvement. Rx: steroids, intralesional or systemic.

Actinic cheilitis Sun damage to the lower lip causes excessive keratin production and ↑ mitotic activity in the basal layer. This disorder is premalignant. Advise sun blocks.

Exfoliative cheilitis Similar to above, but of unknown etiology.

Dry sore lips Except when accompanied by frank cheilitis, this is usually entirely innocent and can be treated symptomatically. Common causes are lip licking, and exposure to wind or sunlight. It is also a manifestation of viral illness. Rx: lip ointment.

Peutz–Jegher syndrome See p. 684.

Herpes labialis See p. 430.

Mucocele See p. 376.

Allergic angioedema Severe type I allergic response affecting lips, neck, and floor of mouth. Usually an identifiable cause. Rx: mild—antihistamine PO; severe—treat as anaphylaxis.

Hereditary angioedema Defect of C_1-esterase inhibitor. Lip, neck, floor of mouth swelling, and swelling of feet and buttocks. Precipitated by trauma. Rx: acute attacks—fresh-frozen plasma (contains C_1-esterase inhibitor). Prophylaxis, stanozalol.

Kawasaki disease occurs in 19 out of every 100,000 children in the United States. It is most common among children of Japanese and Korean descent, but the illness can affect all ethnic groups. Kawasaki disease is an illness that involves the skin, mouth, and lymph nodes, and typically affects children who are under the age of 5. It can be treated if diagnosed early. The criteria include red, dry, cracked lips, strawberry tongue and erythematous oropharyngeal mucosa, bilateral conjunctivitis, cervical lymphadenopathy, generalized rash, and fever. If suspected, refer to a pediatrician.

Salivary gland disease—1

The salivary glands consist of the major glands (the paired sublingual, submandibular, and parotid glands) and the minor salivary glands present throughout the oral mucosa, but particularly dense in the posterior palate and lips.

Xerostomia Dry mouth can be both a sign and a symptom. Note that some patients complain of a dry mouth when, in fact, they have an abundance of saliva. True xerostomia predisposes the mouth, pharynx, and salivary glands to infection and caries. Common causes include irradiation of the head and neck, drugs (e.g., tricyclic antidepressants), anxiety states, and Sjögren's syndrome. Ideally, the management of xerostomia should include identification of the underlying cause. For those whose xerostomia is related to medication use, effective symptomatic treatment may be important to maintain compliance with their medication regime. Symptomatic treatment typically includes increasing existing salivary flow, replacing lost secretions, control of dental caries, and specific measures such as treatment of infections. For example, saliva substitutes (e.g., carboxymethyl solution and Glandosane spray), saliva stimulants, special dentifrices, and certain prescription drugs (e.g., pilocarpine and cevimeline) can be useful.

Sialorrhea/ptyalism Excessive flow of saliva. Rare, although apparent sialorrhea can occur with drooling due to inflammatory conditions of the mouth, or neurological disorders that inhibit swallowing. Rare causes include mercury poisoning and rabies. Rx options include behavioral therapy, surgical therapy, and radiotherapy.

Sialadenitis Inflammation of, usually, the major salivary glands. *Acute bacterial sialadenitis* presents as a painful swelling, usually with a purulent discharge from the duct of the gland involved. It may also develop as an exacerbation of *chronic bacterial sialadenitis*, which often exists as a complication of duct obstruction. Both conditions are almost always unilateral, and common infecting organisms are oral streptococci, oral anaerobe,s and *Staph. aureus*. Rx: exclusion or removal of an obstructing calculus. Radiographs with reduced exposure may reveal calculus, but 50% are radiolucent. Stimulation of salivary flow by chewing or massage helps chronic recurring sialadenitis. Rarely, loculated puss collection within the gland necessitates incision and drainage; USS can localize collection. Once the acute symptoms have resolved, sialography is indicated to define duct structure and may prove therapeutic. Other treatments include irrigating the gland with antibiotics and/or steroids. Recurrent chronic sialadenitis is an indication for removal of the gland.

Viral sialadenitis (↑ serum amylase and lipases) is an acute, infectious viral disease that affects primarily the parotid. It is transmitted by direct contact with droplets of saliva, and usually affects children and young adults with sudden onset of fever, pain, and parotid swelling. Classically, one gland is affected first, although bilateral swelling is the norm. In adults, the disease is more severe, with multisystem problems such as orchitis. Protection is now conferred by the measles, mumps, and rubella vaccine. Rx: isolate patent for 7–10 days. Rarely, sialadenitis can occur as a manifestation of allergy to various drugs, food, or metals.

Sialolithiasis See p. 419.

Recurrent parotitis of childhood Unknown etiology; congenital malformation of portions of ducts, and infections ascending from mouth following dehydration. Ages 5–9; recurrent unilateral parotitis with malaise. Eased by antibiotics. Resolves by puberty. EBV is implicated in etiology, possibly by structural damage to ducts. Rx: antibiotics, duct irrigation.

Salivary duct and salivary gland fistulae Communications between the duct or gland and the oral mucosa or skin may occur post-traumatically or postoperatively. Botox, duct repair, or gland excision may be needed.

Mucocele, ranula See p. 376.

Salivary gland disease—2

Sialosis A noninflammatory, non-neoplastic swelling of the major salivary glands (usually parotids). Of unknown etiology, although linked with endocrine abnormalities, nutritional deficiencies, and alcohol abuse. Sialography is normal. Histology reveals serous acinar cell hypertrophy. Rx: aimed at removing etiological factors. Diagnosis: exclusion of underlying disease by history, hematology, and biochemistry.

Sjögren's syndrome (secondary Sjögren's syndrome) is the expression of an autoimmune process that results in rheumatoid arthritis, xerostomia, and keratoconjunctivitis sicca due to lymphocytic replacement of lacrimal and salivary glands. When the connective tissue component is absent, the condition is called *primary Sjögren's syndrome (sicca syndrome)*. The etiology is probably autoimmune, and there is a 5% risk of malignant lymphomatous transformation of the affected gland. Diagnosis: antinuclear antibodies (70% +ve), SSA (70% +ve), SSB (40% +ve). Rheumatoid factor (70% +ve), ESR (↑), immunoglobulins (↑), and labial gland biopsy show lymphocytic infiltrate. Parotid gland flow, sialography, Schrimer test, and slit-lamp exam are all advocated, but once a diagnosis is established, all that can be done for the patient is symptomatic Rx and an awareness of complications. This includes artificial saliva, artificial tears, meticulous OH, Rx of candida, and patient awareness of the risk of lymphomatous change.

Salivary gland tumors 80% are benign; 80% occur in the parotid, and 80% of these are in the superficial lobe. The majority are *pleomorphic adenomas*, which have a mixed cellular appearance on histopathology. Although benign, the cells lie within the capsule of the tumor and satellite cells may lie outside of the capsule, creating a tremendous propensity for recurrence if simply enucleated. Any tumor in the superficial lobe of the parotid should be removed by superficial parotidectomy, taking a safe margin of normal tissue. *Lymphangiomas and hemangiomas* are the two common tumors found in salivary glands in children. *Adenolymphoma* is found almost exclusively in the parotid, and *adenoid cystic carcinoma* is more commonly found in the minor than the major salivary glands. Tumors of the submandibular, sublingual, and minor salivary glands are more likely to be malignant than those found in the parotid. Pointers to malignant change in salivary gland tumors are fixation to surrounding tissues, nerve involvement (particularly the facial nerve in parotid tumors), pain, rapid growth, and lymphadenopathy.

Rare salivary tumors include mucoepidermoid carcinoma and acinic cell carcinoma, both of which can behave indolently or aggressively. Monomorphic adenomas are benign, with many histological varieties.

Miscellaneous Lymphoepithelial lesion (Mikulicz's disease) is essentially an aggressive form of the Sjögren's syndrome without the eye or connective tissue component. **Note:** Mikulicz's syndrome is salivary enlargement of known cause.

Frey syndrome See p. 682.

Drug-induced lesions of the mouth

Local reactions

Chemical burns, such as from an aspirin tablet being held against the oral mucosa beside a painful tooth, are still seen in some patients. The burns are superficial necrosis of the epithelium and can appear as a transient white patch. Rx: re-education and removal of the irritant. The mucosa will spontaneously heal. Iatrogenic causes include trichloroacetic acid and phenol. Also caused by accidental ingestion of corrosives (e.g., paraquat).

Interference with commensal flora Prolonged or repeated use of antibiotics, particularly topical antibiotics, can lead to the overgrowth of resistant organisms, especially candida. Corticosteroids can cause a similar problem by immunosuppression.

Oral dysesthesia A sore, but normal-appearing, tongue can be caused by certain drugs (e.g., captopril).

Systemic effects

Depressed marrow function There are a wide range of drugs that will depress any or all of the cell lines of the hemopoietic systems and these in turn can affect the oral mucosa (e.g., phenytoin). Long-term use can result in folate deficiency and macrocytic anemia, which can produce severe aphthous stomatitis. Chloramphenicol and certain analgesics can induce agranulocytosis, leading to severe oral ulceration. Chloramphenicol can also induce aplastic anemia, which affects hemostasis, although spontaneous oral purpura and hemorrhage are a rare presentation.

Immunosuppression Steroids and other immunosuppressants predispose to viral and fungal infection.

Lichenoid eruption Classically associated with the use of gold in the Rx of rheumatoid arthritis. NSAIDs, oral hypoglycemics, and beta blockers are commoner offenders.

Erythema multiforme (Stevens–Johnson syndrome) See p. 685.

Fixed drug eruptions A drug eruption that recurs at a particular site or following the administration of a particular drug. These are extremely rare in the oral mucosa.

Exfoliative stomatitis Simply an oral manifestation of the very dangerous drug reaction known as exfoliative dermatitis, in which the skin and other membranes are shed.

Gingival hyperplasia Common in patients on phenytoin, cyclosporin A, nifedipine, and certain other calcium channel blockers. It is characterized by progressive fibrous hyperplasia, and while improved by OHI can reduce the incidence, it can occur even in the presence of meticulous OH. Rx: gingival surgery may be needed.

Oral pigmentation Black lines in the gingival sulcus are described as being a sign of heavy metal poisoning. Chlorhexidine causes a black or brown discoloration of the dorsum of the tongue, and some antibiotics can also do this. Tetracycline discoloration of teeth is well known.

Xerostomia See p. 448.

Allergic reactions Penicillin is a common offender.

There are a host of conditions affecting the oral mucosa that may be ascribed to the use of drugs. However, one has to pay attention to the reason the drug was given in the first place, and it may be that minor oral symptoms have to be tolerated when the drug is essential for the overall well-being of the patient.

Facial pain

Pain is an unpleasant sensory and emotional experience caused by actual or probable tissue damage. It is a complex process, and multiple signs and symptom are involved. The most common source of pain in the region of the face is the tooth pulp.

Trigeminal neuralgia is the most common neurological cause of facial pain. It is an excruciating condition, affecting mainly people over 50. It presents as a shooting, "electric shock" type of pain of rapid onset and short duration, which is often stimulated by touching a trigger point in the distribution of the trigeminal nerve. Patients may refuse to shave or wash the area that stimulates the pain, although strangely, they are rarely woken by it. In the early stages of the disease there may be a period of prodromal pain not conforming to the classical description, and it may be difficult to arrive at a diagnosis; patients often have multiple extractions in an attempt to relieve the symptoms. It is thought to be a sensory form of epilepsy, although some cases are due to vascular pressure intracranially.

Diagnosis is done by the review of history. Carbamezipine can be used for both therapeutic and diagnostic purposes, with an 80% response rate. In addition, injection of LA can break pain cycles and can be a useful diagnostic method. Cryotherapy can induce protracted analgesia, but sectioning the nerve rarely helps. For intractable cases, radiofrequency gangliolysis or decompression of trigeminal nerve intracranially may be required.

Glossopharyngeal neuralgia A similar condition to trigeminal neuralgia, but less common. It affects the glossopharyngeal nerve, causing a sharp, shooting pain on swallowing. There may be referred otalgia. Again, carbamezipine is the drug of choice.

• Patients under the age of 50 presenting with symptoms of cranial nerve neuralgia require full neurological examination and investigation, as these may be the presenting symptoms of an intracranial neoplasm, HIV, syphilis, or multiple sclerosis.

Temporal arteritis (giant cell arteritis) is an inflammatory condition affecting the medium-sized blood vessels that supply the head, eyes and optic nerves. This is a condition affecting older age groups. The pain is localized to the temporal and frontal regions and usually described as a severe ache, although it can be paroxysmal. The affected area is tender to touch. A major risk is involvement of retinal arteries, with sudden deterioration and loss of vision; underlying pathology is inflammatory arteritis. Tongue necrosis following lingual artery involvement has been described. Biopsy shows the arterial elastic issue to be fragmented with giant cells. Diagnosis: artery tenderness or decreased temporal arterial pulse, classical distribution of pain, and increased ESR. Rx: relieve pain and prevent blindness. Rx may involve systemic prednisolone, guided by symptoms and ESR.

Migraine See p. 493.

Periodic migrainous neuralgia (cluster headache) Similar etiology to migraine, but with different clinical presentation. Periodic attacks of severe unilateral pain lasting 30–60 min; located around the eye; associated with watering of eye on affected side; congestion of conjunctiva and nasal discharge are common. Attacks often occur at a particular time of night (early morning "alarm clock wakening"), and they tend to be closely concentrated over a period of time, followed by a longer period of remission. Most sufferers describe alcohol intolerance. Rx: O_2 inhalation, NSAIDs, ergotamine or sumatriptan, or intranasal lidocaine.

Pain associated with herpes zoster See p. 430.

Glaucoma gives rise to severe unilateral pain centered above the eye, with a tense, stony, hard globe. It is due to raised intraocular pressure. Acute and chronic forms are recognized. The acute form presents with pain and responds to acetazolamide. Patient will need ophthalmologist referral.

Myocardial infarction and angina may on occasion radiate to the jaws.

Multiple sclerosis may mimic trigeminal neuralgia or cause altered facial sensation. Eye pain (retrobulbar neuritis) is associated. Diagnosis depends on finding multiple focal neurological lesions, disseminated in time and place.

Atypical facial pain This constitutes a large proportion of patients presenting with facial pain. Classically, their symptoms are unrelated to anatomical distribution of nerves or any known pathological process. These patients have often been through a number of specialists in an attempt to establish a diagnosis and gain relief. This diagnosis tends to be used as a catchall for a large group of patients, with the connecting underlying supposition that the pain is of psychogenic origin. There may be a florid psychiatric history or undiagnosed depression; alternatively, the patient may simply be over-reacting to an essentially minor discomfort or recently noticed anatomical variant as part of a general inability to cope with life. Pointers to a psychogenic etiology include imprecise localization, often bilateral pain or "all over the place," and bizarre or grossly exaggerated descriptions of pain. Pain is described as being continuous for long periods with no change, and none of the usual relieving or exacerbating factors apply. Sleeping and eating are not obviously disturbed, despite continuous unbearable pain. Most analgesics are said to be unhelpful, and many patients refuse to try analgesics. No objective signs are demonstrable, and all investigations are essentially normal. After exclusion of any possible organic cause, the introduction of an antidepressant may (or may not) produce dramatic improvement in the pain.

Oral dysesthesia or burning mouth syndrome is an unpleasant abnormal sensation affecting the oral mucosa in the absence of clinically evident disease. It is five times more common in women aged 40–50 yr than in other groups. It is related to atypical facial pain. Diagnosis: by exclusion of hematological, metabolic, nutritional, microbiological, allergic, and prosthetic causes. With experience, the patient type often becomes obvious.

Bell's palsy is caused by inflammation of cranial nerve VII. Although the main symptom is facial paralysis, pain in or around the ear, often radiating to the jaw, precedes or develops at the same time in ~50% of cases. Rx: steroids and antiviral (acyclovir) drugs improve chance for full recovery if Rx is early (within 3 days of onset). If no Rx, 30% of patients will not completely recover.

Ramsey Hunt syndrome (p. 684) is associated with herpes zoster virus infection of the geniculate nerve ganglion that causes paralysis of the facial muscles on the same side of the face as the infection. Systemic acyclovir, corticosteroid and analgesics are used to manage this syndrome.

Oral manifestations of skin disease

Lichen planus is a chronic inflammatory disease of adults involving skin and mucous membranes. It affects up to 2% of the general population, with 50% of patients with skin lesions having oral lesions, and 25% having oral lesions alone. The oral lesions persist longer than the skin lesions. It affects females more commonly than males at the ratio of 3:2. It is an autoimmune condition mediated by a T-lymphocyte attack on stratified squamous epithelia, which leads to hyperkeratosis with erythema or striations. "Lichenoid eruptions" are an unwanted reaction to some drugs. Usually the oral lesions are bilateral and posterior in the buccal mucosa; it is not seen on the palate, but can affect the tongue, lips, gingiva, and floor of mouth. The most common oral lesion is a lacey reticular pattern of hyperkertotic epithelia seen bilaterally on the buccal mucosa. Other variants include coalesced plaque-like lesions. Six types are recognized: the reticular pattern, papular pattern, plaque-like pattern, erosive pattern, atrophic pattern, and bullous pattern. The skin lesions affect the flexor surfaces of the arms, wrists and legs, and are particularly common on the shin as purple papules with fine white lines (Wickham's striae) overlying them. Histology shows hyperparakeratosis, with elongated rete ridges with a saw-tooth appearance, a prominent granular cell layer, acanthosis, and basal cell liquefaction. There is usually a dense band of lymphocytes directly beneath the epithelium. Lichen planus can last for months or years. It can always be distinguished histologically and usually clinically from leukoplakia.

Lichen planus is essentially benign. Some controversy exists about the risk of malignant transformation; this risk has only really been identified in the erosive forms of lichen planus, and Rx of the erosive form is based on transforming it to the completely benign reticular pattern. Rx: distinction from leukoplakia, systemic lupus erythematosus, or malignancy is needed; if there are lichenoid eruptions, the implicated drugs should be identified and avoided if possible. If the condition is symptomatic, superinfection should be treated or prevented with chlorhexidine mouthwash. The first-line treatments are topical steroids, particularly class I or II ointments. A second choice would be systemic steroids for symptom control and possibly more rapid resolution. Many practitioners prefer intramuscular triamcinolone 40–80 mg every 6–8 weeks.

Dyskeratosis congenita A rare autosomal dominant condition, characterized by oral leukoplakia, dystrophic changes of the nails, and hyperpigmentation of the skin; the oral lesion is prone to malignant change (p. 442).

Vesiculobullous lesions See p. 435.

Oral manifestations of connective tissue disease

Ehlers–Danlos syndrome Rare inherited connective tissue disease characterized by hyperextensible skin, hypermobile joints, and fragile vessels due to mutations in collagen. This results in very easy bruising and bleeding of skin, as well as hypermobility. Oral features include severe early-onset periodontal disease, pulp stones, and occasional hypermobility of the TMJ.

Bleeding during surgery, weak scars, sutures pulling through, and difficulty with root canal Rx are the main practical points. Some types of Ehlers–Danlos syndrome can lead to an ↑ susceptibility to infective endocarditis and significant heart damage due to mitral valve prolapse, and some types are prone to cerebrovascular accident (CVA) due to weakness of intra-cranial blood vessels. Rx: aimed at the symptoms.

Rheumatoid arthritis Main associations are Sjögren's syndrome and rheuma-toid of the TMJ (10% cases), which may cause pain, swelling, and limitation of movement. Rarely, pannus formation within the joint may occur. Rx: three general classes of drugs are commonly used: NSAIDs, corticoster-oids, and remitive agents or disease-modifying antirheumatic drugs (DMARDs)

Systemic lupus erythematosus (SLE) is a chronic disease with many mani-festations. It is an autoimmune disease in which the body's own immune system is directed against the body's own tissues. The association with the presence of antinuclear factor is more common in females. SLE gives rise to skin lesions, classical malar "butterfly" rash, and oral mucosal lesions in 30%, which include ulceration and purpurae. Antinuclear anti-bodies are present. F > M. Arthritis and anemia are frequent.

Chronic discoid lupus erythematosus (DLE) The lesions of this condition are limited to skin and mucosa. It may present as disc-like, white plaques in the mouth and can progress to SLE, although it is more likely to remain a chronic and recurring disorder. Lip lesions in women may be premalig-nant. Rx: SLE—systemic steroids; DLE—topical steroids. Butterfly rash may be present. DLE can be distinguished from SLE by the presence of specific double-stranded DNA antinuclear antibody in serum. Rx: DLE recalcitrant lesions may respond to dapsone or thalidomide.

Systemic sclerosis is a chronic disease characterized by diffuse sclerosis of connective tissues, occurring in F > M. It has an insidious onset and is often associated with Raynaud's phenomenon (painful reversible digital ischemia on exposure to cold). Classically, the face has a waxy mask-like appearance. Eating becomes difficult because of immobility of underlying tissues, and dysphagia occurs from esophageal involvement. Autoantibod-ies are present. Circulating levels of E-selectin and thrombomodulin are useful markers in monitoring disease activity. Rx: combination of cyclo-phosphamide and steroids may help in early disease; penicillamine has always been used, but has numerous unwanted effects.

Polyarteritis nodosa is characterized by inflammation and necrosis of small and medium-sized arteries; necrosis at any site may occur and is seen as ulceration in the mouth. Up to 60% of patients die in the first year; Rx with systemic steroids ↑ the 5-yr survival to 40%.

Dermatomyositis Inflammatory condition of skin and muscles; 15% of cases are associated with internal malignancy. Tenderness, pain, and weakness of the tongue may be an early finding.

Reiter syndrome See p. 684.

Oral manifestations of gastrointestinal disease

Patterson–Brown–Kelly syndrome (p. 684)

Celiac disease This common form of intestinal malabsorption may present with oral ulceration as the only symptom in adults. Although children also present with ulceration, they are more likely to show weight loss, weakness, and failure to thrive. Other findings are glossitis, stomatitis, and angular cheilitis. Rx: hematological and gastrointestinal investigations are required, blood picture, and hematinic assay. ↑ malabsorption. Antibodies (Ab) to gluten, reticulin, and endomysium (antiendomysial Ab is marker for celiac disease); small bowel biopsy required for definitive diagnosis. B12, folate, iron ↓↓ should be corrected. Rx: gluten-free diet.

Ulcerative colitis (gluten-sensitive enteropathy) is a chronic inflammation of the large intestine. Ulcerative colitis is closely related to Crohn's disease. Gastrointestinal symptoms predominate. Arthritis, uveitis, and erythema nodosum also occur. Topical steroids and systemic sulfasalazine are used in Rx; low doses of thyoprine are effective in maintaining remission. Most of these patients are managed by gastrointestinal specialists.

Crohn's disease Chronic inflammatory disease affecting any part of the gut from mouth to anus. Primarily affects the terminal 1/3 of the ileum, although ~1% of cases will present with oral ulceration predating any other symptoms. These tend to affect the gingiva, buccal mucosa, and lips with purplish-red nonhemorrhagic swellings, linear, long-standing ulcers, and granulations. Granulomatous cheilitis is probably a variant. Painful oral lesions seem to respond well to simple excision, but Rx is aimed at the systemic disease.

Orofacial granulomatosis Clinically and histologically identical to oral manifestations of Crohn's disease. Probable etiology is a hypersensitivity response to certain foods, additives such as benzoates in toothpaste, etc. Rx: specific to the local problem; intralesional steroid. Most beneficial Rx is to identify and avoid the irritant factors. Patients who have generalized Crohn's or very severe orofacial granulomatosis may benefit from systemic Rx with sulfasalazine or TNF-α.

Gardener syndrome See p. 682.

Peutz–Jegher's syndrome See p. 684.

Cirrhosis Glossitis occurs in ~50% of patients. Sialosis is another association.

Oral manifestations of hematological disease

Anemia The nutritional deficiencies associated with anemia, iron, B12, and folate are all associated with *recurrent oral ulceration* (p. 434), and specific deficiencies may be present even in the absence of a frank anemia. *Atrophic glossitis* was formerly the most common oral symptom of anemia, but is less often seen now. Red lines or patches on a sore, but normal-looking tongue may indicate B12 deficiency. *Candidiasis* (p. 432) may be precipitated or exacerbated by anemia, particularly iron deficiency, and *angular cheilitis* is a well-recognized association. The sore, clinically normal tongue (*burning tongue*) is sometimes a manifestation or even precursor of anemia.

Patterson–Brown–Kelly syndrome See p. 684.

Leukemia This and other hematological malignancies are associated with a ↓ in resistance to infection. The mouth may be involved, either secondarily to this tendency to infection or as a direct consequence of infiltration of the oral tissues. The oral lesions of leukemia are painful and can lead to difficulty in swallowing. Prevention of superinfection with chlorhexidine mouthwashes and aggressive appropriate Rx of infections are of real help. There is an ↑ tendency to bleed, manifested as fine petechial hemorrhages or bruising around the mouth, and the gingiva may bleed heavily in the presence of only negligible trauma. Management of the bleeding is aimed at the underlying disorder; local techniques include improving OH, avoiding extractions, and using local hemostatic methods. Spontaneous gingival bleeding may be controlled by using impressions as a made-to-measure pressure dressing.

Cyclical neutropenia This condition may manifest as oral ulceration, acute exacerbations of periodontal disease, or necrotizing ulcerative gingivitis (NUG). As the name suggests, it recurs in 3- to 4-week cycles.

Myeloma Macroglossia is an occasional finding. Multiple osteolytic lesions in the skull are a classic appearance. Rarely, similar lesions are seen in jaws. Bisphosphonates are often used in myeloma and are a major risk for jaw osteonecrosis.

Purpura is due to platelet deficiency. It is most common as idiopathic thrombocytopenic purpura (ITP) in children. Palatal petechiae or bruising may be seen. Palatal petechiae are also seen in glandular fever, rubella, HIV, and recurrent vomiting.

Angina bullosa hemorrhagica Oral blood blisters; irritating but of no known significance (p. 436).

Oral manifestations of endocrine disease

Acromegaly Oral signs of acromegaly include enlargement of the tongue and lips, spacing of the teeth, and an ↑ in jaw size, particularly the mandible resulting in a Class III malocclusion. Treatment relates to a normalization of growth hormone levels, with concomitant preservation of normal pituitary function. The most frequently used Rx is transsphenoidal hypophysectomy.

Addison's disease (adrenal cortical insufficiency) may result from adrenal gland infection, autoimmune disease, or idiopathic cause. It classically causes melanotic hyperpigmentation of the oral mucosa, commonly on cheek. There is no Rx indicated for this lesion.

Cushing's syndrome A "moon face" and oral candidiasis are the common head and neck manifestations. Facial acne is also seen. Note a need for steroid prophylaxis.

Hypothyroidism Congenital hypothyroidism is associated with enlargement of the tongue, with puffy, enlarged lips and delayed tooth eruption. In adult hypothyroidism, puffiness of the face and lips also occurs, but there are no particular oral changes. Rx involves daily use of the synthetic thyroid hormone such as levothyroxine.

Hyperthyroidism Although the oral manifestations of this condition are not specific, they are consistent. In children, premature or accelerated exfoliation of deciduous teeth and concomitant rapid eruption of permanent teeth are often noted. In adults, osteoporosis of the mandible and maxilla may be found. Ocular proptosis is characteristic of Graves' disease. Rx consists of thyroid-suppressive drug therapy or radioactive iodine administration.

Hypoparathyroidism is the disease caused by a lack of parathyroid hormone. Facial twitching and paresthesia due to hypocalcemia can be seen. Occasionally delayed eruption and enamel hyperplasia can be seen. The goal of Rx is to restore calcium and mineral balance.

Hyperparathyroidism Rare. Caused by hyperplasia or adenoma of the parathyroid. ↑ parathyroid hormone causes ↑ plasma Ca^{2+} liberated from bone. Appears in the jaws as loss of lamina dura; a "ground-glass" appearance of bone and cystic lesions (often looking multilocular), which contain dark-colored tissue; "brown tumor" histologically indistinguishable from a giant cell granuloma. Surgery is the Rx of choice in most instances.

Diabetes No specific oral changes, although manifestations of ↓ resistance to infection can be seen if poorly controlled (e.g., severe periodontal disease). Xerostomia and thirst are prominent features of ketoacidosis. Sialosis is sometimes seen as a late feature of diabetes. Burning mouth may be a presenting feature, and oral or facial dysesthesia may reflect the peripheral neuropathies seen in diabetics. There is a tendency to slower healing following surgery.

Sex hormones Possible ↑ in the severity and frequency of gingivitis at puberty and in pregnancy. Some females have recurrent aphthae clearly associated with their menstrual cycle, and several symptoms such as burning tongue or mouth or general soreness of the tongue or mouth have been described during the menopause. It should be remembered, however, that there are profound psychological changes at this time of life in many women, and these symptoms may be a manifestation of atypical facial pain rather than a directly hormonally mediated effect. Hormone replacement therapy does not seem to help.

Oral manifestations of neurological disease

Examination of the cranial nerves, p. 492; general concepts of neurological disease, p. 494. Of the cranial nerves, the trigeminal and facial nerves contribute most to disorders affecting the mouth, face, and jaws.

Trigeminal nerve Ophthalmic lesions result in abnormal sensation in skin of the forehead, central nose, upper eyelid, and conjunctivae. Maxillary lesions affect skin of cheek, upper lip and side of nose, nasal mucosa, upper teeth and gingiva, and palatal and labial mucosa. The palatal reflex may be lost. Mandibular lesions affect skin of lower face, lower teeth, gingiva, tongue, and floor of mouth. Lesions of the motor root manifest in the muscles of mastication. Taste sensation is not lost in such lesions, although other sensations from the tongue are lost. Testing is performed by having the patient close their eyes and report on sensations experienced, in comparison to each other, while the areas of superficial distribution of the nerve are stimulated by light touch (cotton wool) and pin-prick (probe or blunt needle). Moving the jaw against resistance tests the motor branch. A blink should be elicited by stimulating the cornea with a cotton swab (corneal reflex).

Facial nerve is motor to the muscles of facial expression and stapedius muscle, is secretomotor to the submandibular and sublingual salivary glands, and relays taste from anterior 2/3 of tongue via the chorda tympani. It is tested by having the patient raise their eyebrows, screw eyes shut, whistle, smile, and show their teeth. Upper and lower motor neuron lesions can be distinguished because the forehead has a degree of bilateral innervation and is relatively spared in upper motor neuron lesions. Taste is tested using sour, salt, sweet, and bitter solutions. If taste is intact, flow from the submandibular duct can be assessed by gustatory stimulation. Test hearing to assess stapedius.

Neurological causes of facial and oral pain See p. 454.

Neurological conditions causing altered sensation 1) *Intracranial*—e.g., CVA, multiple sclerosis, polyarteritis, cerebral tumors, infection, trauma, sarcoidosis; 2) *Extracranial*—nasopharyngeal or antral carcinoma, trauma, osteomyelitis, Paget's disease, viral or bacterial infection, leukemic infiltrate. Psychogenic causes include hyperventilation syndrome and hysteria.

Neurological causes of facial paralysis Upper motor neuron or lower motor neuron; of the former, strokes are the most common. Combination lesions can be caused by amyotrophic lateral sclerosis (ALS) of the cord. Lower motor neuron paralysis can be caused by Bell's palsy (p. 455), trauma, infiltration by malignant tumors, Ramsay Hunt syndrome, or Guillain–Barré syndrome (postviral polyneuritis, may even appear to be bilateral). Apparent paralysis may occur in myasthenia gravis where abnormally ↑ fatigue of striated muscle causes ptosis and diplopia. Therapeutic paralysis may be induced for facial spasm, using botulinus toxin injected locally. Horner syndrome results in ptosis.

Neurological causes of abnormal muscle movement Tetanus is an obvious cause. Muscular dystrophy may present with ptosis and facial paralysis. Hemifacial spasm and other tics may be caused by a tumor at the cerebellopontine angle. Orofacial dyskinesia can be a manifestation of Parkinson disease or an unwanted effect of major tranquillizers. Phenothiazines and metoclopramide are notorious for causing dystonic reactions in young women and children. Bizarre attacks of trismus due to masseteric spasm have been ascribed to metoclopramide.

Oral manifestations of HIV infection and AIDS[1]

AIDS is the terminal stage of infection with the human immunodeficiency virus (HIV), which is recognized as undergoing a number of mutations. The underlying severe immunodeficiency leads to a number of oral manifestations that, although not pathognomonic, should raise the possibility of HIV infection.

Group I (strongly associated with HIV)

Candidiasis is seen in 60% of HIV patients as an early manifestation (p. 432). Erythematous (early), hyperplastic, pseudomembranous (late), and angular cheilitis is seen in young people (most common oral feature of HIV).

Hairy leukoplakia Bilateral white, nonremovable, corrugated lesions of the tongue are unaffected by antifungals, but usually resolved with acyclovir or valacyclovir and are associated with EBV. It is a predictor of poor prognosis and possible development of lymphoma.

Necrotizing periodontal disease (previously known as HIV-associated periodontitis) includes necrotizing uncreative gingivitis and periodontitis.

Linear gingival erythema (previously known as HIV-associated gingivitis) is seen in patients with increased immunosuppression and is not associated with pain, but is considered a potential precursor of necrotizing ulcerative periodontitis.

Kaposi's sarcoma (KS) was the most common malignancy among HIV patients in the 1980s, but is still occasionally seen. Rx: radiotherapy is effective. One or more erythematous/purplish macules or swelling, frequently on the palate.

Non-Hodgkin's lymphoma is similar to the above, and is less common.

With AIDS becoming a chronic illness after HAART, the most prevalent malignancies are anorectal, Hodgkins, melanoma and lung.

Group II (less strongly associated with HIV)

Atypical oropharyngeal ulceration

Idiopathic thrombocytopenic purpura

HIV-associated salivary gland disease (similar to Sjögren's syndrome)

Wide range of common viral infections

Group III (possible association with HIV)

Wide range of rare bacterial and fungal infections

Cat scratch disease

Neurological abnormalities

Osteomyelitis/sinusitis/submandibular cellulitis

Squamous carcinoma

Persistent generalized lymphadenopathy Otherwise inexplicable lymphade-nopathy >1 cm persisting for 3 months, at two or more extrainguinal sites. Cervical nodes are particularly commonly affected. This condition may be prodromal or a manifestation of AIDS.

Rx for AIDS AIDS is currently incurable, however, antiretroviral drugs prolong and improve quality of life. Early detection and Rx of opportunistic infections and neoplasms also have a major impact on quality of life.

Dental Rx for patients with AIDS This group present two risks with regard to dental Rx.

1 To personnel carrying out the Rx. Affected patients carry an infectious disease with no known cure, which is transmitted by blood and blood products. As it is impossible to adequately identify all such patients, routine cross-infection control is now a necessity.

2 As these patients are immunocompromised, any Rx with a known risk of infective complications (e.g., extractions) should be covered with antiseptic and antimicrobial prophylaxis, and any surgery should be as atraumatic as possible. There may also be a slight tendency toward bleeding in these patients, and local hemostatic measures may be needed.

Needlestick injury Combination therapy offers the best chance of preventing HIV seroconversion.[2]

1 S. Challacombe 1991 BDJ **73** 305
2 Consumers Association 1997 *Drug Ther Bull* **39** 25.

Cervicofacial lymphadenopathy

You cannot palpate a normal lymph node, therefore a palpable one must be abnormal. The most important distinction to make is whether this is part of the node's physiological response to infection or whether it is undergoing some pathological change. The finding of an enlarged node or nodes in children is relatively common and can be reasonably managed by watchful waiting. Undiagnosed cervical lymphadenopathy in adults mandates biopsy-establishing definitive diagnosis.

Investigations Routine EO and IO examinations to exclude the common causes: apical and periodontal abscesses, pericoronitis, tonsillitis, otitis, etc. The fundamentals are history and palpation.

History Ask about pain or swelling in the mouth, throat, ears, face, or scalp. Was there any constitutional upset when the lump appeared? Has it been getting bigger progressively or has it fluctuated? Is it painful, and how long has it been present?

Palpation Fully expose the neck and palpate from behind, with the patient's head bent slightly forward to relax the neck. Examine systematically, feeling the submental, facial, submandibular, parotid, auricular, occipital, the deep cervical chain, supraclavicular, and posterior triangle nodes. Differentiating between the submandibular salivary gland and node can be a problem, thus perform bimanual examination; the salivary gland can be felt moving between the external and internal fingers. Supraclavicular nodes are more liable to be due to occult tumor in the lung or upper gastrointestinal tract, whereas posterior triangle nodes are more liable to be hematological or scalp skin in origin.

- If a node is palpable, note its texture, size, and site, and whether it is tender to touch or fixed to surrounding tissues.
- Nodes that are acutely infected tend to be large, tender, soft, and freely mobile.
- Chronically infected nodes are soft to firm and less liable to be tender.
- Metastatic carcinoma in nodes tends to be hard and fixed.
- Lymphomatous nodes are described as rubbery and have a peculiar firm texture.

Supplementary investigations Examine axillary and inguinal nodes, liver, and spleen. Carry out an FBC to look for leukocytosis and a monospot test for glandular fever. Once infection is excluded, it is essential to exclude an occult primary malignancy of the head and neck; the best way to do this is by direct examination, flexible nasendoscopy, and CXR. If examination is limited, examine under anesthesia (EUA). Ultrasound-guided fine-needle aspiration cytology is recommended. MRI and CT scanning will confirm the presence, shape and size of nodes and may reveal occult tumor. MRI and CT cannot, however, confirm the pathological process within the node. If the diagnosis has still not been established, it is reasonable to proceed to excision biopsy of the node, which should be cultured for mycobacteria as well as examined histologically.

Common causes Dental abscesses, pericoronitis, tonsillitis, glandular fever, lymphoma, metastatic deposits, and leukemia.

Rare causes Brucellosis, atypical mycobacteria, TB, AIDS, toxoplasmosis, actinomycosis, sarcoidosis, cat scratch fever, syphilis, drugs (e.g., phenytoin) mucocutaneous lymph node syndrome (Kawasaki disease), and Crohn's disease.

An approach to oral ulcers

Even though oral ulceration is probably the most common oral mucosal disease to be seen, it may also be the most serious. Therefore, it is important to have an approach to the management of oral ulcers established in your mind.

Duration How long has the ulcer been present?
- If >3 weeks, referral for appropriate specialist investigation, including biopsy, is mandatory.
- If of recent onset, ask whether it was preceded by blistering. Are the ulcers multiple? Is any other part of the body affected and have similar ulcers been experienced before? Then look at the site and distribution of the ulcer(s).

Blistering preceding the ulcer suggests a vesiculobullous condition (p. 435) such as herpetic gingivostomatitis. Blistering with lesions elsewhere in the body suggests erythema multiforme, or hand, foot, and mouth disease.

Distribution If limited to the gingiva, consider NUG (p. 190). Unilateral distribution suggests herpes (p. 430). If under a denture or other appliance suggest traumatic ulceration.

Recurrence of the ulcers after apparent complete resolution is characteristic of recurrent aphthae (p. 434).

Pain Its presence or absence is not a particularly useful diagnosis, although the character of the pain may be of value. Pain is often a late feature of oral carcinoma, and the fact that an ulcer may be painless *never* excludes it from being a potential cancer.

Note: For most ulcers of recent onset and a few present for an indeterminate period, a trial of therapy is often a useful adjunct to diagnosis. This is especially useful in recurrent oral ulceration, viral conditions (where Rx is essentially symptomatic), and lesions probably caused by local trauma (Rx being removal of the source of trauma and review after 1 week).

Ulcers that need early diagnosis include the following:
- *Herpes zoster* Early Rx with acyclovir may reduce postherpetic neuralgia.
- *Erythema multiforme* To avoid re-exposure to the antigen.
- *Erosive lichen planus* This may benefit from systemic steroids or other specialist Rx and will require specialist long-term follow-up.
- *Oral squamous cell carcinoma*

Temporomandibular pain—dysfunction/facial arthromyalgia

What is it? The problem being addressed is pain in the preauricular area and muscles of mastication with trismus, with or without evidence of internal derangement of the meniscus. Conditions that can otherwise be classified as facial pain syndromes or other forms of joint disease are excluded and can be found on the relevant pages (pp. 410, 454).

Prevalence Affects ~40% of the population at some time in their lives, with F > M occurrence.

Etiology Idiopathic. Multiple theories have been put forward regarding occlusion, trauma, stress, habits, and joint hypermobility. To date, the concept of stress-induced parafunctional habits (bruxism, clenching) causing pain and spasm in the masticatory apparatus coupled with a ↓ pain threshold has seemed the most reasonable. This is compatible with the observed high association with back pain, headaches, and migraine. It does not explain the cause in those patients who can identify no different levels of stress in their lives, nor does it help explain the high incidence of internal derangement of the meniscus. The discovery of a biochemical marker (tyramine sulfate in the urine) in non-depressed TMJ patients has suggested that these patients are somehow biochemically sensitive to both mediators of damage in the joint, such as neuropeptides, and centrally (via serotonin) resulting in a lowered ability to cope with the local discomfort. The neuropeptide release can explain both joint pain and internal derangement (see Diagram 1).[1]

Clinical features Pain, clicking, locking, crepitus, and trismus are the classical signs and symptoms. Some patients may be clinically depressed, but most are not. Pain is elicited by palpation over the muscles of mastication and/or the preauricular region. Clicking commonly occurs at 2–3 mm of tooth separation on opening and sometimes closing. This is due to the meniscus being displaced anteriorly on translation of the head of the condyle and then returning to its usual position (the click). A lock is when it does not return.

Management Success has been claimed for a wide range of treatments, reflecting confusion over diagnosis, and the multifactorial and self-limiting nature of the condition. Simple conservative Rx within the range of every dentist is successful in up to 80% of cases (see Diagram 2).

1 *Reassurance and explanation* Advice as to the nature of the problem and its benign and frequently self-limiting course is all that many patients require. Do not create a problem where there is none! This is also the time to take a gentle but thorough social and family history to identify clinically depressed patients or those with significant stress.

1 M. Harris 1993 *BDJ* **174** 129.

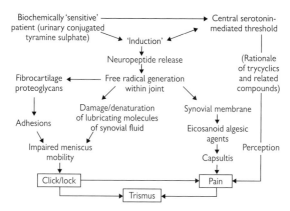

Diagram 1 Biochemical mechanism.

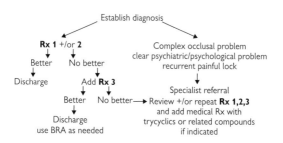

Diagram 2 Practice-based protocol for TMJ patient.

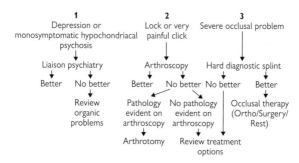

Diagram 3 Specialist-based protocol (once Rx 1, 2 and 3 have been clearly exhausted and tricyclics instituted, residual problem is usually one of three).

2 *Simple analgesia, rest, gentle heat, and remedial exercises* Whether these are performed by the dentist, physiotherapist (in the form of short-wave diathermy and ultrasound), or ancillary staff is unimportant, as the crucial part is that treatment is carried out by the patient at home by taking the analgesics and performing the exercises as instructed.

3 *Splint therapy* Upper/lower, hard/soft have all been used with varying success. The initial aim of a splint is to (a) show that something is being done (placebo); (b) ↓ bruxism and joint load; and (c) ↑ the gap between condyle and fossa, whereby the disc may be freed. A simple, full-coverage upper or lower splint should be worn as often as possible, nights and evenings especially, and reassessed after 4–6 weeks.

Note: These three simple measures should relieve symptoms in ~80% of patients and identify those needing referral to a specialist (Diagram 3). **Do not** persist with ineffective Rx if symptoms have not improved within 3 months.

4 *Drug therapy* There is a natural reluctance among many patients to take drugs. There is also a misconceived reluctance among clinicians to use the tricyclics and related compounds. They are non-addictive, and the common side effects of weight gain, constipation, and dry mouth can be overcome. Benzodiazepines are not recommended, but nortriptyline, dothiapine and related compounds have been demonstrated to have analgesic and muscle relaxant effects independent of their antidepressant effect, and probably work via the central biochemical sensitivity identified by the presence of urinary conjugated tyramine sulfate.

5 *Occlusal adjustment* There are some patients in whom a significant occlusal problem exists. In these cases a hard diagnostic occlusal splint can be constructed for the mandible or for the maxilla and should be made to give multiple even contacts in centric relation and anterior guidance. The patient is told to wear this full-time for up to 3 months. If pain is abolished while wearing the appliance, returns when it is removed, and is abolished on reinstitution, then occlusal adjustment by orthodontic, surgical, or restorative means is a reasonable option.

6 *Surgery for internal derangement* If pain can be abolished by other methods and the patient continues to be bothered by a painful click, particularly with recurrent locking, Rx aimed specifically at the meniscus is justified. The first line that may be useful diagnostically and improve pain due to capsulitis is arthroscopy. This is examination and irrigation of the upper joint space by a rigid endoscope, through which lysis and lavage of adhesions and synovial inflammatory mediators can be performed. Menisci damaged beyond the scope of arthroscopy can be repositioned at open arthrotomy. Consensus dictates that the minimum of interference to the articulatory surfaces and the avascular meniscus is carried out. Rarely, completely ruined joints will benefit from total joint replacement.

Medicine relevant to dentistry

Principal sources: C. Scully 1998 *Medical Problems in Dentistry,* Wright. M. Longmore 2002 *Oxford Handbook of Clinical Medicine,* OUP. Various 1995 *Procedures in Practice, BMJ.* HMSO *Prescribers Journal.* Medicine online BNF 44.

Note: All drug doses relate to fit adult patients ≅70kg (154 lb) in weight. Always check doses for children, the elderly, and those with other medical conditions.

Anemia

Anemia is a ↓ in the level of circulating hemoglobin to below the normal reference range for a patient's age and gender. It indicates an underlying problem and, as such, the cause of the anemia should be diagnosed *before* instituting Rx.

▶ Never rush into transfusing patients presenting with a chronic anemia. Perform basic blood work before giving iron or transfusing. Elective surgery in patients with an Hb <10 g/dl is rarely appropriate.

Clinical features of anemia are notoriously unreliable, but beloved of examiners and include general fatigue, heart failure, angina on effort, pallor (look at conjunctiva and palmar creases, but unreliable), brittle nails and/or spoon-shaped nails (koilonychia), oral discomfort and/or ulceration, glossitis, and classically angular cheilitis.

Syndromes, p. 680.

Types of anemia

Microcytosis (mean corpuscular value [MCV] <78 fl) Iron-deficiency anemia is by far the most common cause, from chronic blood loss (gastrointestinal or menstrual) or inadequate diet. FBC and biochemistry show microcytic, hypochromic anemia with a low-serum iron and a high total iron binding capacity (TIBC). ↑ red blood cell count (RBC) zinc protoporphyrin is a fast and sensitive early test. Thalassemia and sideroblastic anemia are rare causes of microcytosis.

Normocytosis Commonly, anemia of chronic disease. Other causes include pregnancy, hemolytic anemia, and aplastic anemia. Once pregnancy is excluded, the patient needs investigation by an expert. The TIBC is usually ↓.

Macrocytic (MCV >100 fl) Low B12 and/or low folate are the common causes. B12 is ↓ in pernicious anemia (deficit of intrinsic factor), alcohol abuse, small-gut disease, and chronic exposure to nitrous oxide. Low folate is usually dietary, but may be caused by illness (e.g., celiac disease, skin disease) or drugs such as phenytoin, methotrexate, trimethoprim, and cotrimoxazole.

Management In all cases the cause must be sought; this may necessitate referral to a hematologist. Drugs used in iron deficiency: ferrous sulfate 200 mg tid. Transfusion of packed cells covered with furosemide 40 mg PO if elderly or ↓ cardiac function, indicated rarely for severe microcytic anemia. Lifelong IM hydroxycobalamin 1 mg every 3 months is used to treat B12 deficiency, and folic acid 5 mg qid for folate deficiency.

▶ Never use folate alone to treat macrocytosis unless it is proven to be the only deficiency. **Note:** Folic acid is **not** the same as folinic acid.

Note on sickle cell anemia A homozygous hereditary condition causing red cells to "sickle" when exposed to low O_2 tensions, resulting in infarctions of bone and brain. In sickle-cell trait (heterozygous form), the cells are less fragile and sickle only in severe hypoxia. Management: perform hemoglobin electrophoresis (or Sickledex if result is needed urgently) on all Afro-Caribbean (and consider Mediterranean, Middle Eastern, and Indian) patients planned for GA.

Hematological malignancy

Leukemias are a neoplastic proliferation of white blood cells. Acute leukemias are characterized by the release of primitive blast cells into the peripheral blood and account for 50% of childhood malignancy. Acute lymphoblastic leukemia, the most common childhood leukemia, now has an up to 90% cure rate in favorable cases. It may present as gingival hypertrophy and bleeding. Acute myeloblastic leukemia is the most common acute leukemia of adults, but although an 80% remission rate is possible this is rarely maintained. Chronic leukemias have cells that retain most of the appearance of normal white cells. Chronic lymphocytic leukemia is the most common and has a 5-yr survival of >50%. Chronic myeloid leukemia is characterized by the presence of the Philadelphia chromosome, a fact beloved by examiners. It affects patients >40. Rx: interferon and and/or bone marrow transplant (BMT) or stem cell transplantation. Remissions are common, although a terminal blast crisis usually supervenes at some stage.

Myeloproliferative disorders are proliferation of non-leukocyte marrow cells, with a wide range of behavior and presentation, including anemia, bleeding, and infections.

Monoclonal gammopathies such as multiple myeloma are B-lymphocyte disorders characterized by production of a specific immunoglobulin by plasma cells. Multiple myeloma is also a differential Δ of lytic lesions of bone, particularly the skull. Δ: monoclonal paraprotein band on plasma electrophoresis, Bence–Jones proteins in urine.

Lymphomas A group of solid tumors arising in lymphoid tissue. They are divided into Hodgkin's or non-Hodgkin's lymphomas, with the latter carrying a poorer prognosis. Lymphoma should always be considered in the differential Δ of neck swellings.

Cytotoxic chemotherapy has been the mainstay of Rx for these diseases, with supplemental radiotherapy for masses or prior to bone marrow transplant. It is essential to remember that any patient receiving these drugs will be both immunocompromised and liable to bleed.

Hints In hematological malignancy, anemia, bleeding, and infection are the overwhelming risks. Look for and treat anemia. Avoid aspirin, other NSAIDs, trauma, and IM injections. Prevent sepsis, and if it occurs treat very aggressively with the locally recommended broad-spectrum antibacterials and antifungals, e.g., azlocillin 5 g and gentamicin 80mg IV tid plus fluconazole up to 100 mg daily. Consult with hematologist urgently.

Amyloidosis is characterized by deposits of fibrillar eosinophilic hyaline material in a wide range of organs and tissues. There are two types. *Amyloidosis* (AL amyloid), a plasma cell dyscrasia, has signs and symptoms including peripheral neuropathy, renal involvement, cardiomyopathy, xerostomia, and macroglossia. Rx: immunosuppression (rarely helps). 2° *amyloidosis* (AA amyloid) reflects an underlying chronic disease, such as infection, rheumatoid, or neoplasia. It may respond to Rx of underlying disease. Δ: biopsy of rectum or gingiva—stain with Congo red.

Other hematological disorders

For the practical management of a bleeding patient, see p. 355.

Bleeding disorders

Platelet disorders may present as nosebleeds, purpura, or post-extraction bleeding. Remember that aspirin is the most common acquired cause, its effect being irreversible for 1 week. Other causes include diseases such as Von Willebrand's disease; immune thrombocytopenic purpura (ITP); virally associated (especially HIV) thrombocytopenic purpura; thrombocytopenia secondary to leukemia; cytotoxic drugs; or unwanted effects of drugs, notably aspirin and chloramphenicol. Management: ensure platelet levels of >50 × 10^9/l, preferably 75 × 10^9/l for anything more than simple extraction or LA. If patient is actively bleeding, use a combination of local measures (p. 355), tranexamic acid, and platelet transfusion. Platelet transfusions are short-lived and if used prophylactically must be given immediately prior to or during surgery. Consult closely with the lab. The quality of preparation varies by locality. Tranexamic acid mouthwash may ↓ oral bleeding.

Coagulation defects present as prolonged wound bleeding and/or hemarthroses. Causes include the hemophilias, anticoagulants, liver disease, and von Willebrand's disease.

Others Less common causes include hereditary hemorrhagic telangiectasia, aplastic anemia, chronic renal failure, myeloma, SLE, disseminated intravascular coagulation, and isolated deficiency of clotting factors.

Hemophilia A (factor VIII deficiency) The most common clotting defect. Inherited as a sex-linked recessive, it affects males predominantly, but female hemophiliacs can occur. All daughters of affected males are potential carriers. It usually presents in childhood as hemarthroses. Bleeding from the mouth is common. Following trauma, bleeding appears to stop, but an intractable general ooze starts after an hour or so. Severity of bleeding depends on the level of factor VIII activity and degree of trauma.

Hemophilia B (factor IX deficiency) Clinically identical to hemophilia A; also known as Christmas disease.

Von Willebrand's disease A combined platelet and factor VIII disorder affecting males and females. Mucosal purpura are common, hemarthroses less so. Wide range of severity. May improve with age and/or pregnancy.

Management The hemophilias and Von Willebrand's disease should always be managed at specialist centers. Check the patient's warning card for the contact telephone number.

Anticoagulants

Heparin Given IV or high-dose SC for therapeutic anticoagulation. Its effect wears off in ~8 h, although it can be reversed by protamine sulfate in an emergency. Measure in activated partial thromboplastin time (APTT).

Warfarin Given orally; effects take 48 h to be seen. Normal therapeutic range is an International Normalized Ratio (INR) of 2–4. Simple extractions are usually safe at a level within therupeutic range. Avoid attempts to reverse warfarin with vitamin K unless *in extremis*. Use fresh frozen plasma if needed, but consider why the patient is anticoagulated in the first place.

Cardiovascular disease

This is the leading cause of death in the United States, with ~685,000 deaths occurring annually.[1]

Clinical conditions

Hypertension is a consistently raised BP (>160 systolic, >90 diastolic >3 months) and is a risk factor for ischemic heart disease, cerebrovascular accidents, and renal failure. Up to 95% of hypertension has no definable cause: essential hypertension. The other 5% is secondary to another disease such as renal dysfunction or endocrine disorders.

Ischemic heart disease is ↓ of the blood supply to part of the heart by narrowing of the coronary arteries, usually by atherosclerosis, causing the pain of angina pectoris. If occluded, myocardial infarction (MI) occurs (p. 506).

Heart failure is the end result of a variety of conditions, not all of them cardiovascular. Basically, the heart is unable to meet the circulatory needs of the body. In right heart failure, dependent edema and venous engorgement are prominent. In left heart failure, breathlessness is the principal sign. The two often coexist. There is an ever-present risk of precipitating heart failure, even in treated patients, by ↑ the demands on the heart, e.g., by fluid overload or excessive exertion.

Hypovolemic shock is collapse of the peripheral circulation due to a sudden ↓ in the circulating volume. If this is not corrected there can be failure of perfusion of the vital organs, resulting in heart failure, renal failure, and unconsciousness ending in death.

Murmurs are disturbances of bloodflow that are audible through a stethoscope. They may be functional or signify structural disorders of the heart. Echocardiography will differentiate.

---

1 http://www.cdc.gov.

Respiratory disease

Disease of the chest is an everyday problem in developed countries. The principal symptoms are cough, which may or may not be productive of sputum, dyspnea (breathlessness), and wheeze. The coughing of blood (hemoptysis) mandates that malignancy be excluded.

Clinical conditions

Upper respiratory tract infections include the common cold, sinusitis (p. 384), and pharyngitis/tonsillitis (which may be viral or bacterial), laryngotracheitis, and acute epiglottitis. *All* are C/I to elective GA in the acute phase. Penicillin is the drug of choi landular fever may mimic this condition and these drugs will produce ce for a streptococcal sore throat. Avoid amoxicillin and ampicillin, as g a rash of varying severity in such a patient. Epiglottitis is an emergency, and the larynx should NEVER be examined unless expert facilities for emergency intubation are at hand.

Lower respiratory tract infections Both viral and bacterial lower tract infections are debilitating and constitute a C/I to GA for elective surgery. Bear in mind TB and atypical bacteria, e.g., legionella, mycoplasma, and coxiella. Open TB is highly infectious and cross-infection precautions are mandatory (p. 676).

Chronic obstructive pulmonary disease (COPD) is a very common condition usually caused by a combination of bronchitis (excessive mucus production, persistent productive cough >3 months per year for 3 yr) and emphysema (dilation and destruction of air spaces distal to the terminal bronchioles). Smoking is the prime cause and must be stopped for Rx to be of any value. Be aware of possible systemic steroid use.

Asthma Reversible bronchoconstriction causes wheezing and dyspnea. Up to 8% of the population are affected; there is often an allergic component. Patients complain of the chest feeling tight. It may be precipitated by NSAIDs. Penicillin and aspirin allergies are more common. For management of acute asthma, see p. 515.

Cystic fibrosis is an inherited disorder whereby viscosity of mucus is ↑. Patients suffer pancreatic exocrine insufficiency and recurrent chest infections. Δ: by history and sweat sodium measurement.

Bronchial carcinoma Causes 28% of cancer deaths. The principal cause is smoking. ↑ incidence in females. Symptoms are persistent cough, hemoptysis, and recurrent infections. The 5-yr survival is only 13%.[1] Mesothelioma is an industrial disease caused by asbestos exposure.

Sarcoidosis most commonly presents as hilar lymphadenopathy in young adults. Oral lesions can occur. Erythema nodosum is common.

Dental implications

Avoid GA. Use analgesics and sedatives with caution; opioids and sedatives ↓ respiratory drive, NSAIDs may exacerbate asthma. Advise your patients to stop smoking (and if you are a smoker, stop). Refer if symptoms are suspicious, especially in the presence of confirmed hemoptysis.

---

1 http://www.cancer.gov.

Gastrointestinal disease

The mouth and its mucosal disorders and disorders of the salivary glands are covered in Chapter 9.

Esophagus presents symptoms that can be confused with those originating from the mouth, the most important being *dysphagia*. Difficulty in swallowing may be caused by conditions within the mouth (e.g., ulceration), pharynx (e.g., FB), benign or malignant conditions within the esophagus, compression by surrounding structures (e.g., mediastinal lymph nodes), or neurological conditions. It is a symptom that should be taken seriously and investigated by at least CXR, barium swallow, and/or endoscopy. Reflux esophagitis is a common cause of dyspepsia, sore throat, cough, and bad taste.

Peptic ulceration and gastric carcinoma (duodenal malignancy rare) may present with epigastric pain, vomiting, hematemesis, or melena.

Peptic ulceration is commonly due to infection with *Helicobacter pylori* and usually responds to *H. pylori* eradication therapy (combination of proton pump inhibitor, broad-spectrum antibiotic, and anerobicidal, i.e., metronidazole). Other causes include stress ulceration in critically ill or major-surgical patients, and elderly people on NSAIDs. Prophylaxis with sucralfate, a mucosal protectant, is more appropriate than H2 antagonists as the gastric pH barrier is maintained. Symptomatic relief of dyspepsia without significant ulceration is with antacids and alginates. Persisting epigastric pain or other symptoms *must* be investigated, as gastric carcinoma requires early surgery and carries a poor prognosis. ▶ Endoscopic investigation of patients >40 with persisting epigastric symptoms is mandatory.

Nonmalignant, *Helicobacter*-negative ulceration (esophagitis, gastritis, duodenitis) clears with 1 month of proton pump inhibitor Rx (e.g., omeprazole 10–20 mg qd) and can often be maintained with H2 antagonists (ranitidine or cimetidine).

Small bowel This has a multitude of associated disorders that tend to present in a similar manner—namely, malabsorption syndromes, diarrhea, steatorrhea, abdominal pain, anemia, and chronic deficiencies. Celiac disease and Crohn's disease are the best known conditions. Celiac disease is a hypersensitivity response of the small bowel to gluten and treated by strict avoidance. A number of oral complaints are related, typically "cobblestoning" of the mucosa. Crohn's disease may affect any part of the gastrointestinal tract but has a preference for the ileocecal area. It is a chronic granulomatous disease affecting the full thickness of the mucosa and may result in fistula formation. Ulcerative colitis is often mistaken for Crohn's disease initially, but affects the colorectum only. Treatment with systemic steroids and other immunosuppressants is common.

Large bowel Diverticular disease is a condition with multiple outpouching of large bowel mucosa that can become inflamed, causing diverticulitis. The irritable bowel syndrome is a condition associated with ↑ colonic tone, causing recurrent abdominal pain; there may be some psychogenic overlay.

Colon cancer is common in older patients; it may present as rectal bleeding, a change in bowel habit, intestinal obstruction, tenesmus (wanting to defecate but producing nothing), abdominal pain, or anemia. It is treated surgically, with up to 90% 5-yr survival if diagnosed early. Familial polyposis coli is associated with the Gardener syndrome (p. 682). Antibiotic-induced colitis results from overgrowth of toxigenic *Clostridium difficile* after use of antibiotics, commonly ampicillin and clindamycin. It responds to oral vancomycin or metronidazole.

Pancreas Malignancy has the worst prognosis of any cancer and most Rx is essentially palliative.

Acute pancreatitis is often a manifestation of alcohol abuse. The etiology is not entirely clear. It causes acute abdominal pain. Amylase levels are a guide but not infallible. Patients need aggressive rehydration, maintenance of electrolyte balance, and analgesia, in a high-dependency or ICU setting.

Hepatic disease

The main problems presented by patients with liver disease are the potential for increased bleeding, inability to metabolize and excrete many commonly used drugs, and the possibility that they can transmit hepatitis (Hep) B, C, and/or D (Hep A and E are spread by fecal–oral route). The liver is also a site of metastatic spread of malignant tumors. Patients in liver failure needing surgery, especially under GA, are a high-risk group who should have specialist advice on their management.

Jaundice is the prime symptom of liver disease. It is a widespread yellow discoloration of the skin (best seen in good light, in the sclera), caused by the inability of the liver to process bilirubin, the breakdown product of hemoglobin. This occurs either because it is presented with an overwhelming amount of bilirubin to conjugate (e.g., hemolytic anemia), or it is unable to excrete bile (cholestatic jaundice). Cholestatic jaundice in turn may be either intrahepatic or extrahepatic.

Intrahepatic cholestasis represents hepatocyte damage; this is reflected by ↑ aspartate transaminase levels on liver function tests, and results in impaired bile excretion, as indicated by ↑ plasma bilirubin. Causes include alcohol and other drugs, toxins, and bacterial and viral infections. A degree of hepatitis is present with these causes, whereas primary biliary cirrhosis and anabolic steroids cause a specific intrahepatic cholestasis without hepatitis.

Extrahepatic cholestasis is caused by obstruction to the excretion of bile in the common bile duct by gallstones, tumor, clot, or stricture. Carcinoma of the head of the pancreas or adjacent lymph nodes may also compress the duct and must be excluded.

Surgery in patients with liver disease

- Ascertain a Δ for the cause. Do hepatitis serology. Use cross-infection precautions (p. 674).
- Do coagulation screen. Patient may need correction with vitamin K or fresh-frozen plasma.
- **Always** warn the anesthesiologist, as it will affect the choice of anesthetic agents.
- If a jaundiced patient must undergo surgery, correct fluid and electrolyte balance, and ensure a good perioperative urine output by aggressive IV hydration with 5% dextrose and mannitol diuresis to avoid hepatorenal syndrome (see OHCM).
- Do not use IV saline in patients in hepatic failure, as there is a high risk of inducing encephalopathy.

Liver disease patients in dental practice

- Know which disease you are dealing with. If Hep B or C, employ strict cross-infection control (p. 674).
- Be cautious in prescribing drugs (consult the PDR) and with administering LA.
- **Do not** administer GA.
- Take additional local precautions against postoperative bleeding following simple extractions (p. 355). A clotting screen should be obtained for anything more advanced, and in all patients with severe liver disease.

Renal disorders

The most common urinary tract problems, infections, are of relevance only to those who manage inpatients. Rarer conditions such as renal failure and transplantation are, surprisingly, of more general relevance because these patients are at ↑ risk from infection, bleeding, and iatrogenic drug overdose during routine Rx.

Urine This is tested in all inpatients. "Multistix" will test for glycosuria (diabetes, pregnancy, infection), proteinuria (diabetes, infection, nephrotic syndrome), ketones (diabetic ketoacidosis), hematuria (infection, tumor), and bile as bilirubin and urobilinogen (cholestatic jaundice).

Urinary tract infections A common cause of toxic confusion in elderly in-patients, especially females. Send a mid-stream urine (MSU) for culture and sensitivity, then start trimethoprim 200 mg bd PO or ampicillin 250 mg qid PO and ensure a high fluid intake. Minimal investigations of renal function are U&Es, creatinine, and ionized Ca^{2+}.

Nephrotic syndrome A syndrome of proteinuria (>3.6 g/day), hypoalbuminemia, and generalized edema. Facial edema is often prominent. Glomerulonephritis is the major precipitating cause and investigations should be carried out by a physician with an interest in renal medicine.

Acute renal failure (ARF) A medical emergency causing a rapid rise in serum creatinine, urea and K^+. It may follow surgery or major trauma and is usually marked by a failure to pass urine (PU). *Remember* the most common causes of failing to PU postoperatively are underinfusion of fluids and urinary retention. Rx: ↑ IV fluid input and catheterize (p. 523). If ARF is suspected get urgent U&Es, ECG, and blood gases. Obtain aid from a physician. Control of hyperkalemia, fluid balance, acidosis, and hypertension are the immediate necessities.

Chronic renal failure Basically the onset of uremia after gradual but progressive renal damage, commonly caused by glomerulonephritis (inflammation of the glomeruli following immune complex deposits), pyelonephritis (small scarred kidneys due to childhood infection, irradiation, or poisoning), or adult polycystic disease (congenital cysts within Bowman's capsule). It has protean manifestations, starting with nocturia and anorexia, progressing through hypertension and anemia to multisystem failure. Continuous ambulatory peritoneal dialysis, hemodialysis, and transplants are the mainstays of Rx.

Main problems relevant to dentistry
- ↑ risk of infection, worsened by immunosuppression
- ↑ bleeding tendency
- ↓ ability to excrete drugs
- Veins are sacrosanct; **never** use their AV fistula.
- Bone lesions of the jaws (renal osteodystophy, 2° hyperparathyroidism)
- Generalized growth impairment in children
- Potential carriage of Hep B, HIV

Renal transplantation is an increasingly common final Rx of renal failure, and when successful renal function may reach near-normal levels. Kidneys are, however, immunosuppressed and at greatly ↑ risk from infection. They may share the problems associated with chronic renal failure depending on the level of function of the transplant.

Hints
- Take precautions against cross-infection (p. 674).
- Treat all infections aggressively and consider prophylaxis.
- Use additional hemostatic measures (p. 355).
- Be cautious with prescribing drugs (p. 546).
- Never subject these patients to outpatient GA.
- Remember veins are precious.
- Try to perform Rx just after dialysis if possible.

Endocrine disease

Addison's disease 1° hypoadrenocorticism. Atrophy of the adrenal cortices causes failure of cortisol and aldosterone secretion. 2° hypoadrenocorticism is far more common, due to steroid therapy or ACTH deficiency (p. 531). All need steroid cover.

Conn syndrome Primary hyperaldosteronism causes hypokalemia and hypernatremia with hypertension.

Cushing's disease and Cushing syndrome These are due to excess corticosteroid production. The disease refers to 2° adrenal hyperplasia due to ↑ ACTH, whereas the syndrome is a 1° condition, usually due to therapeutic administration of synthetic steroid or adenoma. Classical features are obesity (moon face, buffalo hump) sparing the limbs, osteoporosis, skin thinning, and hypertension.

Diabetes insipidus Production of copious dilute urine due to ↓ antidiuretic hormone (ADH) secretion or renal insensitivity to ADH. May occur temporarily after head injury.

Diabetes mellitus Persistent hyperglycemia due to a relative deficiency of insulin (p. 514).

Gigantism/acromegaly Excess production of growth hormone, before and after fusion of the epiphyses, respectively.

Goiter A large thyroid gland, of whatever cause.

Hyperthyroidism Symptoms of heat intolerance, weight loss, and sweating occur. Signs are tachycardia (may have atrial fibrillation), lid lag, exophthalmos, and tremor. The most common cause is Graves' disease (p. 682). Functioning adenomas are another cause.

Hypothyroidism Can be 1° due to thyroid disease, or 2° to hypothalamic or pituitary dysfunction. 1° disease is often an autoimmune condition. Symptoms are poor tolerance of cold, loss of hair, weight gain, loss of appetite, and poor memory. Signs are bradycardia and a hoarse voice.

Hyperparathyroidism 1° form is caused by an adenoma. 2° form is a response to low plasma Ca^{2+}, e.g., in renal failure, and 3° form follows 2° hyperparathyroidism when the parathyroids continue ↑ production, even if Ca^{2+} is normalized.

Hypoparathyroidism Usually 2° to thyroidectomy, when parathyroid glands are inadvertently removed. Plasma Ca^{2+} ↓, resulting in tetany. Chvostek's sign is +ve if spasm of facial muscles occurs after tapping over the facial nerve.

Hypopituitarism Can lead to 2° hypothyroidism or 2° hypoadrenocorticism.

Inappropriate ADH secretion Caused by certain tumors (e.g., bronchial carcinoma), head injury, and some drugs. Hyponatremia, overhydration, and confusion occur.

Lingual thyroid May be the only functioning thyroid the patient has; do not excise lightly. Do preoperative isotope scan.

Pheochromocytoma A very rare tumor of the adrenal medulla, secreting adrenaline and noradrenaline. Symptoms are recurring palpitations and headache with sweating. Simultaneous hypertension with a return to baseline on settling of symptoms is a good marker.

Pituitary tumors May erode the pituitary fossa (seen on lateral skull X-ray) and can cause blindness via optic chiasma compression.

Endocrine-related problems

▶ Always ask yourself "Is she, or can she be, pregnant?"

Pregnancy A C/I to elective GA, the vast majority of drugs (p. 546), and nonessential radiography. The most vulnerable period is in the first trimester. Elective Rx is best performed in the second trimester. Oral infections should be treated immediately. Elective treatment should be postponed until after delivery.

Menopause The end of a woman's reproductive life and her periods. It is often associated with hot flushes and other relatively minor physical problems. Emotional disturbances may coexist, and the incidence of psychiatric disorders increases at this time.

Related problems

Succinylcholine sensitivity Around 1:3000 people have an inherited defect of plasma cholinesterase. These families are absolutely normal in every respect except in their ability to metabolize suxamethonium. This leaves them unable to destroy the drug that, normally wearing off in 2–4 min, produces prolonged muscle paralysis. This paralysis requires ventilatory support until the drug wears off, which, in the homozygote, may take as long as 24 h.

Malignant hyperthermia A rare, potentially lethal reaction to, usually, an anesthetic agent. Characterized by ↑ pulse, muscle rigidity, and ↑ temperature.

Rare endocrine tumors

Glucagonoma Secretes glucagon causing hyperglycemia.

Insulinomas Secrete insulin. Cause sporadic hypoglycemic episodes.

Gastrinomas Secrete gastrin causing duodenal ulcers and diarrhea (Zollinger–Ellison syndrome).

Multiple endocrine neoplasia (MEN) syndromes A rare group of endocrine tumors. MEN IIb is medullary thyroid cancer, pheochromocytoma, and oral mucosal neuromas.

Bone disease

Pathology of the bones of the facial skeleton is covered in Chapter 8.

Osteogenesis imperfecta (brittle bone disease) An autosomal dominant type 1 collagen defect. Multiple # following slight trauma with rapid but distorted healing is characteristic. Associated with blue sclera, deafness, and dentinogenesis imperfecta (p. 69). The jaws are *not* particularly prone to # following extractions.

Osteopetrosis (marble bone disease) There is an ↑ in bone density and brittleness, and a ↓ in blood supply. Patient is prone to infection that is difficult to eradicate. Bone pain, #, and compression neuropathies may occur. Anemia can complicate severe disease. Facial characteristics are frontal bossing and hypertelorism.

Achondroplasia An inherited defect in cartilaginous bone formation, usually autosomal dominant. Causes a "circus dwarf" appearance with skull bossing; many have no other problems.

Cleidocranial dysostosis An inherited defect of membraneous bone formation, usually autosomal dominant. Skull and clavicles are affected. Multiple unerupted teeth with retention of 1° dentition are characteristic.

Disorders of bone metabolism

Rickets/osteomalacia Failure of bone mineralization in, respectively, children and adults. Either can be caused by deficiency, failure of synthesis, malabsorption, or impaired metabolism of vitamin D, and hypophosphatemia or ↑ Ca^{2+} requirement in pregnancy.

Osteoporosis A lack of both bone matrix and mineralization. Important causes are steroid therapy, postmenopausal hormone changes, immobilization, and endocrine abnormalities. Hormone replacement therapy (HRT) in postmenopausal women appears helpful. Results in ↑ incidence of #, especially femoral neck and wrist.

Fibrous dysplasia Replacement of a part of a bone or bones by fibrous tissue with associated swelling. It usually starts in childhood and ceases with completion of skeletal growth. This condition is termed *monostotic* if one bone is affected, *polyostotic* if more than one bone, and *Albright syndrome* if associated with precocious puberty and café-au-lait areas of skin hyperpigmentation.

Cherubism A bilateral variant of fibrous dysplasia.

Paget's disease of bone A common disorder of the elderly, where the normal, orderly replacement of bone is disrupted and replaced by a chaotic structure of new bone, causing enlargement and deformity. The hands and feet are spared. Complications include bone pain and cranial nerve compression, or, more rarely, high-output cardiac failure or osteosarcoma.

Diseases of connective tissue, muscle, and joints

Connective tissue diseases

These are mainly vasculitidies (inflammation of vessels).

Cranial arteritis (temporal arteritis) Giant cell vasculitis of the craniofacial region. The presenting symptom is unilateral throbbing headache. Signs are high ESR with a tender, pulseless artery. Major complication of temporal arteritis is optic nerve ischemia causing blindness, so start high-dose steroids (60 mg prednisolone PO od) and monitor using ESR. Biopsy confirms this condition.

Polymyalgia rheumatica More generalized vasculitis affecting proximal axial muscles. It accounts for 25% of cases of cranial arteritis, and responds to steroids, with gradual improvement over time.

Disease of muscles

Muscular dystrophy A collection of inherited diseases characterized by muscle degeneration. Most are fatal in early adulthood.

Myotonic disorders Distinguished by delayed muscle relaxation after contraction. They are genetically determined in a complex fashion.

Polymyositis A generalized immune-mediated inflammatory disorder of muscle. If a characteristic rash is present the condition is known as dermatomyositis and has an association with occult malignancy.

Joint disease

Osteoarthritis 1° degeneration of articular cartilage, cervical and lumbar spine, hip and knee joints, commonly affected by or 2° to trauma or other joint disease, resulting in pain and stiffness. Osteophyte formation and subchondral bone cysts, which collapse leading to deformity, are characteristic. Physiotherapy, weight loss, and analgesia are the mainstays of Rx. Joint replacement is definitive Rx.

Rheumatoid arthritis Immunologically mediated disease in which joint pain and damage are the most prominent symptoms. Morning pain and stiffness in the hands and feet, usually symmetrical, are characteristic. There may be systemic upset and anemia. Ulnar deviation of the fingers is pathognomonic. Rx includes NSAIDs, steroids, and physiotherapy. Second-line or disease-modifying antirheumatic drugs may favorably influence outcome at the expense of unwanted effects, e.g., penicillamine, antimalarials, immunosuppressants. Dry eyes and mouth may be associated with rheumatoid arthritis (Sjögren syndrome, p. 685). TMJ symptoms are rare in rheumatoid arthritis, although up to 15% of patients have radiographic changes in the joint.

Juvenile rheumatoid arthritis Rarer form of the disease that affects children. It can be much more severe than the adult condition and can cause TMJ ankylosis.

Psoriatic arthritis Associated with the skin condition and affects the spine and pelvis. It is milder than rheumatoid arthritis and has no serological abnormalities. The TMJ can be affected, but symptoms are usually mild despite some isolated case reports to the contrary.

Gout Urates are deposited in joints, causing sudden, severe joint pain, often in the big toe. Affected joints are red, swollen, and very tender. Gout 2° to drugs, radiotherapy, or hematological disease is more common than that caused by an inborne error of metabolism.

Ankylosing spondylitis Affects the spine, usually in young men. Inflammation involves the insertion of ligaments and tendons. It is associated with HLA-B27. Later, kyphotic deformity and increased risk of cervical fractures occur.

Reiter syndrome Seronegative arthritis, urethritis, and conjunctivitis, usually in response to an infection. Oral lesions are often present. There are genital and intestinal variants.

Legg Calve Perthes' disease Osteochondritis with avascular necrosis of the femoral head in, mainly, boys aged 3–11 yr. There are no systemic implications.

Neurological disorders

Cranial nerves

- **Olfactory** Sense of smell is rarely tested, although damage is quite common following head and/or mid-face trauma.
- **Optic** Examine the pupils for both direct and consensual reflex; assess the visual fields; check visual acuity and examine the fundus with an opthalmoscope (p. 10).
- **Oculomotor** The motor supply to the extraocular muscles *except* lateral rectus and superior oblique. It supplies the ciliary muscle, the constrictor of the pupil, and levator palpebre superioris. A defect ∴ causes impairment of upward, downward, and inward movement of the eye, leading to diplopia, drooping of the upper eyelid (ptosis), and absent direct and preserved consensual reflexes.
- **Trochlear** Supplies superior oblique, paralysis of which causes diplopia; worst on looking downward and inward.
- **Trigeminal** Major sensory nerve to the face, oral, nasal, conjunctival, and sinus mucosa, and part of the tympanic membrane. It is motor to the muscles of mastication. Sensory abnormalities are mapped out using gentle touch and pin-prick. Motor weakness is best assessed on jaw opening and excursion.
- **Abducens** Supplies lateral rectus. A defect causes paralysis of abduction of the eye.
- **Facial** Motor to the muscles of facial expression. It supplies taste from the anterior 2/3 of the tongue (via chorda tympani) and is secretomotor to the lacrimal, sublingual, and submandibular glands. It innervates the stapedius muscle in the middle ear. The lower face is innervated by the contralateral motor cortex, whereas the upper face has bilateral innervation. Assess by demonstrating facial movements.
- **Vestibulocochlear** Is sensory for balance and hearing. Deafness, vertigo, and tinnitus are the main symptoms.
- **Glossopharyngeal** Supplies sensation and taste from the posterior 1/3 of the tongue, motor to stylopharyngeus, and secretomotor to the parotid. Lesions impair the gag reflex in conjunction with vagus.
- **Vagus** Has a motor input to the palatal, pharyngeal, and laryngeal muscles. Impaired gag reflex, hoarseness, and deviation of the soft palate to the unaffected side are seen if damaged. The vagus has a huge parasympathetic output to the viscera of the thorax and abdomen.
- **Accessory** Is motor to sternomastoid and trapezius, causing weakness on shoulder shrugging and on turning the head away from the affected side.
- **Hypoglossal** Motor supply to the tongue. Lesions cause dysarthria (impaired speech) and deviation toward the affected side on protrusion.

Headache

The vast majority of headaches are benign; the secret is to pick out those that are not.

Tension headache Most common type, due to muscle tension in occipitofrontalis. It is usually worse as the day progresses, and may feel "band-like." It responds to reassurance, anxiolytics, and analgesics.

Migraine A distinct entity characterized by a preceding visual aura (fortification spectra). It is a severe, usually unilateral headache with photophobia, nausea, and vomiting. Migraine is thought to be due to cerebral vasoconstriction, followed by reflex vasodilation (the latter is the cause of the pain). F > M incidence, the oral contraceptive being a contributing factor. There are many variants of classical migraine.

Migrainous neuralgia Rarer than migraine and causes localized pain, usually around the eye, with associated nasal stuffiness. M > F incidence. There is a typical time of onset, often in early morning, which recurs for several weeks, called "clustering." Alcohol is a common precipitant.

Raised intracranial pressure (ICP) A cause of headache demanding urgent further investigation. Pointers are headache, which is worse on waking, irritation, ↓ level of consciousness, vomiting, sluggish or absent pupillary reflexes, and bulging of the optic disc (papilledema). *Rising BP and slowing pulse* are late premorbid signs of ↑ ICP.

Medication misuse headache Affects up to 1:50. It presents as a daily headache due to excessive or regular use of over-the-counter (OTC) analgesics (especially codeine-containing) and some antimigraine preparations. Pain pathways may be altered and after withdrawal of the drug the headache may be slow to resolve.

Rare and wonderful headaches Ice-cream headache, postcoital headache, needle-through-eye headache, and many other distinctive and benign headaches are described.

More neurological disorders

Central nervous system (CNS) infections

Bacterial meningitis Must be considered in the differential Δ of headache with photophobia and neck stiffness. Organisms are *Hemophilus influenza*, *Neisseria meningitidis* (meningococcus), *N. gonorrhea*, and *Streptococcus pneumonia*. In children, the meningococcus is especially important and classically associated with a non-blanching purpuric rash. This is one of the very few indications for instituting immediate blind antibiotic therapy (parenteral penicillin).

Viral meningitis Usually mild and self-limiting. Distinguished from bacterial meningitis by lumbar puncture.

Herpetic encephalitis A rare manifestation of infection with the herpes simplex virus. Can be distinguished from drunkenness or dementia by history and rapid onset. Parenteral aciclovir can be curative.

CNS tumors Most brain tumors are 2° deposits. Although both benign and malignant primary tumors are found, they are rare. Despite this, they are the most common cause of cancer death in children after leukemia.

Epilepsy An episodic outflow from the brain causing disturbances of consciousness, motor, and sensory function. Most causes are idiopathic, but those with onset in adult life must be investigated for local or general cerebral disease. Major or *grand mal* epilepsy is characterized by an aura and loss of consciousness, and followed by tonic and clonic phases. Incontinence is a good guide to a genuine seizure. The seizure rarely lasts >5 min; if it does, the patient has entered status epilepticus (p. 513).

Petit mal (absence attacks) Epileptic attacks usually confined to children, taking the form of a short absence when movement, speech, and attention cease.

Temporal lobe epilepsy Characterized by hallucinations of the special senses.

Localized (Jacksonian) epilepsy Affects limbs in isolation. Patients with established epilepsy (once any treatable cause has been excluded) must be maintained on adequate levels of antiepileptic drugs.

Febrile convulsions Fits, usually in children >5 years old, 2° to pyrexia.

Cerebrovascular accidents (CVA; strokes) A very common cause of death in the elderly. A stroke is basically death of part of the brain following cerebral ischemia, due to either bleeding into the brain or occlusion of vessels. It is often clinically difficult to distinguish these different types of stroke. CT scanning is of value when Rx is to be attempted to decide if there is an infarct or hemorrhage, but wait 24 h after symptoms to allow infarct to become visible on scan. Cerebral angiography defines the source of subarachnoid bleeds.

Multiple sclerosis[1] A disorder characterized by demyelination in multiple "plaques" throughout the CNS. Symptoms are multiple and disseminated in both time and place. It is the most common neurological disease of young adults. MRI helps in Δ but is not specific. Currently there is no cure; hyperbaric therapy and interferon remain controversial. Progress, although relentless, is widely variable.

Myasthenia gravis[2] Muscle weakness due to inadequate response to, or levels of, acetylcholine. Extraoccular muscles are often first affected. MG is diagnosed using the edrophonium or tensilon test.

Parkinson disease[3] A disease that results from a loss of dopamine producing cells. It is characterized by tremor, rigidity, and bradykinesis with a shuffling gait.

1 https://www.ninds.nih.gov/disorders/multiple_sclerosis
2 https://www.myasthenia.org
3 https://www.parkinson.org

Skin neoplasms

▶ The skin of the face is the most common site of curable skin cancers, so look and think.

Basal cell carcinoma (BCC; epithelioma, rodent ulcer) An indolent skin cancer that very rarely metastasizes. If it kills it does so by local destruction. Chronic exposure to sunlight is a major etiological factor. There are various forms, the most common being an ulcerated nodule with raised pearly margins and a telangiectatic surface. Rx: excision (micrographic or conventional), radiotherapy (especially electron beam), cryotherapy, curretage, and electrodessication.

SCC of the skin is surprisingly indolent in comparison to SCC of mucosa. It presents as an ulcerated lesion with raised edges. Keratin horns may be present, and it may arise in areas of previously sun-damaged skin or in gravitational leg ulcers. Surgical excision or radiotherapy are the Rx of choice.

Malignant melanoma This condition is being increasingly diagnosed, with a doubling of the incidence in the last 20 yr. The prognosis is dependent primarily on the depth of the tumor, as the thicker the lesion the poorer the prognosis. Early metastasis is common. Sunlight is a major etiological factor, possibly due to burning at early age. Suspect it if a pigmented lesion rapidly enlarges, bleeds, ulcerates, shows "satellite" lesions, or changes color. Prompt referral for specialist management is needed.

Nevi Areas of skin containing a disproportionate number of melanocytes.

Lentigo simplex A freckle.

Dysplastic nevi Premalignant lesions often found in patients with malignant melanoma. They should be excised and patients advised to use high-factor sunscreens.

Lentigo maligna A premalignant, pigmented lesion of the elderly.

Carcinoma in situ Presents as a scaly, red plaque. It is basically a squamous carcinoma that has not yet penetrated beyond the basal layer.

Actinic keratosis Persistently sun-damaged areas of skin in which cancer may arise.

Kaposi's sarcoma A purple, vascular, multifocal malignant tumor typically seen in AIDS and other immunocompromised patients. Also seen intraorally.

Metastatic deposits to the skin occur most frequently from breast, kidney, and lung, but skin secondaries from oral cancer are being seen increasingly.

Dermatology

Psoriasis A common, relapsing, proliferative inflammatory skin disease. It appears as a red plaque with silvery scale, chiefly on extensor skin of the knees and elbows, although any area can be affected. It can be associated with systemic disease, particularly arthropathy (p. 490). Rx is mainly topical: steroids, coal tar, dithranol, and/or UVB radiation can be used.

Eczema Also called dermatitis. It has several variants according to etiology.

Atopic eczema Starts in the first year of life with a red symmetrical scaly rash. Emulsifying ointments help prevent fissuring, although steroids are sometimes needed. Up to 90% of patients grow out of it by age 12.

Exogenous eczema Can be produced in anyone exposed to a sufficient irritant. The hands are the usual target, with blistering, erythema, and cracking of skin.

Allergic contact eczema A genuine allergic response, e.g., to nickel.

Seborrheic eczema A fungal infection mainly affecting the scalp ("cradle cap") in neonates.

Skin infections Fungal infections are particularly common, causing angular cheilitis, athlete's foot, paronychia, vaginitis, etc. Furuncles are staphylococcal boils. Erysipelas is a streptococcal cellulitis. Viruses cause herpes zoster and simplex infections, molluscum contagiosum, and warts.

Infestations of the skin bring a shudder to most people, but they are also a hazard of working closely with patients! Head lice respond to malathion. Flea bites, as well as being unpleasant, can spread plague, among other serious diseases. Scabies is an infestation with a mite that creates a characteristic itchy burrow in the finger webs.

Acne Acne vulgaris is characterized by the blackhead (comedone), and is an inflammatory condition caused by increased sebum secretion. Acne is hormone dependent, although superinfection with the acne bacillus is a contributing factor. It tends to scar. After proprietary lotions, low-dose tetracyclines help. The RetiN-A is useful in severe and late-onset acne unresponsive to other Rx.

The skin and internal disease

The skin, like the mouth, acts as an outside indicator for many internal diseases.

Erythema nodosum Painful, red, nodular lumps on the shins.

Erythema multiforme Circular target lesions.

Erythema marginatum Vanishing and recurring pink rings. These are all nonspecific markers for a variety of diseases.

Vitiligo An autoimmune hypopigmentation, associated with other autoimmune conditions.

Pyoderma gangrenosum Blue-edged ulcers, especially on the legs. They are associated with ulcerative colitis and Crohn's disease.

Granuloma annulare Subcutaneous circular thickening and *necrobiosis lipoidica* (yellow plaques on the shins) are associated with diabetes.

Dermatitis herpetiformis Vesicular rash of knees, elbows, and scalp. It is associated with celiac disease.

Pretibial myxedema Red swellings above the ankle. It is associated with hyperthyroidism.

Skin diseases associated with malignancy are *acanthosis nigricans* (rough, pigmented, thickened areas of skin in axilla or groin) and *thrombophlebitis migrams* (tender nodules within blood vessels that move from site to site).

Psychiatry

One way of coming to grips with a new subject—and to virtually all dentists, psychiatry as opposed to psychology is new—is to categorize. The major adult psychiatric diagnoses are listed in order of severity. The *Diagnostic and Statistical Manual of Mental Disorders* (DSM) is the standard classification of mental disorders used by mental health professionals in the United States. The DSM consists of three major components: the diagnostic classification, the diagnostic criteria, and the descriptive text. Each disorder in the DSM has a set of inclusion criteria as well as exclusion criteria for each diagnosis. The most recent revision, DSM-IV-TR (fourth edition, text revision), was published in July 2000. The following do not strictly follow DSM-IV but are a few basic groups of psychiatric illness.

Organic brain syndromes

Acute organic reaction (delirium, toxic confusion) Clouding of consciousness and disorientation in time and place are major symptoms. Mood swings are common, and visual hallucinations, rare in other psychiatric conditions, can be present.

▶ There is an underlying, frequently treatable cause to this condition (infection, hypoxia, drugs, dehydration, alcohol withdrawal, etc.). Rx: find the cause and correct it, using sedation until the cause is identified and Rx has taken effect.

Chronic organic reaction (dementia) A global intellectual deterioration highlighted by worsening short-term memory. *Never* label someone as demented until all other possible causes, including depression, have been excluded by a psychiatrist. Alzheimer disease and multi-infarct dementia are the most common causes. There is no cure, although effective support services can improve the quality of life considerably. Anticholinesterase inhibitors, e.g., donepezil, may slow the rate of cognitive decline.

Mental disabilities, p. 48.

Psychosis

Contact with reality is lost and normal mental processes do not function. There is loss of insight. If an organic condition is excluded, the Δ is one of three.

Schizophrenia A disorder in which the victims live in an incomprehensible world full of vivid personal significance. First-rank symptoms are a good guide to Δ: delusions, thought insertion, broadcasting and withdrawal, passivity feelings, visual and auditory hallucinations.

Affective disorders Mania, hypomania, manic-depressive psychosis, and depression. Mania and hypomania are characterized by euphoria, hyperactivity, overvalued ideas or grandiose delusions, and pressure of speech. They differ only in degree. Cyclical mania and depression is known as bipolar affective disorder. Rx is with major tranquillizers and prophylaxis with lithium carbonate.

Depression May be either psychotic or a disorder. Markers of major depressive illness are anhedonia (failure to find pleasure in things that once did please), anorexia, especially with weight loss, early morning wakening, tearfulness, inability to concentrate, feelings of guilt and worthlessness, and suicidal ideation.

Paranoid states are psychoses in which paranoid symptoms predominate and, despite lack of insight, other diagnoses do not apply.

▶ The commonly abused drugs can all mimic or precipitate psychotic states, as can giving birth—puerperal psychosis.

Disorders
A disorder is a maladaptive psychological symptom in the absence of organic or psychotic causes of the symptom and after exclusion of a psychopathic personality. Insight is present.

Anxiety disorder frequently coexists with depression. These patients often have physical symptoms for which there is no physical explanation.

Obsessive-compulsive disorder Intrusive thoughts or ideas that the subject recognizes as coming from within themselves, but resents and is unable to stop. May be associated with *compulsive behavior* in which repeated purposeless activity is carried out because of an inexplicable feeling that it must be done.

Phobia is the generation of fear or anxiety out of proportion to the stimulus. Numerous stimuli exist, including dentists.

Anorexia nervosa/bulimia nervosa
The development of weight reduction as an overvalued idea. Associated with weight ↓ of >25% of ideal body weight and obsessive food avoidance. Most common in females, it is also associated with amenorrhea. It has a significant mortality rate; binge-eating followed by vomiting and/or laxative abuse can occur. To binge without weight loss is bulimia nervosa. Dental effects, p. 276.

Personality disorders
These are not illnesses but extremes of normal personality traits, e.g., obsessional, histrionic, schizoid (cold, introspective). The most important is the psychopathic (sociopathic) individual who has no concept of affection, shame, or guilt, and is characterized by antisocial behavior. They are often superficially personable, highly manipulative, and irresponsible. They have insight and are responsible for their own actions (bad not mad).

The immunocompromised patient

There is a group of individuals who present special problems because of defects in, or suppression of, their immune system. The condition with the highest profile among these is AIDS.

The chief effect of being immunocompromised is an ↑ susceptibility to infection, often due to opportunistic organisms. Anything that changes the host environment in favor of opportunistic pathogens (e.g., surgery, broad-spectrum antibiotics) can lead to potentially fatal infection with rare or otherwise innocuous organisms.

Drugs that suppress the immune response, such as corticosteroids, cyclo-porin A, azathioprin, cytotoxics, etc., are now in common use therapeutically. For cross-infection, see p. 674. Aggressive Rx of infections and antimicrobial prophylaxis are needed (p. 528).

Congenital immunodeficiency states There are at least 18 of these. The most common is selective IgA deficiency, which affects ~1:600; it has a wide spectrum of severity but may remain asymptomatic.

Acquired immunodeficiency

Autoimmune disease e.g., SLE, rheumatoid arthritis, carry a minor ↑ risk of infection.

Chronic renal failure (p. 484) Moderately ↑ risk.

Deficiency states e.g., anemia. Carry a minor ↑ risk.

Diabetes mellitus is common and carries a moderately ↑ risk of infection.

Infections Severe viral infections, TB, AIDS (specific defect).

Neoplasia All hematological malignancies have a severely ↑ risk of infection.

AIDS

AIDS is an increasingly common disease caused by HIV (HIV-1, HIV-2). CD4 T-lymphocyte defect ensues with failure of (mostly) cell-mediated immunity. Although HIV exposure produces antibody response, the virus remains infective in the presence of antibody; it must ∴ be regarded as a marker of infectivity. Absence of HIV antibody *does not*, however, guarantee that that person is not infected with HIV. HIV antibody +ve patients are at risk of developing AIDS, usually after a prolonged latent period during which CD4 cells ↓ in number. AIDS-related complex, which includes cervical lymphadenopathy, oropharyngeal candidiasis, and "hairy leukoplakia," is precursor to full-blown AIDS. Infections characteristic of AIDS are *Pneumocystis carinii* pneumonia and disseminated mycobacterial infection. Kaposi's sarcoma was the tumor most often associated with the condition in the 1980s; now these are anorectal and lung cancer, Hodgkin's disease, and melanoma.

The mode of transmission is (traumatic) anal or vaginal sex, being a recipient of contaminated blood or blood products, or from HIV-positive mother to fetus. The main risk groups in the developed world are IV drug abusers and male homosexuals, although transmission through the heterosexual population is increasing. Transfusion recipients and hemophiliacs, who were at risk prior to screening of blood products, now have a minimal risk.

In the developing world, heterosexual spread is common and mother-to-fetus transmission is creating a huge ↑ in HIV +ve children. Antenatal testing for HIV is crucial, as is avoiding breastfeeding. Zidovudine (AZT) therapy and delivery by cesarean section dramatically ↓ vertical transmission.[1] While there is no cure or vaccination, numerous symptom-reducing and life-prolonging Rx are available, with mixed results. Combination therapy, especially triple therapy including a protease inhibitor, can prolong survival and delay disease progression.[2] Increasing numbers of HIV +ve patients have virus that is resistant to most or all of the available drugs. Patients with resistant strains are being placed on "salvage therapy". In June 2006 the U.S. Food and Drug Administration (FDA) granted accelerated approval to the protease inhibitor darunavir (Prezista®), administered with ritonavir (Norvir®) for treatment of these patients.[3] Psychological and social supports are the most helpful options after preventive advice. Prophylaxis consists of screening blood products and avoidance of unprotected sexual activities and shared needles. For oral manifestations of AIDS, see p. 464. There are practical procedures for control of cross-infection (p. 674).

Prophylaxis after needlestick injury depends on estimation of the likely HIV exposure risk. Triple-therapy guidelines exist in the United States.

1 Editor *BMJ* 1998 **316**.
2 *Drug and Therapeutics Bulletin*, 1997 **35** 28.
3 http://www.fda.gov

Useful emergency kit

Every practice should possess apparatus for delivering O_2, or at least air. In addition, the facility to deliver nitrous oxide and O_2 mixture, e.g., via an anesthetic or relative analgesia machine, can be invaluable. State boards vary on regulations licensing for conscious sedation, deep sedation, GA, nitrous oxide-oxygen sedation, and the permits required for each level of administration. In some cases, the minimum drug and equipment content required for an emergency kit are determined by the licensing board. Consult the rules that govern your local jurisdiction.

The following are guidelines for what should be available:

- suction
- monitoring equipment (including stethoscope and sphygmomanometer)
- equipment capable of delivering oxygen under positive pressure
- gas delivery machines must have an oxygen fail-safe system, adequate waste gas scavenging, and should be checked and calibrated periodically
- automated external defibrillator (AED)
- a protocol for management of emergencies should be developed and emergency drills must be carried out and documented
- all emergency equipment and drugs must be maintained on a scheduled basis
- an adequate supervised recovery area must be available
- epinephrine
- an antihistamine
- an anticonvulsant
- vasodilator (e.g., nitroglycerine)
- an antihypoglycemic agent
- a bronchodilator
- a corticosteroid
- vasopressor
- equipment for the insertion and maintenance of an IV infusions
- a pulse oximeter
- a narcotic antagonist
- a muscle relaxant
- atropine
- lidocaine
- sodium bicarbonate

Ideally, all public areas should have access to an AED, as this is the most valuable single piece of equipment for a cardiac arrest (p. 508).

▶ If you buy something learn how to use it!

Fainting

Fainting (vasovagal syncope) is innocuous, provided it is recognized. It is easily the most common cause of sudden loss of consciousness, with up to 2% of patients fainting before or during dental Rx. The possibility of vasovagal syncope while under GA, and hence failure to recognize the condition and correct cerebral hypoxia, is the major reason for recommending the supine position.

Predisposing factors are pain, anxiety, fatigue, relative hyperthermia, and fasting. Characteristic signs and symptoms are a feeling of dizziness and nausea; pale, cold, and clammy skin; a slow, thin, thready pulse that rebounds to become rapid, and loss of consciousness with collapse, if unsupported.

A faint may mimic far more serious conditions, most of which can be excluded by a familiarity with the patient's PMH. These include strokes, corticosteroid insufficiency, drug reactions and interactions, epileptic fit, heart block, hypoglycemia, and MI.

Prevention
- Avoid predisposing factors.
- Treat patients in the supine position unless specifically contraindicated (e.g., heart failure, pulmonary edema).

Management
- Lower the head to the level of, or below, the heart (Trendelenberg position). This is best achieved by laying the patient flat with legs slightly elevated.
- Open airway.
- Monitor pulse and blood pressure.
- Use ammonia inhalant.
- If bradycardia persists with no evidence of recovery to rapid full pulse, administer O_2 via facemask dose of atropine (0.5 mg IV q 3–5 min total dose of 0.03 mg/kg).

Acute chest pain

Severe, acute chest pain is usually the result of ischemia of the myocardium. The principal differential is between angina and MI. Both exhibit severe retrosternal pain described as heavy, crushing, or band-like. It is classically preceded by effort, emotion, or excitement, and may radiate to the arms, neck, jaw, and, occasionally, the back or abdomen. Angina is usually rapidly relieved by rest and nitrostat (0.4 mg) given sublingually, which most patients with a history of angina carry with them. If pain persists, give aspirin 325 mg.

Failure of these methods to relieve the pain, and coexisting sweating, breathlessness, nausea, vomiting, or loss of consciousness with a weak or irregular pulse suggest an infarct.

Management depends on your immediate environment, but always ensure that the patient is placed in a supported upright position if conscious, as the supine position increases pulmonary edema and, hence, breathlessness.

Management

In dental practice Summon help (call 911). Administer O_2 via face mask. Monitor BP, P, R. Don't panic. Be prepared should cardiac arrest supervene. Give aspirin 325 mg PO. Give dose of nitrostat 0.4 mg sublingual. Tell emergency medical technicians what you have done and when.

Cardiorespiratory arrest

▶ Don't await "expertise." **ACT**.

Ninety percent of deaths from cardiac arrest occurring outside the hospital are due to ventricular fibrillation (VF). This is also the most common arrest pattern seen in the hospital. It is potentially reversible by prompt (<90 sec) defibrillation. The most common underlying cause is ischemic heart disease, but other causes may exist, especially in younger people. Acute asthma, anesthesia, drug overdose, electrocution, immersion, or hypothermia often precipitate pulseless electrical activity (PEA) arrests. These are treatable conditions and potentially reversible.

In certain instances properly performed cardiopulmonary resuscitation (CPR) can sustain life for up to an hour while a precipitating condition is being treated.

Diagnosis and management These proceed simultaneously.

Approach and assess Protect yourself! Do not become another casualty, whether in the street, practice, or hospital environment. Gently "shake and shout" to assess the person's level of consciousness. If there is no response, call for help 911 and get AED (and ask whoever goes for help to come back to tell you if help is coming). Place patient in recovery position. **Then:**

- *Airway* Carry out a head tilt chin lift. Remove loose dentures, but retain if they are well fitting (it gives a better mouth seal). Give one breath and watch for the chest to rise.
- *Breathing* Look, listen, and feel for breathing for 5 sec but not more than 10 sec. If there is none, check circulation.
- *Circulation* Feel for a carotid pulse. If it is present, provide 10 breaths per minute, checking the pulse for 10 sec every 10 breaths. **If no pulse** commence chest compression, at the middle of the lower half of the sternum, depressing 1 1/2–2 in (4–5cm) **100** times per minute. Use a ratio of 30 compressions to 2 breaths. Perform 5 cycles of compressions and ventilations (30:2 ratio).
- *Defibrillation* Attach AED and use it if it detects a shockable rhythm. Remember, statistically the patient's best chance at survival once absence of breathing is confirmed is defibrillation, therefore getting early help may be the most useful thing you can do.

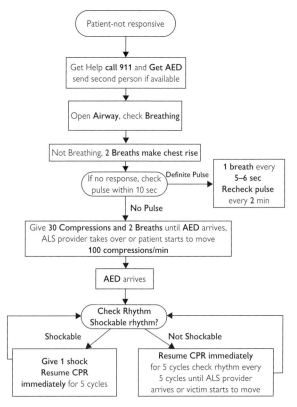

Adult BLS Algorithm, American Heart Association, 2006. Reproduced with permission. Basic Life Support for Healthcare providers. © 2006, American Heart Association.

Rates of compression/ventilation
- Ventilation only (good cardiac output): 10 breaths per minute.
- CPR, single and two rescuers: 30 compressions to 2 breaths for an adult, 15:2 for a child.
- Aim for 100 compressions per minute.

Anaphylactic shock and other drug reactions

Penicillins are the most common offender, but it is worth remembering that there is a 10% crossover in allergic response between penicillins and cephalosporins.

An anaphylactic reaction is not an all-or-nothing response, and grades of severity are seen. **Caution**: the quicker the onset of an anaphylactic reaction the more severe it is likely to be.

Principal symptoms are facial flushing, itching, numbness, cold extremities, nausea, and sometimes abdominal pain. Signs include wheezing, facial swelling and rash, and cold, clammy skin with a thin, thready pulse. Loss of consciousness may occur, with extreme pallor that progresses to cyanosis as respiratory failure develops.

It can be difficult to distinguish anaphylaxis from acute asthma in, e.g., an asthmatic person given an NSAID they are allergic to. Don't panic, just go through management for acute asthma, then start on management for anaphylaxis. Epinephrine is a bronchodilator anyway.

Angioedema is sudden onset, with severe face and neck allergic swelling. The airway is at risk and ∴ should be managed as for anaphylaxis.

Management
- Place patient supine with legs raised, if possible.
- 0.5 ml of 1:1000 epinephrine IM or SC. Repeat after 5–10 min as needed, then every 10 min until improved. Do not give IV in this concentration as it will induce ventricular fibrillation.
- 50–100 mg Solu-Cortef
- 25–50 mg benadryl
- O_2 by mask
- Monitor BP, P, R.

Other drug reactions and interactions

While there are a multitude of drug interactions that the dental surgeon should be aware of as a prescriber, the drugs most liable to present an emergency problem to the dentist are those administered as LA.

Although it is possible to achieve toxic levels of lidocaine, epinephrine, or prilocaine, without intravascular injection, this generally requires a particularly cavalier attitude to the administration of LA. Commonly, this effect is due to intravascular injection of a substantial proportion of a cartridge of LA. Confusion, perioral tingling, drowsiness, agitation, seizures, or loss of consciousness may occur. Do not use more than 13×1.8 ml cartridges of lidocaine 1:100,000 epinephrine (7 mg/kg up to 500 mg). In practice, you will rarely consider coming near this amount.

Management
- Stop procedure! (They won't be numb.)
- Place supine.
- Maintain airway, give O_2.
- Await spontaneous recovery (in 30 min) unless, tragically, a serious event such as MI supervenes, in which case treat as indicated.

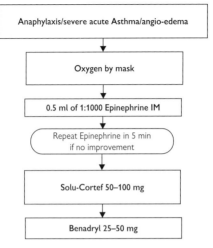

Albuterol inhaler-2 puffs for Asthmatic
IV fluids as necessary. Check PDR for children's doses

Treatment for anaphylaxis algorithm

Collapse in a patient with a history of corticosteroid use

The use of corticosteroids therapeutically or otherwise for whatever cause may suppress the adrenal response to stress. The longer the course of Rx and the higher the dose used, the more likely this is to occur.

The primary aim is to prevent the occurrence of stress-induced collapse; if patients have received steroids in the past year or are on steroids at present, cover any stressful procedure, anesthetic, infection, or episode of trauma with 50–100 mg Solu-Cortef IM. It is a fallacy to believe you are reducing the risk of undesired steroid effects by trying to avoid giving prophylactic steroids. Doubling the oral dose may work but is rather hit and miss. Calculating an "exact" dose is unnecessarily complicated and risks people "forgetting." Stick to giving them 100 mg Solu-Cortef IM unless you have a very valid reason to change this.

In patients presenting acutely, treat immediately. If collapse occurs in such a patient, Δ is established by pallor, rapid, thin pulse with a profound and sudden ↓ in BP, and loss of consciousness.

Management
- Place in supine position. Maintain airway. Give O_2. Obtain IV access.
- Administer up to 500 mg hydrocortisone IV immediately.
- Call 911 for help.
- Exclude other causes of collapse.

Seizures

Most epileptic seizures do not require active intervention as the patient will usually recover spontaneously. All that is needed is sensible positioning to prevent the patient from injuring themselves. Seizures may be precipitated in a known epileptic by starvation, flickering lights, certain drugs such as tricyclics, alcohol, or menstruation. They may also follow a deep faint.

Diagnosis Many epileptics have a preceding aura followed by sudden loss of consciousness with a rigid extended appearance and generalized jerking movements. Frequently, they are incontinent of urine and may bite their tongue. There is a slow recovery, with the patient feeling sleepy and dazed. There may be a *cause* for the seizure: trauma, tumor, and alcohol withdrawal are common. There are numerous others; any adult should have a first seizure fully investigated.

▶ Should the seizure repeat, the patient has entered the state of status epilepticus. This is an emergency and requires urgent control.

Management In a simple major seizure the patient should be placed in the recovery position when practicable and allowed to recover. If they enter status epilepticus, IV lorazepam 4 mg or IV diazepam 10–20 mg (in 5 mg boluses, 2 min between boluses) usually aborts the seizure; beware of respiratory depression. Assess cardiorespiratory function; clear and maintain airway, and give O_2. It is worthwhile considering placing an IV cannula or a butterfly in any epileptic patient with less than perfect control, as stress is an important precipitant. Status epilepticus should not be allowed to continue for more than 20 min, as the mortality rate (up to 30%) and chance of permanent brain damage ↑ with the length of attack.

Hypoglycemia

Hypoglycemia is the diabetic emergency most likely to present to the dentist. It is an acute and dangerous complication of diabetes and may result from a missed meal, excess insulin, or increased calorific need due to exercise or stress. Most diabetics are expert in detecting the onset of hypoglycemia themselves; however, a small number may lose this ability, particularly if changed from porcine to human insulin. Recognition of this state is essential and an acutely collapsed diabetic should be assumed hypoglycemic until proven otherwise, e.g., by "BM" sticks or blood-glucose levels.

Diagnosis Disorientation, irritability, increasing drowsiness, excitability, or aggression in a known diabetic suggest hypoglycemia. They often appear to be drunk.

Treatment

- If conscious, give glucose orally in any available form.
- If unconscious, protect airway, place in recovery position, establish IV access, and give up to 50 ml of 20–50% dextrose. If available, 1 mg of glucagon IM may be used. Call 911 for help.

Acute asthma

An acute asthmatic attack may be induced in a patient predisposed to bronchospasm by exposure to an allergen, infection, cold, exercise, or anxiety. Characteristically, the patient will complain of a tight chest and shortness of breath. Examination will reveal breathlessness, with widespread expiratory wheezing. The accessory muscles of respiration may be used to support breathing. If the patient is unable to talk, you are dealing with a potentially fatal episode.

Management Make use of the patient's own antiasthmatic drugs, such as albuterol inhalers. A do-it-yourself nebulizer can be fabricated from the patient's own inhaler pushed through the base of a paper cup. Repeated depressions of inhaler plunger will create an aerosol inside the cup that the patient can inhale. This will relieve most reversible airways obstruction. Steroids should be administered either as oral prednisolone, if the patient carries these with them, or as IV hydrocortisone up to 200 mg IV. This combination of albuterol, steroids, and O_2 will often completely resolve an attack; however, in individuals who do not respond, an urgent hospital admission is required. Patients who are only partially responsive must have underlying irritants such as a chest infection either excluded or treated.

▶ Be aware of the possibility of anaphylaxis mimicking acute asthma. Remember epinephrine 0.5 ml 1:1000 SC.

Management in dental practice
- Keep the patient upright.
- Administer albuterol inhaler.
- Give O_2.
- Give steroids.

If a complete response takes place it is reasonable to allow the patient to return home. If there is any doubt, arrange for the patient to be seen at the nearest emergency department.

Inhaled foreign bodies

The combination of delicate instruments and the supine position of patients for many dental procedures inevitably ↑ the risk of a patient inhaling a FB. Two basic scenarios are likely, depending on whether or not the item impacts in the upper or lower airway.

Upper airway This will stimulate the cough reflex, which may be sufficient to clear the obstruction. A choking subject should be bent forward to aid coughing. If the obstruction is complete or there are signs of cyanosis in the

- *Conscious patient* Carry out abdominal thrusts (Heimlich) by encircling victim with your arms from behind and deliver a sharp upward and inward squeeze to create sudden expulsion of air. Repeat up to 5 times.
- *Unconscious patient* Finger sweep to try to remove foreign body. Deliver abdominal thrusts with victim supine.[1]

If all else fails, cricothyroid puncture may preserve life if the obstruction lies above this level.

Lower airway As only a segment of the lungs will be occluded, this presents a less acute problem. It is also easier to miss. Classically, this involves a tooth or tooth fragment slipping from the forceps and being inhaled. With the patient in a semi-upright position the object ends up in the right posterior basal lobe. Should this happen, inform the patient and arrange to have a chest radiograph taken ASAP. If the offending item is in the lungs, removal by a pulmonary specialist using fiber-optic bronchoscopy is indicated, as this is inevitably followed by collapse and infection distal to the obstruction. Rarely, lobectomy may be needed. See plate 4.

If in doubt

When presented with a suddenly collapsed patient the first thing to assess is your own response. Don't panic. You are only of value to the patient if you can function rationally. If presented with a case of sudden loss of consciousness, in the absence of an obvious change, the following steps should be followed:

- **Maintain the airway** and provide O_2 if available.
- **Place in supine position.** If the patient has simply fainted they will recover virtually immediately.
- **Are they breathing?** If not, begin artificial respiration (p. 508).
- **Feel for the pulse.** If it is absent, there has been a cardiac arrest (p. 508). If it is present:
- Establish IV access and give up to 20 ml 20–50% dextrose IV.
- Give hydrocortisone up to 200 mg IV.
- If unable to get access, use glucagon 1 mg IM.

These measures will usually resolve most cases of sudden, nontraumatic loss of consciousness.

If the patient is acutely distressed and breathless they should be treated in an upright position and given O_2 while you try to differentiate between an acute asthmatic attack, anaphylaxis, and heart failure, and treat as indicated.

Always ensure that someone has requested assistance by calling 911.

Immediately after resolution of an emergency there tends to be a period of numb inactivity among the staff involved. Use this period to review your management of the situation and carefully document what happened. If the patient has been transferred to the hospital or another department, a brief, legible account of proceedings must accompany them. Include drugs used, their dosages, and when they were given. Try to ensure that a friend or relation of the patient is aware of the situation.

Management of the dental inpatient

The vast majority of inpatients will experience considerable anxiety on being admitted for an operation, including about those procedures which are in themselves "routine." In addition, as dentists have little in-hospital training, there is a substantial risk of compounding an already stressful situation by being overly stressed yourself. Minimize this by preparation. Learn about the setting you will work in before taking a position. Never be afraid to ask assisting staff if you are unsure, and try to know a day in advance what cases are coming in.

Preoperative

All patients attending as inpatients for operation must (a) be examined and "clerked," and (b) have consented to surgery. In addition, many will require a variety of preoperative investigations; these vary widely from consultant to consultant, so get to know the local variations. Common investigations and their indications are listed below. For sampling techniques, see p. 520; samples, p. 12.

(a) Clerking This basically consists of taking a complete medical and dental history from the patient, including any drugs that they are taking at present, a family history for inherited disease, and a social history for problems related to smoking, alcohol, drug abuse, and ability to cope at home postoperatively. This is followed by a systematic clinical examination (p. 9). Any special consultations are then arranged, and the results of these should be seen before the patient goes to the operating room. Any problems uncovered should be relayed to the anesthesiologist, who is the only person capable of saying whether or not the patient is fit for anesthesia. Any required pre-, peri-, or postopertive drugs are written up (p. 546).

(b) Consent All patients undergoing GA or sedation must give written, informed consent. It is advised that patients receiving interventions under LA also do so. Every hospital has its own surgical consent form that must be completed. After having the procedure and its likely potential risks explained, the patient also signs the form. It is essential that you are happy in your own mind that you understand what the operation entails; if in doubt, ask your senior staff. Obtain consent only for procedures with which you are familiar. No one should wake up with scars without being previously warned.

Findings (p. 12)

Complete blood count Elderly patients. Any suspicion of anemia.

Sickle cell test All Afro-Caribbeans for GA. Consider also those of Mediterranean, Arabic, or Indian origin.

Urea and electrolytes All patients needing IV fluids, on diuretics, who are diabetics, or have renal disease. They have a low threshold for doing this test.

Coagulation screen All major surgery, any past history of bleeding disorders, liver disease, or history of ↑ alcohol, anticoagulants.

Liver function tests Liver disease, alcohol, major surgery.

Group and save/cross-match Major surgery, trauma, shock, anemia.

ECG Heart disease, all major surgery, most patients >50.

CXR Trauma, active chest disease, possible metastases.

Hepatitis B and C, HIV markers Varies; usually at-risk groups only; pretest counseling is now considered mandatory. Check local hospital policy.

Postoperation

Immediately postoperatively, patients are resuscitated in a recovery room adjacent to the operating room, with a nurse monitoring cardio-respiratory function. Once recovered, unless they are to be monitored in the ICU they will be returned to the ward. In all patients, ensure a patent airway and consider the following factors.

Analgesia may take the form of LA (should be given postanesthetic/pre-surgery), oral or parenteral NSAIDs, or oral or parenteral opioids. Immediately postoperatively, analgesia is best given parenterally. Antiemetics should be given if nausea or vomiting is present.

Antimicrobials are given in accordance with the selected regimen (p. 528). Certain patients may benefit from corticosteroids pre- and postoperatively to ↓ edema; regimens vary.

Nutrition is a problem principally for patients undergoing major head and neck cancer surgery (p. 420), but it is worthwhile reminding nursing staff to order soft diets for all oral surgery patients who can feed by mouth and to have blenders available for patients in IMF.

Fluid balance is covered on p. 521. Special consideration needs to be given to patients in IMF and those with tracheostomies. Although the use of immediate postoperative IMF is rare, it is still required, and postoperative elastic IMF is common. These patients need to be specially attended by a nurse looking after that patient only, for the first 12–24 h. Lighting, suction, and the ability to place the patient head-down if they vomit, are mandatory.

Venipuncture and arterial puncture

Venipuncture To become proficient in the skills of venipuncture you must practice the art in all its forms. To develop the skill of placing IV cannula, cultivate a sympathetic anesthesiologist, as anesthetized patients are venodilated and will not feel pain! When carrying out cannulations and arterial punctures on patients in the ward, a drop or two of 2% plain lidocaine deposited SC with a fine needle will aid both your peace of mind and the patient's comfort.

Tools of the trade Tourniquet, alcohol wipes, cotton wool. Green (21G) needles and butterflies are commonly used. Many hospitals have adopted sealed "vacutainer" systems that are convenient but fiddly to use. Learn the basics first, then your hospital's system. Sometimes finer needles or butterflies are needed, e.g., blue (23G). Patients who are difficult to cannulate can have fluids and certain drugs through fine (20G) or even 22G IV cannula; most have 18G. Shocked patients or those needing blood should have at least a 16G and preferably a 14G cannula inserted. Note that gauges and colors are not consistent between needles and cannulas.

Sites of puncture

For sampling First choice is the cubital fossa. Inspect and palpate; veins you can feel are better than those you can only see. Insert the needle at a 30–40° angle to the skin and along the line of the vein. If no veins are found in the cubital foss,a try the back of the hand with a butterfly and use a similar approach. The veins of the dorsum of the foot are a last resort before the femoral vein lying just medial to the femoral artery in the groin.

For infusion Single-bolus injections; use a 21G butterfly in a vein on the back of the hand.

• For IV fluids or multiple IV injections place an 18G IV cannula in a straight segment of vein in the forearm, hand, or just proximal to the "anatomical snuffbox." Try to avoid crossing a joint as the cannula tissues more quickly if subjected to repeated movements. When inserting the cannula ensure that the skin overlying the vein is fixed by finger pressure; pierce the skin, and move the stillete along the line of the vein until it enters the vein and blood flows into the cannula. As soon as you enter the vein, pull the stillete back into the cannula to minimize the risk of going through the vein. Insert the full length of the cannula into the vein and secure. Keep patent with heparinized saline.

Arterial puncture Whenever possible, obtain an arterial sampling syringe. Use LA unless patient is anesthetized. The syringe and needle must be flushed with heparin. Use radial, brachial, or femoral arteries. Palpate, prepare area with alcohol wipe, and insert needle at 30–60° to skin. When the needle enters the artery, blood pulsates into the syringe. Only 1–2 ml is needed. Remove needle and place in a bag with ice, contact the hematology lab, and treat as an urgent specimen. The puncture site needs to be firmly pressed on for 2–3 min to prevent formation of a painful hematoma.

Intravenous fluids

Principles Maintain daily fluid requirements plus replace any abnormal loss by infusion of (usually) isotonic solutions. Normal requirements are ~2.5–3 l in 24 h. This is lost via urine (normal renal function needs an absolute minimum of 30 ml/h, but aim for 60 ml/h), fecal loss, and sweating. Where possible, replace with oral fluids; IV fluids are second best.

Common IV regimens 1 l normal saline (0.9%) and 2 l 5% dextrose in 24 h, or 3 l dextrose/saline solution in 24 h. Add 20 mmol potassium chloride/l after 36 h, unless U&Es suggest otherwise. Hartmann's solution is more expensive but most physiological crystalloid (aka Ringer's lactate).

Increase the above in the presence of abnormal losses, burns, fever, dehydration, and polyuria, and in the event of hemorrhage or shock.

Special needs
- For burns, start with Hartmann's and be guided by the local burns unit.
- For fever, use saline.
- For dehydration or polyuria, use 5% dextrose, unless hyponatremic. An exception is ketoacidosis: use saline.
- Hemorrhage demands replacement by whole blood if available; packed cells are second best, and shock needs blood, crystalloid challenge, and control of hemorrhage. Be guided by the pulse, BP, urine output, hemoglobin, hematocrit, and U&Es.

↓ the above in heart failure, and avoid saline. Shock and dehydration are rare complications of maxillofacial trauma or any other condition principally presenting to the dentist; ∴ in their presence, consider damage to other body systems and seek appropriate advice.

Polyuria Postoperatively, this is usually due to overtransfusion. Review anesthetic notes, and if this is the case, simply catheterize and observe.

Oliguria Postoperatively, this is usually due to undertransfusion or dehydration pre- or perioperatively. First, palpate abdomen for ↑ bladder and listen to chest to exclude pulmonary edema. Then catheterize the patient to exclude urinary retention and allow close monitoring of fluid balance. Then ↑ rate of infusion of fluid (**max** 1 l/h) **unless** the patient is in heart failure or bleeding. The former needs specialist advice, the latter needs blood or an operation. In an otherwise healthy postoperative patient, if this does not produce a minimum of 30 ml/h of urine, a diuretic (20–40 mg furosemide PO/IV) may be tried. Take care when using IV fluids, as failure to PU makes it possible to fluid overload the patient quickly. Review fluid balance and U&Es over several days for an overview.

Blood transfusion

▶ Group and save: you won't get blood; group and cross-match: you will get blood in ~1 hr; type-specific group: you will get blood urgently. Blood may be required for patients in an acute (e.g., traumatized) situation, electively (e.g., perioperatively) during major surgery, or to correct a chronic anemia (p. 474). In practice, the former two are much more commonly encountered by junior dental staff.

Whole blood is indicated in patients who have lost >20% blood volume, exhibit signs of hypovolemic shock, or in whom this appears inevitable.

▶ Remember that maxillofacial injuries *alone* only rarely result in this degree of blood loss (p. 397).

Always take blood for grouping in severely traumatized patients, and proceed to cross-match as indicated by the clinical signs. Always use cross-matched blood, except in utter extremis when O Rhesus –ve blood can be used. Massive transfusions create problems with hyperkalemia, thrombocytopenia, and low levels of clotting factors; ∴ in patients with severe hemorrhage, simultaneous fresh-frozen plasma (4–6 units) and platelets (6 units) will be needed. Most labs only provide packed cells.

Autologous blood is blood donated by a patient prior to elective surgery for use only on themselves. It avoids risks of cross-infection but requires a specially interested hematology department, so check locally. Autotransfusion is sometimes used in vascular surgery.

Packed cells are used for the correction of anemia if too severe for correction with iron, or if needed prior to urgent surgery. This ↓ the fluid load to the patient, but elderly individuals and those in heart failure should have their transfusion covered with 40 mg furosemide PO or IV.

Useful tips

- Cross-match one patient at a time and be sure you are familiar with local procedures.
- The nurse will perform regular observations of temperature, pulse, respiration, and urine output during transfusion—watch them!
- Except in shock, transfuse slowly (1 unit over 2–4 h; >4 h the cannulas start to clog).
- 1 unit of blood raises the Hb by 1 g/dl = 3% hematocrit.

Complications

- ABO incompatibility. Causes anaphylaxis; manage accordingly (p. 510)
- Cross-infection
- Heart failure can be induced by over-rapid transfusion.
- Milder allergic transfusion reactions are the most common problem; Rx by slowing the transfusion. If progressive or temperature >40°C, stop transfusion and inform lab to check cross-matching. IV hydrocortisone 100 mg and benadryl 50 mg are useful standbys.
- Citrate toxicity is a hazard of very large transfusions and can be countered by 10 ml calcium gluconate with alternate units.

Catheterization

This is not a topic normally covered by the dental syllabus, but the dental graduate may find him- or herself confronted with a patient needing urethral catheterization if working on an oral and maxillofacial surgical ward. The only procedure they are likely to need to be able to perform is temporary urethral catheterization. This is indicated for urinary retention (almost always postop), for precise measurement of fluid balance, or, rarely, to avoid use of a bedpan or bottle. Avoid catheterization if a history of pelvic trauma is present, as an expert is needed. Catheters are associated with a high incidence of UTIs, and presence of a UTI is a relative C/I.

Equipment You should have a tube of local anesthetic gel, a dish with some aqueous chlorhexidine, swabs, a waterproof sheet with a hole in the middle, sterile gloves, a 10 ml syringe filled with sterile water, and a drainage bag. In most cases a 14–16 French gauge Foley catheter will suffice. Use a silicone catheter if you anticipate it being in situ for more than a few days.

Procedure Explain what you are going to do and why. If catheterizing for postop fluid balance, do it in the anesthetic room after intubation (ask the anesthetist first!). The operating room is the best place to learn. The procedure can be made both aseptic and aesthetic by wearing two pairs of disposable gloves; one pair is discarded after achieving analgesia, which is done by instillation of lidocaine gel (also acts as a lubricant). Find the urethral opening and, using the nozzle supplied, squeeze in the contents of the tube. In females, finding the opening is the only significant problem; most women are catheterized by female nursing staff. In males, it is necessary to massage the gel along the length of the penis and leave *in situ* for several minutes before progressing. Once analgesia is obtained, the female urethra is easily catheterized; if you have been unable to find the meatus to instil LA you should not proceed but get help. In the male, hold the penis upright and insert the tip of the catheter; pass it gently down the urethra until it reaches the penoscrotal junction, pull the penis down so that it lies between the patient's thighs, thereby straightening out the curves of the urethra, and advance the tip into the bladder until urine flows.

Once urine flows, the catheter balloon can be inflated with sterile water. In the conscious patient it should be painless; if not, deflate the balloon and reposition the catheter. In the anesthetized patient, insert the catheter all the way, inflate, then pull back. Connect the drainage bag and remember to replace the foreskin over the glans to avoid a paraphimosis.

▶ If, in the presence of adequate analgesia, you are unable to pass the catheter, **do not** persist, but get expert assistance.

Enteric and parenteral feeding

The main role for this type of feeding, as far as dental staff are concerned, is in the care of debilitated patients and those undergoing surgery for head and neck cancers. In view of the latter, it is worthwhile having a basic understanding of the subject.

Enteric feeding is providing liquid, low-residue foods either **1** by mouth, or **2** more commonly, by fine-bore nasogastric tube. A range of proprietary products are available for these feeds. Be guided by the dietitian, who has expertise in this area, which you will lack. The major problem is osmotic diarrhea, which can be ↓ by starting with dilute solutions.

Fine-bore nasogastric tubes are the mainstay in enteric nutrition for patients undergoing major oropharyngeal surgery. In many institutions, nurses are not allowed to pass these tubes, although they are allowed to pass standard nasogastric tubes for aspirating stomach contents. You can ∴ find yourself asked to pass such a tube by someone who is more proficient but forbidden to do so.

Technique Wear gloves. Explain the procedure to the patient and have them at 50–60° upright with neck in neutral position. Place a small amount of lidocaine gel in the chosen nostril after ensuring it is patent. Keep a small drink of water handy. Select a tube; check that the guidewire is lubricated and does not protrude. If a tracheostomy tube is present the cuff should be deflated to allow passage of the tube. Lubricate the tube and introduce it into the nostril; pass it horizontally along the nasal floor. There is usually a little resistance as the tube reaches the nasopharynx; press past this and ask the patient to swallow (use the water if this helps). The tube should now pass easily down the esophagus, entering the stomach at 40 cm. Secure the tube to the forehead with sticky tape and only now remove the guidewire, being careful to shield the patient's eyes. Inject air into the tube and listen for bubbling over the stomach. Confirm position with a CXR. (Some systems require leaving a radiopaque guidewire in prior to X-ray: check the tube you are using.)

Problems

- *Nasal patency* Select the least narrow nostril, use a lubricant, and, if necessary, a smaller tube and topical vasoconstrictor.
- *Gagging/vomiting* Press ahead; all sphincters are open.
- *Tube coiling into mouth* Cooling the tube makes it more rigid and often helps. As a last resort, topical anesthesia and direct visualization with a laryngoscope or nasendoscope, while an assistant passes the tube, may be necessary.
- *Tube pulled out by patient* If they must have the tube, consider a septal suture or stitch to soft tissue of the nose.

Parenteral feeding is extremely hazardous and expensive. It requires a central venous line and considerable expertise if your patient is to survive. Avoid if at all possible.

Percutaneoeous endoscopic gastrostomy (PEG) Feeding tube is placed directly in the stomach through the abdominal wall at endoscopy.

Radiologically inserted gastrostomy (RIG) Ultrasound version of PEG. Needs nasogastric tube (NGT) in place to inflate stomach.

Pain control

LA (p. 572); RA (p. 578); IV sedation (p. 584).

The aim of pain control is to relieve symptoms while identifying and removing the cause; the exception is when the cause is not treatable, as in terminal care. Then the approach is to deal with the symptoms to enable the patient to have comfort to the end of their life.

Acute and postoperative pain may often be well controlled by LA (p. 572), but it is often necessary to use systemic analgesics. Useful analgesics in this situation include acetaminophen (1000 mg PO/PR q 4–6h) and ibuprofen (400–600 mg q 8h). Both of these can be combined with codeine (8–30 mg). Also, NSAIDs are useful. These drugs are all simple analgesics and, with the exception of acetaminophen, have the advantage of an anti-inflammatory action that is at least as important as their central analgesic effect. In *postoperative* pain, opioid analgesics are helpful when used parenterally and short term. Morphine 10 mg 3–4 hourly combined with an antiemetic such as metoclopramide (10 mg IM/IV) is useful in the immediate postoperative period. PCA systems (see below) after major surgery are commonly used. They are set up and maintained by the anesthesiologists.

Pain following maxillofacial trauma is a problem, as these patients must be assessed neurologically for evidence of head injury that C/I opioids. The addition of codeine phosphate (60 mg IM) to an NSAID is often effective and does not significantly interfere with neurological observations. There is often a hospital pain management team who will be happy to advise in difficult cases.

Facial pain not of dental or iatrogenic origin is covered on p. 454. These conditions often require the use of co-analgesics such as antidepressants, antiepileptics, and anxiolytics.

Pain control in terminal disease is an important subject in its own right. Points to note include the following: aim for continuous control using oral analgesia; use regular, not on-demand, analgesia titrated to the individual; diagnose the cause of each ↑ pain and prescribe appropriately (e.g., steroids for liver secondaries or ↑ intracranial pressure, NSAIDs and/or radiotherapy for bone metastases, co-analgesics for nerve root pain, etc.). Remember that psychological dependence is very rare in advanced cancer patients using long-term opioids, and analgesic tolerance is slow to develop. When starting patients on opioid analgesia, always consider using an antiemetic (p. 554) and a laxative. OH may be incredibly difficult for patients with oral cancer or following head and neck surgery. Use of chlorhexidine gluconate and metronidazole (200 mg bd) ↓ the smell associated with wound infection or tumor fungation even when there is no prospect of eliminating it entirely. Patients rarely develop the disulfiram reaction to metronidazole on this regimen that occurs with higher doses.

Pre-emptive analgesia Surgery is painful. Providing LA (consider the long-acting agent bupivocaine) or systemic analgesia before surgery begins may ↓ overall requirements for analgesia.

Patient-controlled analgesia is the optimal technique for severe postoperative pain. A small machine delivers a bolus (1–2 mg morphine) when the patient presses a button. This can be repeated as needed.

There are two variables: **1** bolus dose; **2** "lock-out time" time during which the machine will not respond (allows time for opioid to achieve maximum effect and prevents overdosage).

Prophylaxis

Prophylaxis is the prevention of an occurrence. Prophylaxis used to prevent the occurrence of bacterial infection is quite different from treating an established infection. There are two broad categories of patients requiring antibiotic prophylaxis: **1** those who have it to prevent a minor local bacteremia causing a serious infection out of all proportion to the procedure, e.g., people at risk from IE, or the immunocompromised; **2** those who receive it to prevent local septic complications of the procedure, e.g., third-molar prophylaxis.

Principles of prophylaxis The regimen should be short, high dose, and appropriate to the potential infecting organisms. The aim is to prevent pathogens establishing themselves in surgically traumatized or otherwise at-risk tissues, ∴ the antimicrobial must be in those tissues prior to damage or exposure to the pathogen. It must not, however, be present too long before this, as there is then a risk of pathogen resistance and damage to commensal organisms. The regimen should ∴ start 30–60 min preoperatively.

Examples

Not all total joint prostheses need to receive prophylaxis—e.g., those older than 2 years with no complications (except in the presence of immunocompromising diseases).

Immunocompromised patients should be prophylaxed (e.g., severe leukopenia).

Dentoalveolar surgery Simple extractions need not be covered but third-molar surgery often is.

Prophylactic anticoagulation Prevention of DVT and/or pulmonary embolus in susceptible patients (e.g., women on the pill, prolonged surgery, iliac crest grafts) can be achieved using 5000 units heparin SC bd. TED antiembolism stockings will also ↓ DVT. Low-molecular-weight heparins given SC od are now favored. There are many different types. Check which one your hospital favors. Rx of pulmonary embolus, see p. 532.

Cardiac conditions for which prophylaxis is recommended – highest risk

A) Prosthetic cardiac valve

B) Previous IE

C) Congenital heart disease (CHD)*

- Unrepaired cyanotic CHD, including palliative shunts and conduits

- Completely repaired congenital heart defect with prosthetic material or device, whether placed by surgery or catheter intervention, during the first 6 months after the procedure. (Prophylaxis is recommended because endothelialization of prosthetic material occurs within 6 months)

- Repaired CHD with residual defects at the site or adjacent to the site of a prosthetic patch or prosthetic device

D) Cardiac transplantation recipients who develop cardiac valvulopathy

*Except for the conditions listed above, antibiotic prophylaxis is no longer recommended for any other form of CHD.

Adapted by W. Wilson et al. Prevention of infective endocarditis: Guidelines for the American Heart Association 2007 JADA **138**(6) 739–60. and W. Wilson et al. April 19, 2007 Circulation American Heart Association online: http://circ.ahajournals.org.

Prophylactic regimens*

Standard

• Amoxicillin	• Adults: 2.0 g
	• Children: 50 mg/kg 30–60 min prior to procedure

Unable to take oral medication

• Ampicillin	• Adults 2 g IM or IV
or	• Children 50 mg/kg IM or IV
• Cefazolin or ceftriaxone	• Adult 1 g IM or IV
	• Children 50 mg/kg IM or IV

Penicillin allergic

• Clindamycin	• Adults: 600 mg
	• Children: 20 mg/kg 30–60 min prior to procedure
• Or cephalexin** or ceftriaxone**	• Adults: 2.0 g
	• Children: 50 mg/kg 30–60 min prior to procedure
• Or azithromycin or clarithromycin	• Adults: 500 mg/kg
	• Children: 15 mg/kg 30–60 min prior to procedure

Unable to take oral medication

• Cefazolin or ceftriaxone**	• Adult 600 mg IM or IV
	• Children 50 mg/kg IM or IV
• Clindamycin	• Adult 600 mg IM or IV
	• Children 20 mg/kg IM or IV

* Total children's dose should not exceed adult dose.

** Cephalosporins should not be used in individuals with immediate-type hypersensitivity reaction (urticaria, angioedema, and anaphylaxis) to penicillins.

Adapted by W. Wilson et al. Prevention of infective endocarditis: Guidelines for the American Heart Association 2007 JADA **138**(6) 739–60.

Management of the diabetic patient undergoing surgery

▶ Hospitals have diabetic teams who will advise you on the management of these patients. Find out if this happens in your locality and make use of them.

Guidelines
- Know the type and severity of the diabetes you are dealing with.
- Inform the anesthesiologist (and diabetic team if available).
- Remember that these patients are more likely to have occult heart disease, renal impairment, and ↓ resistance to infection, so get an ECG and U&Es, and use antibiotics prophylactically.
- If nursing staff are experienced with blood glucose estimation using BM sticks or similar, 2–4 hourly BMs will suffice for monitoring control. Otherwise pre-, peri-, and postoperative blood glucose estimation is needed.
- Always have diabetics first on the operating list, in the morning if possible. Admit to the hospital the day before surgery if an insulin regimen is to be used.

Management: non-insulin-dependent

If doing anything other than a minor, short procedure, treat as insulin dependent. If random blood glucose is >15 mmol/l, treat as insulin dependent.

Patients being treated under LA, or LA and sedation should maintain their carbohydrate intake and any oral hypoglycemic drugs as normal. Plan surgery to fit their regular mealtimes. Have carbohydrate readily at hand if needed, and ensure adequate postoperative analgesia, as pain or trismus can easily interfere with their usual intake. Remember antibiotic prophylaxis.

Patients for GA should have a consult by the endocrine specialist/anesthesiologist prior to surgical treatment.

Management: insulin-dependent

Admit 24–48 h preoperatively to optimize control. If glycemic control is poor, involve the diabetic team. Examine the patient carefully. Get an ECG, FBC, U&Es, and random blood glucose. Look for heart and respiratory disease, leucocytosis indicating infection, anemia, hypo- or hyperkalemia, and renal impairment. If these are acceptable, normal insulin/carbohydrate intake up to and including the evening meal the day before surgery is acceptable. Omit long-acting insulin on the day before surgery. Starve following this, and place on an IV infusion of *glucose* (*dextrose* 5–10% 500 ml), with *potassium* (10 mmol K^+ injected into bag of dextrose) infused via a controlled-rate device over 5 h, i.e., 100 ml/hr.

Once the patient can eat and drink, resume normal insulin regimen and discontinue infusion as BM levels normalize.

Management of patients requiring steroid supplementation

Principle These patients are unable to respond to the stress of surgery because of depletion or absence of their endogenous corticosteroid response.

Groups Patients with Addison's disease, patients prescribed corticosteroids for modulation of the immune system, and steroid abusers from various 'sports'.

Addison's disease These patients belong to the rarest of these groups but require the most aggressive supplementation, as sufferers are entirely reliant on prescribed steroids. Minor surgery can safely be covered with IM hydrocortisone sodium succinate 100 mg qid the day of surgery. Major surgery should be covered for 3 days using the same regimen. IV administration is kinder over the longer period.

Patients prescribed steroids Do you know why they are on these drugs? Consider the underlying disease and whether it has any bearing on your Rx plan; e.g., a patient receiving steroids as part of a cytotoxic regimen will also be at risk from bleeding and infection. In an uncomplicated case before minor surgery, all that is needed is a single IM injection of hydro-cortisone 100 mg 30 min prior to the procedure. Alternatives are an IV injection immediately preoperative followed by double the normal oral dose of steroid; or relying on the patient to take a double dose on the day of the operation, normal dose plus 50% the day after, and normal plus 25% on the third day, thereafter returning to their usual dose. Those undergoing major surgery should have the IM/IV regimen over 24 h or longer.

Steroid abusers Unfortunately, these are a real and ↑ problem. Although these drugs are taken for their androgenic effect, few athletes have access to appropriate advice or drugs and many users will have a degree of sup-pressed steroid response. It is probably safest to cover procedures using the IM regimen as for those on prescribed steroids, although this could be considered overkill. Remember the risk of shared needles.

Common postoperative problems

General

Pain Use appropriate analgesia (p. 550).

Fever A small physiological ↑ in temperature occurs postoperatively. Other causes: atelectasis, infection (wound, chest, urine), DVT, incompatible transfusion, allergic reactions.

Nausea and vomiting Antiemetics.

Sore throat Common after intubation; patient needs reassurance and simple analgesia. Cold water ↓ symptoms.

Muscle pain Often follows suxamethonium use in anesthetic induction. Again, reassurance and simple analgesics.

Hypotension Usually caused by autonomic suppression by a GA. Treat by placing head-down. If necessary, speed up IV infusion for a short while.

Chest infection CXR, culture sputum, and start on antibiotics.

Confusion A symptom, ∴ look for the cause, e.g., infection, electrolyte imbalance, alcohol withdrawal, hypoxia, or dehydration, and correct. Only consider sedation, e.g., haloperidol 1–5 mg (care in the elderly), after action has been taken to deal with the cause and the patient constitutes a threat to themselves or others.

Rarer general complications

Urinary retention Comparatively rare, even after major maxillofacial surgery. Early mobilization and adequate analgesia help; if not, use temporary catheterization (p. 523).

Superficial vein thrombosis follows "tissued" cannula or irritant IV injections. Observe for infection, treat pain, and consider supportive strapping.

DVT Signs are painful, shiny, red, swollen calf, usually unilaterally but may be bilaterally. At risk are immobile patients, especially following pelvic surgery, patients with cancer, women on the pill, the elderly, and the obese. Confirm by Doppler ultrasound or ascending venography. Prevent by using a low-molecular-weight heparin (dalteparin, enoxaparin) preoperatively and 5 days postop and/or pressure stockings, and ensure early mobilization. Stop use of contraceptive pill prior to any major surgery. Rx: bed rest, leg strapping and elevation, analgesia, and heparinization (give 5000 units stat IV followed by 50,000 units in 50 ml normal saline by syringe driver infusion starting at 1000 units/h (1 ml/h) and adjust according to the KCT/APTT, keep between 1.5 and 2.5 times the control values). The major risk of DVT is development of pulmonary embolus. This classically presents 10 days postoperatively when the patient has been straining at stool and may occur despite no apparent DVT. Symptoms are pleuritic chest pain, dyspnea, cyanosis, hemopytisis, and an ↑ jugular venous pressure. Signs of shock are often present, ranging from very little in the young, who can compensate, to cardiac arrest! Usually a clinical Δ, confirmed after heparinization, analgesia, and O_2 have been instituted, by CXR, blood gases, spiral CT, or lung ventilation–perfusion scan and/or pulmonary angiography. ECG will sometimes show deep S waves in I, pathological Q waves in III, and inverted T waves in III (SI, QIII, TIII). Must be followed up by 3–6 months anticoagulation with warfarin, so involve a hematologist.

Less serious but more common are *post-phlebitic limb*, varicose veins, limb swelling, and skin discoloration. These may lead to varicose eczema.

Local complications following oral surgery

Local pain, swelling, infection, and trismus are the most common. Antral complications may follow maxillary surgery. These are considered in the relevant chapters.

Therapeutics

Relevant chapters and pages: Chapter 10 Medicine relevant to dentistry; Chapter 12 Analgesia, anesthesia, and sedation; asepsis and antisepsis, p. 350; antiseptics and antibiotics in periodontal disease, p. 198; fluorides, p. 28; sugar-free medications, p. 118.

Generic Pharmaceutical name.

Brand Trade name.

Depending on patents, a generic drug may have more than one brand name.

Poison control centers

United States Poison Control (800) 222-1222

American Association of Poison Control Centers
US Poison Control Certified Center Members
Updated August 2006

Alabama

Alabama Poison Center
2503 Phoenix Drive
Tuscaloosa, AL 35405
Emergency Phone: (800) 222-1222

Regional Poison Control Center
Children's Hospital
1600 7th Avenue South
Birmingham, AL 35233
Emergency Phone: (800) 222-1222

Alaska

Oregon Poison Center
Oregon Health Sciences University
3181 SW Sam Jackson Park Road,
CB550 Portland, OR 97201
Emergency Phone: (800) 222-1222

Arizona

Arizona Poison & Drug Info Center
Arizona Health Sciences Center, Room 1156
1501 North Campbell Avenue
Tucson, AZ 85724
Emergency Phone: (800) 222-1222

Banner Poison Control Center
901 East Willetta Street
Room 2701
Phoenix, AZ 85006
Emergency Phone: (800) 222-1222

Arkansas

Arkansas Poison & Drug Info Center
College of Pharmacy
University of Arkansas for Medical Sciences
4301 W. Markham, Mail Slot 522-2
Little Rock, AR 72205
Emergency Phone: (800) 222-1222

California

California Poison Control System—Fresno/Madera Division
Children's Hospital Central California
9300 Valley Children's Place, MB 15
Madera, CA 93638-8762
Emergency Phone: (800) 222-1222

California Poison Control System—Sacramento Division
UC Davis Medical Center
2315 Stockton Boulevard
Sacramento, CA 95817
Emergency Phone: (800) 222-1222

California Poison Control System—San Diego Division
University of California, San Diego, Medical Center
200 West Arbor Drive
San Diego, CA 92103-8925
Emergency Phone: (800) 222-1222

California Poison Control System—San Francisco Division
UCSF Box 1369
San Francisco, CA 94143-1369
Emergency Phone: (800) 222-1222

Colorado
Rocky Mountain Poison & Drug Center
777 Bannock Street
Mail Code 0180
Denver, CO 80204-4028
Emergency Phone: (800) 222-1222

Connecticut
Connecticut Poison Control Center
University of Connecticut Health Center
263 Farmington Avenue
Farmington, CT 06030-5365
Emergency Phone: (800) 222-1222

Delaware
The Poison Control Center
34th & Civic Center Blvd.
Philadelphia, PA 19104-4303
Emergency Phone: (800) 222-1222

District of Columbia
National Capital Poison Center
3201 New Mexico Avenue, NW
Suite 310
Washington, DC 20016
Emergency Phone: 1-800-222-1222
TTY/TDD: (202) 362-8563 (TTY)

Florida
Florida Poison Information Center—Jacksonville
655 West Eighth Street
Jacksonville, FL 32209
Emergency Phone: (800) 222-1222

Florida Poison Information Center—Miami
University of Miami, Dept. of Pediatrics
P.O. Box 016960 (R-131)
Miami, FL 33101
Emergency Phone: (800) 222-1222

Florida Poison Information Center—Tampa
Tampa General Hospital
P.O. Box 1289
Tampa, FL 33601
Emergency Phone: (800) 222-1222

Georgia

Georgia Poison Center
CHOA at Hughes Spalding
Grady Health System
80 Jesse Hill Jr. Drive, SE
P.O. Box 26066
Atlanta, GA 30335-3801
Emergency Phone: (800) 222-1222

Hawaii

Rocky Mountain Poison and Drug Center
777 Bannock Street
Mail code 0180
Denver, CO 80204-4028
Emergency Phone: (800) 222-1222

Idaho

Rocky Mountain Poison & Drug Center
777 Bannock Street
Mail Code 0180
Denver, CO 80204-4028
Emergency Phone: (800) 222-1222

Illinois

Illinois Poison Center
222 S. Riverside Plaza, Suite 1900
Chicago, IL 60606
Emergency Phone: (800) 222-1222

Indiana

Indiana Poison Center
Methodist Hospital, Room AG373
Clarian Health Partners
I-65 at 21st Street
Indianapolis, IN 46206-1367
Emergency Phone: (800) 222-1222

Iowa

Iowa Statewide Poison Control Center
Iowa Health System and University of Iowa Hospitals & Clinics
401 Douglas St., Suite 402
Sioux City, IA 51101
Emergency Phone: (800) 222-1222

Kansas

Mid-America Poison Center
University of Kansas Medical Center
3901 Rainbow Blvd., Room B-400
Kansas City, KS 66160-7231
Emergency Phone: (800) 222-1222

Kentucky

Kentucky Regional Poison Center
Medical Towers South, Suite 847
234 East Gray Street
Louisville, KY 40202
Emergency Phone: (800) 222-1222

Louisiana

Louisiana Poison Center
1521 Wilkinson Street
Shreveport, LA 71103
Emergency Phone: (800) 222-1222

Maine

Northern New England Poison Center
Serving Maine, New Hampshire, and Vermont
22 Bramhall Street
Portland, ME 04102
Emergency Phone: (800) 222-1222

Maryland

Maryland Poison Center
University of MD at Baltimore
School of Pharmacy
20 North Pine Street, PH 772
Baltimore, MD 21201
Emergency Phone: (800) 222-1222

National Capital Poison Center
3201 New Mexico Avenue, NW
Suite 310
Washington, DC 20016
Emergency Phone: (800) 222-1222

Massachusetts

Regional Center for Poison Control and Prevention
Serving Massachusetts and Rhode Island
Children's Hospital Boston
300 Longwood Avenue
Boston, MA 02115
Emergency Phone: (800) 222-1222

Michigan

Children's Hospital of Michigan
Regional Poison Control Center
4160 John R Harper Professional Office Bldg, Ste. 616
Detroit, MI 48201
Emergency Phone: (800) 222-1222

DeVos Children's Hospital
Regional Poison Center
1300 Michigan, NE, Suite 203
Grand Rapids, MI 49503
Emergency Phone: (800) 222-1222

Minnesota

Hennepin Regional Poison Center
Hennepin County Medical Center
701 Park Avenue
Minneapolis, MN 55415
Emergency Phone: (800) 222-1222

Missouri

Missouri Regional Poison Center
7980 Clayton Road, Suite 200
St. Louis, MO 63117
Emergency Phone: (800) 222-1222

Montana

Rocky Mountain Poison & Drug Center
777 Bannock Street
Mail Code 0180
Denver, CO 80204-4028
Emergency Phone: (800) 222-1222

Nebraska

Nebraska Regional Poison Center
8401 West Dodge Road, Suite 115
Omaha, NE 68114
Emergency Phone: (800) 222-1222

Nevada

Oregon Poison Center
Oregon Health Sciences University
3181 SW Sam Jackson Park Road, CB550
Portland, OR 97201
Emergency Phone: (800) 222-1222

Rocky Mountain Poison & Drug Center
777 Bannock Street
Mail Code 0180
Denver, CO 80204-4028
Emergency Phone: (800) 222-1222

New Hampshire

Northern New England Poison Center
Serving Maine, New Hampshire, and Vermont
22 Bramhall Street
Portland, ME 04102
Emergency Phone: (800) 222-1222

New Jersey

New Jersey Poison Information and Education System
University of Medicine and Dentistry at New Jersey
140 Bergen Street
Newark, NJ 07101
Emergency Phone: (800) 222-1222

New Mexico

New Mexico Poison & Drug Information Center
MSC 09 5080
1 University of New Mexico
Albuquerque, NM 87131-0001
Emergency Phone: (800) 222-1222

New York

Central New York Poison Center
750 East Adams Street
Syracuse, NY 13210
Emergency Phone: (800) 222-1222

The Ruth A. Lawrence Poison and Drug Information Center Serving
Finger Lakes
University of Rochester Medical Center
601 Elmwood Avenue, Box 321
Rochester, NY 14642
Emergency Phone: (800) 222-1222

Long Island Regional Poison and Drug Information Center
Winthrop University Hospital
259 First Street
Mineola, NY 11501
Emergency Phone: (800) 222-1222

New York City Poison Control Center
NYC Bureau of Public Health Labs
455 First Avenue
Room 123, Box 81
New York, NY 10016
Emergency Phone: (800) 222-1222

North Carolina

Carolinas Poison Center
P.O Box 32861
Charlotte, NC 28232
Emergency Phone: (800) 222-1222

North Dakoka

Hennepin Regional Poison Center
Hennepin County Medical Center
701 Park Avenue
Minneapolis, MN 55415
Emergency Phone: (800) 222-1222

Ohio

Central Ohio Poison Center
700 Children's Drive, Room E 263
Columbus, OH 43205
Emergency Phone: (800) 222-1222

Cincinnati Drug & Poison Information Center
3333 Burnet Avenue
Vernon Place - 3rd Floor
Cincinnati, OH 45229
Emergency Phone: (800) 222-1222

Oklahoma

Oklahoma Poison Control Center
Children's Hospital at OU Medical Center
940 N.E. 13th Street, Room 3510
Oklahoma City, OK 73104
Emergency Phone: (800) 222-1222

Oregon

Oregon Poison Center
Oregon Health & Science University
3181 SW Sam Jackson Park Road, CB550
Portland, OR 97239
Emergency Phone: (800) 222-1222

Pennsylvania

Pittsburgh Poison Center
Children's Hospital of Pittsburgh
3705 Fifth Avenue
Pittsburgh, PA 15213
Emergency Phone: (800) 222-1222

The Poison Control Center
at The Children's Hospital of Philadelphia
34th & Civic Center Blvd
CHOP North Suite 985
Philadelphia, PA 19104-4303
Emergency Phone: (800) 222-1222

Rhode Island

Regional Center for Poison Control and Prevention
Serving Massachusettes and Rhode Island
300 Longwood Avenue
Boston, MA 02115
Emergency Phone: (800) 222-1222

South Carolina
Palmetto Poison Center
College of Pharmacy
University of South Carolina
Columbia, SC 29208
Emergency Phone: (800) 222-1222

South Dakota
Hennepin Regional Poison Center
Hennepin County Medical Center
701 Park Avenue
Minneapolis, MN 55415
Emergency Phone: (800) 222-1222

Tennessee
Tennessee Poison Center
501 Oxford House
1161 21st Avenue South
Nashville, TN 37232-4632
Emergency Phone: (800) 222-1222

Texas
Central Texas Poison Center
Scott and White Memorial Hospital
2401 South 31st Street
Temple, TX 76508
Emergency Phone: (800) 222-1222

North Texas Poison Center
at Parkland Memorial Hospital
5201 Harry Hines Blvd.
Dallas, TX 75235
Emergency Phone: (800) 222-1222

South Texas Poison Center
University of Texas Health Science Center—San Antonio
Department of Surgery
Mail Code 7849, 7703 Floyd Curl Drive
San Antonio, TX 78229-3900
Emergency Phone: (800) 222-1222

Southeast Texas Poison Center
University of Texas Medical Branch
3.112 Trauma Center
901 Harborside Drive
Galveston, TX 77555-1175
Emergency Phone: (800) 222-1222

Texas Panhandle Poison Center
1501 S. Coulter
Amarillo, TX 79106
Emergency Phone: (800) 222-1222

West Texas Regional Poison Center
Thomason Hospital
4815 Alameda Avenue
El Paso, TX 79905
Emergency Phone: (800) 222-1222

Utah

Utah Poison Control Center
585 Komas Drive, Suite 200
Salt Lake City, UT 84108-1208
Emergency Phone: (800) 222-1222

Vermont

Northern New England Poison Center
Serving Maine, New Hampshire, and Vermont
22 Bramhall Street
Portland, ME 04102
Emergency Phone: (800) 222-1222

Virginia

Blue Ridge Poison Center
University of Virginia Health System
PO Box 800774
Charlottesville, VA 22908-0774
Emergency Phone: (800) 222-1222

National Capital Poison Center
3201 New Mexico Avenue, NW, Suite 310
Washington, DC 20016
Emergency Phone: (800) 222-1222

Virginia Poison Center
Medical College of Virginia Hospitals
Virginia Commonwealth University Medical Center
P.O. Box 980522
Richmond, VA 23298-0522
Emergency Phone: (800) 222-1222

Washington

Washington Poison Center
155 NE 100th Street, Suite 400
Seattle, WA 98125-8011
Emergency Phone: (800) 222-1222

West Virginia

West Virginia Poison Center
3110 MacCorkle Avenue, S.E.
Charleston, WV 25304
Emergency Phone: (800) 222-1222

Wisconsin

Wisconsin Poison Center
Children's Hospital of Wisconsin
P.O. Box 1997, Mail Station 677A
Milwaukee, WI 53201-1997
Emergency Phone: (800) 222-1222

Wyoming

Nebraska Regional Poison Center
8200 Dodge Street
Omaha, NE 68114
Emergency Phone: (800) 222-1222

Prescribing

The following pages are a brief guide to the clinical use of some commonly used and useful drugs in dental practice. Doses are for healthy adults.

Prescribing in general dental practice Extremely useful information is available in the Physicians' Desk Reference (PDR), which is updated annually. Use this as primary reference when unsure about any topic concerning drugs. Use this to check dose alterations in children and the elderly, and for more details on drug interactions, C/I, and undesirable side effects. Controlled substances can be prescribed, in the United States, by a licensed dentist with State and Federal Drug Enforcement Administration (DEA) registration with a DEA number included on the prescription.

Good prescribing Avoid abbreviations and write drug names legibly, using the generic whenever possible. Always describe the strength and quantity to be dispensed. When describing doses use the units micrograms, milligrams, or milliliters when possible. Do not abbreviate the term microgram or unit, as these are easily misinterpreted. By not using abbreviations the potential for errors in drug dispensing is minimized.

Controlled drugs Each prescription must show, in the prescriber's own handwriting in ink, the name and address of the patient, the form, strength, dose, and total quantity of the drug to be dispensed, in both words and numbers.

Prescribing in the elderly Doses may need to be altered in elders who present with chronic diseases that may result in reductions in physiologic capacity. Increasing numbers of patients are routinely taking multiple pharmaceuticals. Drug interactions must always be considered.

Prescribing for children Children differ markedly from adults in their response to drugs, especially in the neonatal period when all doses should be calculated in relation to body weight. Older children can usually be prescribed for in age ranges, usually up to 1 yr, 1–6 yr, and 6–12 yr. All details of dosages should be checked in the PDR.

Prescribing in liver disease (p. 482) Use caution when prescribing for patients with severe liver disease and be aware of the route of drug elimination to avoid drug toxicity.

Prescribing in renal impairment (p. 484) Doses almost always need to be adjusted and some drugs are C/I completely.

Drug Schedules[1]
Schedule I
- Drug has a high potential for abuse
- Drug has no currently accepted medical use in treatment.
- Drug lacks accepted safety for use under medical supervision.

Drugs such as heroin, MDA, Ecstasy, marijuana, and mescaline are included in this category.

Schedule II

- Drug has a high potential for abuse.
- Drug has a currently accepted medical or a currently accepted medical use with severe restrictions.
- Abuse may lead to severe psychological or physical dependence.
- Available by written prescription only, oral prescription only in an emergency.
- Production quotas set by DEA.

Drugs such as amphetamines, cocaine, codeine, fentanyl, hydrocodone, and meperidine are included in this category.

Schedule III

- Drug has a reduced potential for abuse compared to substances in schedules I and II.
- Drug has a currently accepted medical use in treatment.
- Abuse may lead to moderate or low physical dependence or high psychological dependence relative to drugs in schedule II.

Drugs such testosterone, codeine combinations, and hydrocodone combinations are included in this category.

Schedule IV

- Drug has a low potential for abuse relative to substances in schedule III.
- Drug has a currently accepted medical use in treatment.
- Abuse of the drug may lead to limited physical dependence or psychological dependence relative to drugs in schedule III.

Drugs such as benzodiazepines, phenobarbital, and chloral hydrate are included in this category.

Schedule V

- Drug has a low potential for abuse relative to other substances in schedule IV.
- Drug has a currently accepted medical use in treatment.
- Abuse of the drug may lead to limited physical dependence or psychological dependence relative to the other drugs in schedule IV.

Drugs such as antitussives with small amounts of opiod derivatives, and antidiarrheals are included in this category.

Food and Drug Administration (FDA) pregnancy categories[1]

A	Adequate, well-controlled studies in pregnant women have not shown an increased risk of fetal abnormalities.
B	Animal studies have revealed no evidence of harm to the fetus, however, there are no adequate and well-controlled studies in pregnant women.
	or
	Animal studies have shown an adverse effect, but adequate and well-controlled studies in pregnant women have failed to demonstrate a risk to the fetus.
C	Animal studies have shown an adverse effect and there are no adequate and well-controlled studies in pregnant women.
	or
	No animal studies have been conducted and there are no adequate and well-controlled studies in pregnant women.
D	Studies, adequate well-controlled or observational, in pregnant women have demonstrated a risk to the fetus. However, the benefits of therapy may outweigh the potential risk.
X	Studies, adequate well-controlled or observational, in animals or pregnant women have demonstrated positive evidence of fetal abnormalities. Use of the product is contraindicated in women who are or may become pregnant.

Prescribing

For prescribing during pregnancy evaluate FDA pregnancy category and avoid if possible.

For prescribing in terminal care, see p. 526.

Dose and route abbreviations

Dose	Route
qd every day	**IM** intramuscular
bid twice daily	**INH** inhalation
tid three times daily	**IV** intravenous
qid four times daily	**PO** by mouth
prn as required	OTC over the counter
q4h every 4 hours	SC subcutaneous
q6h every 6 hours	SUB sublingual
	TOP topical

1 U.S. Food and Drug Administration. http://www.fda.gov/fdac/features/2001/301_preg.html

Analgesics in dental practice

Consult PDR for dosages in children. See also p. 546. Most dental pain is inflammatory in origin and hence is most responsive to drugs with an anti-inflammatory component, e.g., aspirin and the NSAIDs.

Of the peripherally acting analgesics in the PDR, aspirin, acetaminophen, and ibuprofen are available OTC from pharmacies.

Acetaminophen Used in mild to moderate pain. Acetaminophen has no anti-inflammatory action and is a moderate antipyretic. Does not cause gastric irritation or interfere with bleeding times. Overdose can lead to liver failure. *Dose:* PO 325–650 mg q4h, do not exceed 4g/day.

Ibuprofen Popularly used for mild to moderate pain; has a moderate antipyretic action. Risks and side effects are similar to that of aspirin but less irritant to the gut. *Dose:* PO 200–800 mg qid, do not exceed 3.2g/day.

Aspirin Used in mild to moderate pain, it is also a potent antipyretic, which should *not* be used in children <12 yr (because of the rare but serious risk of Reye syndrome). Avoid in bleeding diathesis, gastrointestinal ulceration, and concurrent anticoagulant therapy. Ask about aspirin allergy, particularly in asthmatics. Often causes transient gut irritation (as do all NSAIDs). *Dose:* PO 325–650 mg q4h, do not exceed 4 g/day.

Note that all NSAIDs *may* exacerbate asthma and there is a higher incidence of NSAID allergy in asthmatics, this *does not* constitute a C/I for the use of these valuable analgesics. Frank allergy to NSAIDs or proven exacerbation of asthma *is* a C/I.

Narcotic Analgesics

Narcotic analgesics are Schedule II controlled substances and are only available by written prescription and by oral prescription in emergency situations. Schedule II prescriptions cannot be refilled.

Hydromorphone HCL is a synthetic narcotic analgesic used for moderate to severe pain PO 1–10 mg q3–6h prn pain (Dilaudid®).

Meperidine is a synthetic narcotic analgesic used for moderate to severe pain (international generic name pethidine) PO 50–150 mg q4h prn pain. (Demerol®).

Oxycodone is a synthetic opioid analgesic used for moderate to severe pain. PO in combination with acetaminophen or aspirin (OxyContin®).

The addition of codeine to the minor analgesics, while never being proven to be of advantage, may have marginal benefits in some cases. Some of the more commonly used combinations are Tylenol® with codeine.

- Tylenol with Codeine No. 2 = 300 mg acetaminophen + 15 mg codeine phosphate
- Tylenol with Codeine No. 3 = 300 mg acetaminophen + 30 mg codeine phosphate
- Tylenol with Codeine No. 4 = 300 mg acetaminophen + 60 mg codeine phosphate

The addition of hydrocodone bitartrate to the minor analgesics:
- Vicodin®, Lorcet®, Lortab® 5/500, Margesic H®, 500 mg acetaminophen + 5 mg hydrocodone bitartrate
- Vicodin® ES 750 mg acetaminophen + 7.5 mg hydrocodone bitartrate
- Vicodin® HP 660 mg acetaminophen + 10 mg hydrocodone bitartrate
- Vicoprofen® 200 mg ibuprofen + 10 mg hydrocodone bitartrate

Opioid analgesics

The opioids act centrally to alter the perception of pain, but have no anti-inflammatory properties. They are of value for severe pain of visceral origin, postoperatively (acting partly by sedation), and in terminal care. However, they all depress respiratory function and interfere with the pupillary response, and are C/I in head injury. All opioids cause cough suppression, urinary retention, nausea, constipation by a ↓ in gut motility, and tolerance and dependence. The risk of addiction is, however, greatly overstated when these drugs are used for short-term postoperative analgesia and in the terminal care context. Fear of creating addicts should **never** cause you to withhold adequate analgesia.

Codeine phosphate A moderate opioid analgesic useful for short-term analgesia and less likely to mask a head injury; 30–60 mg 4 hourly IM/PO. There may be some advantage when used in combination (8/15/30 mg) with simple analgesics or NSAIDs.

Morphine In oral form (tablets, elixir, or slow-release tablets) it is the drug of choice in management of terminal pain. Always prescribe a laxative. *Dose:* depends on previous analgesia, but often starts at 10 mg morphine q4h or 10–20 mg PO slow release q24 h. When used SC/IM, 2.5–10 mg q4h prn, or IV for acute or postoperative pain: 10–20 mg 2–4 hourly; give an antiemetic.

Buprenorphine A mixed agonist/antagonist with similar problems to meperidine and pentazocine. Primary use is in the treatment of opioid dependence and pain.[1]

---

1 http://www.buprenorphine.samhsa.gov/

Anti-inflammatory drugs

These are among the groups of drugs that may be either analgesics or co-analgesics (drugs that are not analgesic in themselves but may aid pain relief either directly or indirectly). The two major groups are the NSAIDs (p. 550) and the corticosteroids.

Steroids are used in various forms, topical, oral, intralesional, and parenteral, and all have uses in dentistry.

Topical steroids

- *Hydrocortisone, hydrocortisone acetate, hydrocortisone buteprate, hydrocortisone butyrate, hydrocortisone valerate* are used for eczema, psoriasis, dermatitis, and pruritis, available in concentrations from 0.5 to 2.5% topical creams sprays and ointments. Used TOP qd–qid applied to affected area.
- *Triamcinolone acetonide* is used to treat nonviral inflammatory oral lesions, including aphthous stomatitis, lichen planus, and cicatricial phemphigoid. Available as 0.025%, 0.1%, 0.5% ointment, cream and lotion for TOP application to affected area bid–qid.

Intra-articular steroids

These can be used to induce a chemical arthroplasty in arthrosis of the TMJ (p. 410).
- *Hydrocortisone acetate* 5–10 mg single injection
- *Triamincinolone* Can be used intra-articularly

Systemic steroids

The main indication is prophylaxis in those with actual or potential adrenocortical suppression. Occasionally they are used in erosive lichen planus, severe aphthae, e.g., Behçet syndrome (p. 680), or arteritis (p. 490).
- *Hydrocortisone sodium succinate* is used for prophylaxis; dose 50–100 mg IM 30 min preoperatively.
- *Prednisolone* 5–60 mg PO as enteric-coated tablets given with food. Regimen depends on the condition being treated.
- *Methylprednisolone* 40 mg/ml. Various regimens are described for control of edema, post major surgery.
- *Dexamethasone* 4 mg/ml. Various regimens are described for control of edema, post surgery.

Other immunosuppressants

Azathioprine (Imuran®) is used in transplant centers and to treat pemphigus and phemphigiod, chronic ulcerative cholitis, Crohn's disease, and Behçet's syndrome. Topical *tacrolimus* is used for erosive lichen planus.

Antidepressants

This is another group of drugs that can be used as co-analgesics. In conditions such as atypical facial pain they may be used as the sole "analgesic."

In the past, there has been considerable debate about the potential interactions between the most commonly used antidepressants, the tricyclics, and the monoamine oxidase inhibitors (MAOIs), and epinephrine contained in LA (which constitutes the most commonly professionally administered drug anywhere). To date, there is *no clinical evidence* of dangerous interactions between the epinephrine in LA preparations commonly used in dentistry and the tricyclics or the MAOIs.[1]

Amitriptyline Use with caution in patients with cardiac disease (as arrhythmias may follow the use of tricyclics) and avoid in diabetics, epileptics, and pregnant or breast-feeding women. It can precipitate glaucoma, heighten the effect of alcohol, and cause drowsiness (which can impair driving). In common with other tricyclics it can cause sedation, blurred vision, xerostomia, constipation, nausea, and difficulty with micturition, although tolerance to these side effects tends to develop as Rx progresses. There is often an interval of 2–4 weeks before these drugs reach a level that exhibits a clinically evident antidepressant effect. *Dose:* 50–75 mg either as a single bedtime dose or in divided doses, maximum 150–200 mg daily. For children prescribe half-dose.

Nortriptyline A less sedating tricyclic. *Dose:* 10–30 mg; note: can be increased.

Tranylcypromine A MAOI that may be of value in treating facial pain unresponsive to tricyclics. *Dose:* 10 mg tid before 4 p.m.[2]

Selective serotonin reuptake inhibitors (SSRIs) are much less sedative antidepressants, given as single dose a.m. Fluoxetine (Prozac) is best known (20 mg daily) and also abused (overprescribing and used to prolong effects of MDMA or Ecstasy). Paroxetine 20 mg qd in a.m. and sertraline 50 mg qd a.m. are similar.

1 DPF 2000–02. In *BNF* **40** 2000.
2 M. Harris 1993 *BDJ* **174** 129.

Antiemetics

Antiemetics are an essential part of inpatient prescribing. The common indication is the control of postoperative nausea and vomiting, which may be due to the procedure, anesthetic, postoperative analgesia, or blood in the stomach.

Prochlorperazine A phenothiazine antiemetic that acts as a dopamine antagonist and blocks the chemoreceptor trigger zone. Avoid in small children as the drug's major side effect, the production of extrapyramidal symptoms, is especially common in this group. *Dose:* 5–10 mg IM q4h, PO 5–10 mg tid.

Metoclopramide has both peripheral and central modes of action. It ↑ gut motility, thus emptying the stomach. Acute dystonic reactions may occur, especially in young women and children; a bizarre acute trismus is sometimes seen as one of the manifestations. *Dose:* 10 mg tid PO, 10 mg IM 8 hourly. High-dose intermittent and continuous IV regimens are used for antiemesis in centers using cytotoxic chemotherapy.

Ondansetron *HCL* A selective 5-HT$_3$ antagonist that is very effective in prevention and Rx of postoperative nausea and vomiting. *Dose:* 4 mg single IV dose or 8 mg PO.

Antihistamines, and major tranquillizers all have antiemetic properties but are rarely indicated. If unable to control emesis with one agent use two, acting at separate sites *after* excluding intestinal obstruction, e.g., due to opioid constipation.

Do not forget the benefits of a nasogastric tube in preventing nausea and vomiting from a distended or irritated stomach. Constipation can also cause nausea—remember to exclude it as a cause.

Anxiolytics, sedatives, hypnotics, and tranquillizers

The short-term control of fear and anxiety associated with dental Rx is an entirely appropriate use of the benzodiazepines. It should not be confused with the long-term control of anxiety, which may present problems of dependence and drug withdrawal. A benzodiazepine may also be a valuable adjunct in the management of TMPDS, where it acts as both a muscle relaxant and an anxiolytic (p. 470). For IV and oral sedative techniques prior to surgery, see p. 582.

Diazepam has a long half-life and is cumulative on repeated dosing. Like all benzodiazepines, it can cause respiratory depression, therefore patients should be warned not to drive or operate machinery while on this drug. *Dose for anxiety/TMPDS*: 2 mg tid, maximum 30 mg in divided daily doses. Paradoxical disinhibition may occur in children and its use in those <16 yr is not advised.

Midazolam A water-soluble benzodiazepine of about double the potency of diazepam. Its main use is in IV sedation (p. 582). It is also popular as a pediatric sedative for suture removal.

Temazepam Shorter-acting hypnotic. *Dose:* 7.5–30 mg at bedtime. Main indication is preop or as premedication.

Chlordiazepoxide Sometimes used instead of diazepam in TMPDS. It has the same side-effect profile. *Dose:* 10 mg tid, increasing to maximum of 100 mg daily, in divided doses. It is the drug of choice in stabilization of alcohol-dependent inpatients.

Lorazepam Sometimes used as a premedication by anesthetists. *Dose:* 2–6 mg qd, 2 mg 1 h preoperatively. Alternative to diazepam in epileptics.

Flumazenil A specific benzodiazepine reversal agent (p. 582). Caution is required when there is impaired hepatic and renal function.

Chloral hydrate (Chloral Elixir, pediatric) 20–50 mg/kg PO used as a sedative for pediatric patients.

Antibiotics

When prescribing, consider **1** the patient, **2** the likely organisms, and **3** the best drug. Patients influence choice, in that they may be allergic to various drugs, have hepatic or renal impairment, be immunocompromised, be unable to swallow, be pregnant or breast-feeding, or taking an oral contraceptive; consider also patient age and severity of the infection. The infecting organism should ideally be isolated, cultured, and its sensitivity to antibiotics determined. In reality, most infections are treated blind, therefore it is essential to know the common infecting organisms and their sensitivities. You also need to know the drugs' modes of action, absorption, unwanted effects, development of resistance, interactions, and techniques available for delivery. The best drug is one that is safe in that patient and specific to the infecting organism, and can be given in a reliable, convenient form. Remember prophylaxis (p. 528) differs from Rx with antibiotics, and antibiotics do not replace the drainage of pus in abscesses.

Penicillin G benzathine Inactive orally and only used IM or IV. *Dose:* IM 1.2 million units. It is the drug of choice in treating streptococcal infections. Like all penicillins, it is bactericidal: it interferes with cell-wall synthesis. It has good tissue penetration except for CSF. Its most important unwanted effect is hypersensitivity, which is usually manifested as a rash, rarely as fatal anaphylaxis. Patients allergic to one penicillin will be allergic to all; 10% will be allergic to cephalosporins as well. A history of atopy (e.g., asthma) increases risk.

Penicillin V potassium Oral equivalent of above. Dose: 250–500 mg qid PO. It has a narrow spectrum, and is now largely superseded by amoxicillin.

Amoxicillin Has a broad spectrum similar to that of ampicillin, but is better absorbed and achieves higher tissue concentrations. *Dose:* PO 250–500 mg q8h. Both ampicillin and amoxicillin cause a maculopapular rash in patients with glandular fever, lymphatic leukemia, or possibly HIV infection (this is *not* true penicillin allergy). Amoxicillin is drug of choice in prophylaxis against infective endocarditis (p. 528). It may interfere with the action of oral contraceptives. All penicillins decrease excretion of methotrexate, therefore increase risk of toxicity.

Tetracycline One of a group of broad-spectrum antibiotics with a problem of increasing bacterial resistance. It is likely to promote opportunistic infection with *Candida albicans*, particularly when used topically, as has been recommended for the Rx of aphthae. Other problems are the deposition of tetracyclines in growing bone and teeth, causing staining and hypoplasia (∴ avoid in children <12 yr and pregnancy) and erythema multiforme. It is also particularly likely to render the oral contraceptive ineffective. *Dose:* PO 250–500 mg q6h, 1 h before or 2 h after meals. Absorption is inhibited by chelation with milk, etc. It may be of value in periodontal disease (p. 198). Doxycycline PO 100 mg q12h day 1, then 100 mg qd.

Erythromycin Has a similar spectrum to that of penicillin, but bacteriostatic binds 50s ribosomal subunits, suppressing protein synthesis. It is active against penicillinase-producing organisms. It was formerly an alternative to amoxicillin for endocarditis prophylaxis (superseded by clindamycin). Nausea is a major problem. *Dose:* PO/IV 250–500 mg q6h.

Oral cephalosporins, cephalexin PO 250–500 mg q6h. Clindamycin binds to 50s ribosomal subunits to inhibit protein synthesis. PO 150–450 mg q6h.

Clindamycin Should be used cautiously in management of dental infections, because of the risk of antibiotic-induced colitis. It is useful in staphylococcal osteomyelitis in conjunction with metronidazole (which inhibits overgrowth with *Clostridium difficile*). It has replaced erythromycin for single-dose prophylaxis of infective endocarditis (p. 528).

Metronidazole A direct-acting amebicide/trichomonacide binds and degrades DNA. PO 250 mg tid. It is an anaerobicidal drug, and as such is effective in treating many acute dental and oral infections. The classic dose for NUG is 200 mg tid PO 3 days. For other anaerobic infections it is more often used as 400 mg bid/tid (depending on severity) PO. Available in tablets, IV infusion, or suppository. Its main problem is severe nausea and vomiting if taken in conjunction with alcohol (disulfiram reaction). Remember, it is NOT effective against aerobic bacteria.

Gentamicin A bactericidal aminoglycoside antibiotic, active mainly against gram-negative organisms. It is complementary to the penicillins and available as a topical (opthalmic use) IV or IM. Its major problem is dose-related ototoxicity and nephrotoxicity (monitor levels if used for >24 h). *Dose:* up to 5 mg/kg monitored use per local guidelines.

Vancomycin A unique bactericidal antibiotic. It is ototoxic, nephrotoxic, and prone to cause phlebitis at infusion sites, and it makes people feel generally unwell; therefore, it is not to be used lightly.

Antifungal and antiviral drugs

Antifungals

The main fungal pathogen in the mouth is *Candida albicans* (p. 432).

Amphotericin B use to treat oral fungal infections by *Candidia albicans*. Oral suspension 100 mg/ml qid.

Nystatin Available as tabs, lozenge, or oral suspension. *Dose:* 400,000–600,000 units qid oral supension or by sucking lozenge 200,000–400,000 4–5qd or using 1 ml of the mixture and holding it in the mouth before swallowing.

Miconazole A useful drug, particularly in management of angular cheilitis, as it is active against streptococci, staphylococci, and candida. Miconazole oral gel 2% is of use for chronic mucocutaneous and chronic hyperplastic candidosis. *Dose:* Miconazole cream is used topically for angular cheilitis.

Fluconazole Available in tabs, oral, and IV formulations for severe mucosal candidosis in both normal and immunocompromised patients as a second line to topical preparations. Avoid use in pregnancy. *Dose:* 100–400 mg qd, 200–400 mg IV qd. Itraconazole and tioconazole are other new antifungal drugs.

Ketoconazole Treats systemic candida, coccidioidomycosis, and histo-plasmosis infections with 200 mg tabs, 2% cream. *Dose:* 200 mg qd PO.

There are recognized potentially serious interactions between miconazole, fluconazole, and related drugs and antibacterials, anticoagulants, antidia-betics, antiepileptics, antihistamines, anxiolytics, cisapride, cyclosporin, and theophylline. Check what your patient is currently taking. Candidal resistance to fluconazole is now recognized—get culture and sensitivity if Rx is not working.

Antivirals

Most viral infections are treated symptomatically. One drug is available for the Rx of orofacial viral diseases.

Acyclovir Active against herpes simplex and zoster; relatively nontoxic and can be given systemically or topically. *Dose:* herpes labialis: apply aciclovir cream to site of prodromal or early lesion q3h for 7 days; her-petic stomatitis: 200 mg (400 mg in immunocompromised) PO 5 times daily for 10 days; herpes zoster: 800 mg PO q4h for 7–10 days.

Antihistamines and decongestants

Antihistamines

These are rarely used in the usual range of dental practice. They are sometimes indicated in the management of allergy, especially hay fever, for premedication and sedation in children, occasionally as antiemetics, possibly in the management of overactive gag reflex, and as part of the emergency Rx of angioedema and anaphylaxis (p. 510). The main differences between the antihistamines are duration of action and degree of accompanying sedation and antimuscarinic effects.

Chlorpheniramine A sedative antihistamine. *Dose:* 4 mg qid PO.

Promethazine Also a sedative antihistamine. *Dose:* 10 mg qid PO or 20–30 mg at bedtime when used as a hypnotic.

The sedative effects of these drugs potentiate alcohol and ↓ ability to drive or operate machinery safely. They should be used with caution in glaucoma, prostatic hypertrophy, and epilepsy.

A wide range of non-sedating antihistamines are available as OTC generics to the public, e.g., cetirizine, loratadine.

Decongestants

These are valuable in the management of sinusitis and particularly in the closure of oroantral fitstulae.

Ephedrine nasal drops produce vasoconstriction of mucosal blood vessels and ↓ the thickness of nasal mucosa, thus relieving obstruction. Avoid use in patients taking MAOIs. Other problems: prolonged use leads to a rebound vasodilatation and a recurrence of nasal congestion, and long-term use results in tolerance and damage to nasal cilia. *Dose:* ephedrine nasal drops 0.5–1%, 1–2 drops into the relevant nostril qid for 7–10 days. For symptomatic nasal decongestion and as an adjunct to management of oroantral fistulae (p. 384), inhalation of menthol and eucalyptus is valuable. *Dose:* 1 teaspoonful of menthol and eucalyptus inhalation BP is added to a pint of hot water, and the warm, moist air is inhaled with a towel over the head.

Oxymetazoline nasal drops and spray 0.05% is a more potent alternative to ephedrine, but are more likely to cause a rebound effect. Systemic decongestants are of dubious value and contain sympathomimetics. They do not, however, cause rebound. For prescribed, short-term use, thereby avoiding risk of rebound, oxymetazoline is the drug of choice; spray into relevant nostril tid.

Miscellaneous

A number of drugs not fitting into any specific category are important in managing oral and dental disease. These include:

Carbamazepine Primarily an antiepileptic drug of considerable value in the management of trigeminal and glossopharyngeal neuralgia. It is C/I in those sensitive to the drug, patients with atrioventricular conduction defects, porphyria, and should be used with extreme caution in patients on MAOIs, who are pregnant, or who have liver failure. It may interfere with oral contraceptives. Common unwanted effects are gastrointestinal disturbances, dizziness, and visual disturbances. Rarely, rashes may occur, as can leukopenia. Do a FBC soon after starting carbamezipine: blood dyscrasias usually occur in the first 3 months. *Dose:* 100–200 mg bid; this can be increased gradually to 200 mg tid. Maximum 1600 mg daily in divided doses. It is important to be sure of your diagnosis before starting patients on carbamazepine (p. 454). A slow-release preparation with fewer unwanted effects is available.

Vitamins There is no indication for first-line Rx with vitamins in dental practice. Deficiency due to inadequate dietary intake in the United States is exceedingly rare. Although it can occur in the elderly and alcoholics, these people should be fully investigated and not treated empirically. Severe gingival swelling, stomatitis, glossitis, or pain should be fully investigated before using vitamin supplements.

Vitamin B compound tablets, strong A combination of nicotinamide 20 mg, pyridoxine 2 mg, riboflavine 2 mg, thiamine 5 mg. *Dose:* 1–2 tablets tid.

Ascorbic acid tablets BP (vitamin C ↑ iron absorption and prevents scurvy.

Artificial saliva Valuable adjunct in management of xerostomia, especially after radiotherapy and in Sjögren syndrome. This is a slightly viscous, inert fluid that may have a number of additives, such as antimicrobial preservatives, fluoride, flavoring, etc. Useful preparations such as Biotene. aerosol sprays are sprayed sublingually 4–6 times per day. Regular sips of water may be of more practical long-term help.

Topical anesthetics There are two main uses:
- For preparation of a site prior to injection, e.g. of LA. Lidocaine 5% ointment or spray is the most useful. Benzocaine 20% pastes are available. Tetracaine ointment 1%, cream 2%, gel 2%.
- Can be used on mucosa for topical anesthesia of inflamed or irritated tissues. Viscous lidocaine 2% 5–15 ml q4h, or spray 10% to affected area prn.

Fluorides Fluoride supplementation is discussed on p. 33. It is important when using rinses, and particularly gels, that the fluid is not swallowed, since there is a risk of toxicity (p. 29).

Alarm bells

When prescribing any drug for patients already compromised by concomitant disease or drug therapy, it is essential to exclude possible interactions. This can be achieved fairly quickly by consulting the PDR.

Interactions with the most commonly given drug (LA) are covered on p. 572.

Common drugs with relative contraindications in liver disease	Common drugs with relative contraindications in renal failure
Aspirin	Acyclovir (decrease dose)
All benzodiazepines	All penicillins (decrease dose)
All opioids	All opioids
All sedatives	Cephalosporins (decrease dose)
All antihistamines	Benzodiazepines (decrease dose)
All NSAIDs	NSAIDs
Erythromycin	Tetracyclines
Metronidazole (decrease dose)	Amphotericin
Tetracyclines	

Common drugs with relative contraindications in pregnancy	Common drugs with relative contraindications in breast-feeding
Aspirin	Antihisamines
Benzodiazepines	Aspirin
Carbamazepine	Benzodiazepines
All opioids	Carbamazepine
Cotrimoxazole	Cotrimoxazole
NSAIDs	Metronidazole
Metronidazole	Tetracyclines
Tetracyclines	

These lists are not comprehensive and some of the drugs mentioned can be used in suitably modified doses or under specific circumstances. These tables are designed to ring alarm bells, and encourage you to think and consult the PDR.

Adverse reactions

Almost any drug can produce these, and many are missed. Try to avoid polypharmacy, and never prescribe without being aware of a patient's full medical history. Always enquire about drugs, including self-prescribed medication.

Report suspected adverse reactions to the U.S. Food and Drug Administration at http://www.fda.gov/medwatch/report or call 1-800-FDA-1088 to report by telephone.

Emergency drugs	
Oxygen	Cylinder regulator valve, flow-meter, tubing, and oxygen mask (positive pressure mask or ambu bag)
Epinephrine	1 mg in 1 ml (1:1000) solution for IM injection, preloaded syringes
Diphenhydramine HCL (Benadryl®)	Histamine blocker 50 mg/ml
Hydrocortisone sodium succinate (Solu-Cortef)	100 mg powder, plus 2 ml water for IM injection
Glucose or sugar	Drink, tablets, or gel (PO administration)
Albuterol	90 mcg/spray bronchodialator INH
Nitroglycerin	0.5 tablets or 0.4 mg per dose spray SUB administration
Aspirin	300 mg tablets PO administration

Analgesia, anesthesia, and sedation

The status of general anesthesia in dental practice and, inevitably, the medicolegal aspects of anesthesia and sedation in the United States have changed over the years. The regulations on the use of various levels of anesthesia and sedation differ from state to state. They also vary widely from country to country. The general principles, however, remain the same. Check the rules that govern your local jurisdiction first.

Principal sources: J. Meechan 1998 *Pain and Anxiety Control for the Conscious Dental Patient*, OUP. *Department of Health Working Party on General Anaesthesia and Sedation in Dentistry* (Poswillo Report) 1990.

Relevant pages in other chapters: Local anesthesia for children, p. 78; emergencies in dental practice, p. 504.

Definitions

General anesthesia (GA) A controlled state of unconsciousness, accompanied by a partial or complete loss of protective reflexes, which may include inability to maintain an airway independently and to respond purposefully to physical stimulation or verbal command.

Deep sedation A controlled state of depressed consciousness, from which the patient is not easily aroused. It may be accompanied by a partial loss of protective reflexes, including the inability to continually maintain a patent airway independently and respond appropriately to physical stimulation or verbal command.

Conscious sedation Sedation in which protective reflexes are normal or minimally altered. The patient remains conscious and maintains the ability to independently maintain an airway and respond appropriately to verbal command. Conscious sedation also includes the use of other sedative agents and/or premedication in combination with nitrous oxide-oxygen.

Nitrous oxide-oxygen sedation Conscious sedation accomplished solely by the use of nitrous oxide-oxygen.

Analgesia The loss of the sense of pain, without the loss of consciousness.

Anesthesia The loss of feeling or sensation, especially the loss of the sensation of pain.

Indications, contraindications, and common sense

When dealing with LA, GA, and sedatives, techniques, indications, and contraindications are often relative, and the following should be thought of as guidelines rather than immutable laws.

LA The technique of choice for simple procedures or when a GA is C/I. LA is C/I in

- uncooperative patients (of any description);
- infection around the injection site;
- patients with a major bleeding diathesis; and
- most major surgery.

Adverse reaction to LA is a C/I, but in reality once allergy to preservatives in the solution is excluded, LA allergy probably does not exist.

Conscious sedation

This is an extension of LA technique using drugs and patient-management techniques. It is of benefit to anxious or mildly uncooperative patients and is a kind supplement to apicoectomy or third-molar removal. C/I include the following:

- Cardiorespiratory, renal, liver, or psychiatric pathology
- An unescorted patient or one unable to conform to the requirements of conscious sedation (p. 582)
- A demonstrated adverse reaction to sedative agents
- Pregnancy, during which benzodiazepines should be avoided

GA Indicated when LA or LA and sedation is ineffective or inappropriate (as above). C/I include the following:

- All those for conscious sedation
- Presence of food or fluid in the stomach (most anesthesiologists require at least 4 h between last feed and GA)

The anesthesiologist usually prefers hospital admission for patients with the following:

- Cardiovascular or respiratory disease (especially MI <6 months ago)
- Uncorrected anemia, sickle cell trait or disease
- Severe liver or renal impairment
- Uncontrolled thyrotoxicosis or hypothyroidism
- Poorly controlled diabetes, adrenocortical suppression
- Malignant hyperthermia
- Pregnancy
- Neurological disorders, e.g., myopathy or multiple sclerosis
- Cervical spine pathology such as rheumatoid arthritis or cervical spondylosis

- Certain drugs, e.g., steroids, antihypertensives, MAOIs, anticoagulants, narcotic analgesics, antiepileptics (need to avoid using methohexitone), lithium, and alcohol. Malignant hyperthermia, succinylcholine apnea, and other unwanted reactions to anesthetic agents
- Causes of upper airway obstruction such as angioedema, submandibular cellulitis, Ludwig's angina, and bleeding diathesis affecting the neck (In fact, these are indications to secure the upper airway.)
- Previous problems with anesthesia

Ask about previous GA and any problems. Note drugs used, as repeated administration of halothane may induce hepatitis and should be avoided within a 3-month period. While all these conditions create problems with anesthesia, they may not preclude it absolutely within the hospital setting. They do, however, indicate the need for careful assessment and early prior consultation with the anesthesiologist.

Local anesthesia—tools of the trade

While any disposable-needle and syringe system can be used to give LA, the vast number of LAs given in dental practice (>50,000/dentist/lifetime) has led to some very useful modifications.

LA cartridges Supplied in 1.8 ml capsules, they are presterilized. The most common solution used is lidocaine 2% with epinephrine 1:100,000. A latex-free version is available for patients with latex allergy.[1]

Cartridge syringes Use with above, they are sterilizable and used with disposable needles. Needles are available in 25ga-long, 25ga-short, 27ga-long, 27ga-short, 30ga-short, 30ga-x-short (x-short = 1/2 in, short = 1 in, long = 13/8 in). Their major advantage is the ability to perform controlled aspiration during LA injection.

Lidocaine/epinephrine The most commonly used preparation (2% lidocaine 1:100,000 epinephrine), it gives effective pulpal anesthesia for 1.5 h and altered soft-tissue sensation for up to 3 h. It is extremely safe; the maximum dose (adult) is 7 mg/kg or up to 500 mg (13 × 1.8 ml cartridges). It is also available in ampules 1% + 2% lidocaine plain or 1:200,000 epinephrine. There are theoretical criticisms that the maximum dose is too high, but these have not been borne out in practice.

Prilocaine Similar but of slightly less duration and effect than that of lidocaine/epinephrine. It is available as 4% prilocaine plain or 4% prilocaine 1:200,000 epinephrine. It may cause methemoglobinemia in excess. The maximum safe dose (adult) is 8 mg/kg or up to 500 mg (8 × 1.8 ml cartridges). In reality, there are few hard indications for the use of prilocaine over lidocaine.

Mepivacaine Available in two forms, 2% with levonordefrin 1:20,000 and 3% plain. Short-acting LA is advocated for restorative work but has not really caught on. The maximum safe dose is 6.6 mg/kg or up to 400 mg (11 × 1.8 ml cartridges or 7 × 1.8 ml cartridges, if plain).

Bupivacaine Long-acting LA available as 0.5% with 1:100,000 epinephrine (5–7 h), useful as a postoperative analgesic. The maximum safe dose is 2 mg/kg up to 200 mg (10 × 1.8 ml cartridges).

Articaine Available as 4% articaine with 1:100,000 epinephrine. The maximum dose is 7 mg/kg or up to 500 mg in adults, and 5 mg/kg in children.

Articaine and prilocaine have been reported as being more likely than other anesthetics to be associated with paresthesia. The difference was statistically significant when their level of use was taken into account.[2]

Topical anesthetics Lidocaine is the only really useful topical anestheic among the above. It is available as a spray or an ointment applied to mucosa several minutes prior to injecting. There is a high incidence of contact eczema in people frequently exposed to these preparations, so do not apply with bare fingers. Benzocaine in lozenge or paste form is used for mucosal anesthesia. Cocaine 4% solution is used as a nasal mucosal anesthetic and vasoconstrictor.

1 Astra Pharmaceuticals.
2 D. Haas 1995 *J Can Dent Assoc* **4** 319.

A mix of lidocaine and prilocaine is an invaluable skin topical analgesic, used prior to venepuncture in children.

Handling equipment Use one cartridge and needle per patient. Discard cartridge if a precipitant is seen in the solution or if air bubbles are present. Store in a cool, dark place and use before expiration date. Warm cartridge to reduce discomfort and load into the syringe immediately prior to use. Aspirate before injecting. The ↑ risk associated with needle-stick injuries has spawned a number of devices to aid in safely recapping needles. The Centers for Disease Control and U.S. Department of Labor Occupational Safety and Health Administration (OSHA) have been concerned about the potential risk for disease transmission presented by the recapping of needles. OSHA requires that health-care facilities (including dental offices) continually evaluate and consider the uses of new devices developed to address this concern.

Local anesthesia—techniques

The inferior alveolar dental block and local infiltrations are the mainstay of LA technique; however, numerous others are available as alternatives, supplements, and fallbacks.

IAB (inferior alveolar block) Technique of choice for mandibular molars; also effective for mandibular premolars, canines, and incisors (the latter if supplemented by infiltration). The aim is to deposit solution around the inferior alveolar nerve as it enters the mandibular foramen underneath the lingula. The patient's mouth must be wide open. Palpate the landmarks of external and internal oblique ridges and note the line of the pterygomandibular raphe. With the palpating thumb lying in the retromolar fossa, insert the needle at the midpoint of the tip of the thumb slightly above the occlusal plane lateral to the pterygomandibular raphe. The needle is inserted ~0.5 cm and if a *lingual nerve block* is required, 0.5 ml of LA is injected at this point. The syringe is then moved horizontally ~40° across the dorsum of the tongue and advanced to make contact with the lingula. Once bony contact is made, the needle is withdrawn slightly and the remainder of the LA injected. It should never be necessary to insert the needle up to the hub. Note that the mandibular foramen varies in position with age (for children, see p. 78). In the edentulous, the foramen, and hence the point of needle insertion, is relatively higher than in the dentate.

Gow–Gates technique Blocks sensation in Vc by depositing LA at head of condyle.[1] Akinosi approach: LA is deposited above the lingua.[2]

Long buccal block The long buccal nerve is anesthetized by injecting 0.5–1 ml of LA posterior and buccal to the last molar tooth.

Mental nerve block The mental nerve emerges from the mental foramen lying apical to and between the first and second mandibular premolars. LA injected in this region will diffuse in through the mental foramen and provide limited anesthesia of premolars and canine and, to a lesser degree, incisors on that side. It will provide effective soft-tissue anesthesia. Place the lip on tension and insert the needle parallel to the long axis of the premolars angling toward bone, and deposit the LA. **Do not** attempt to inject into the mental foramen as this may traumatize the nerve. LA can be encouraged in by massage.

Sublingual nerve block An anterior extension of the lingual nerve can be blocked by placing the needle just submucosally lingual to the premolars; use 0.5 ml of LA.

Posterior superior alveolar block An infrequently indicated technique. The needle is inserted distal to the upper second molar and advanced inward, backward, and upward close to bone for ~2 cm. LA is deposited high above the tuberosity after aspirating to avoid the pterygoid plexus.

1 G. A. Gow–Gates 1973 *Oral Surg Oral Med Oral Pathol* **36** 321.
2 J. O. Akinosi 1977 *Br J Oral Surg* **15** 83.

Nasopalatine block Profound anesthesia can be achieved by passing the needle through the incisive papilla and injecting a small amount of solution. This is extremely painful (for hints on how to overcome pain on palatal injections see below).

Infraorbital block Rarely indicated. Palpate the inferior margin of the orbit as the infraorbital foramen lies ~1 cm below the deepest point of the orbital margin. Hold the index finger at this point while the upper lip is lifted with the thumb. Inject in the depth of the buccal sulcus toward your finger, avoid your finger, and deposit LA around the infraorbital nerve.

Infiltrations The aim is to deposit LA supraperiosteally in as close proximity as possible to the apex of the tooth to be anesthetized. The LA will diffuse through periosteum and bone to bathe the nerves entering the apex. Reflect the lip or cheek to place mucosa on tension and insert the needle along the long axis of the tooth aiming toward bone. At the approximate apex of tooth, withdraw slightly and deposit LA slowly. For palatal infiltrations, achieve buccal anesthesia first and infiltrate interdental papillae; then penetrate palatal mucosa and deposit small amount of LA under force.

Intraligamentary anesthesia Individual teeth can be rendered pain-free by injecting small amounts of LA along the periodontal membrane via a specially designed system (high-pressure syringe and ultra-fine needles). This has the advantage of rapid onset and specific anesthesia to isolated teeth; it is a useful adjunct to conventional LA and in some hands may replace it for minor procedures. Disadvantages include post-injection discomfort due to temporary extrusion and an apparent ↑ incidence in dry socket.

Electronic dental anesthesia (EDA) An aggressively marketed technique based on the principles of transcutaneous electric nerve stimulation (TENS). Uses electrodes, buccally and lingually, which carry a minute electrical current to interfere with local nerve conduction and hence pain appreciation. This technique may be of value in restorative procedures and others not requiring the profound anesthesia or vasoconstrictive effects of LA.

Intraosseous anesthesia A recently reintroduced technique that produces profound single-tooth anesthesia. Specialized equipment and technique are needed (e.g., Stabident System, Fairfax Dental; X-Tip, Dentsply). The procedure involves choosing a suitable site for a lateral perforation of the alveolar bone. A site distal to the area to be anesthetized, approximately 2 mm apical to the gingival margin between the roots of the teeth, is ideal. The soft tissue of the perforation site is infiltrated with a small dose of LA. A bone perforator is then used in a contra-angle handpiece to perforate the cortical bone. A short needle is used to slowly deposit LA into the bone perforation.

▶ When developing LA technique there is no alternative to seeing, doing, and doing again.

Local anesthesia—problems and hints

Failure of anesthesia

There are enormous differences in individual response to a standard dose of LA—in the speed of onset, duration of action, and the depth. Soft-tissue anesthesia is more easily obtained, needing a lower degree of penetration of solution into nerve bundles than anesthesia from pulpal stimulation. A numb lip does not ∴ indicate pulpal anesthesia.

Causes of failure include the following:

- Poor technique and inadequate volume of LA
- Injection into a muscle (will result in trismus, which resolves spontaneously).
- Injection into an infected area (which should not be done anyway as this risks spreading the infection)
- Intravascular injection; clearly of no anesthetic benefit. Small amounts of intravascular LA cause few problems. For toxicity, see p. 510.
- Dense compact bone can prevent a properly given infiltration from working. Counter by using intraligamentary, intraosseous, or regional LA.
- Infrequently, anastomosis from either aberrant or normal nerve fibers not transmitted with a blocked nerve bundle

Pain on injection

This is to a certain degree inevitable, but can be ↓ by patient relaxation; application of topical LA; stretching the mucosa; and slow, skilful, accurate injection of slightly warmed solution in reasonable quantities. Causes of pain include the following:

- Touching the nerve when giving blocks, resulting in "electric shock" sensation and followed by rapid anesthesia (it is extremely rare for any permanent damage to occur)
- Injection of contaminated solutions (particularly by copper ions from a preloaded cartridge). Avoid by loading the cartridge immediately prior to use.
- Subperiosteal injections are painful and unnecessary, ∴ avoid.

Other problems with administration

Lacerated artery May be followed by an area of ischemia in the region supplied, or painful hematoma. Rare.

Lacerated vein Followed by a hematoma, which resolves fairly quickly.

Facial palsy Can be caused by incorrect distal placement of the needle tip, allowing LA to permeate the parotid gland. The palsy lasts for the duration of the LA.

Post-injection problems

Lip and cheek trauma Tell patient to avoid smoking, drinking hot liquids, and biting lip or cheek. Assure them that the sensation will pass in a few hours and that their face is not swollen (whether adult or child). If the advice goes unheeded and they return with traumatized mucosa, treat with antiseptics or antibiotics and simple anesthesia.

Needle-tract infection Rare. Use broad-spectrum antibiotic if needed.

General points

Thick nerve trunks require more time for penetration of solution and more volume of LA. In nerve trunks autonomic functions are blocked first, then sensitivity to temperature, followed by pain, touch, pressure, and motor function. Concentration of anesthesia ↑ rapidly around the nerve at first and provides soft tissue anesthesia; however, this is reached substantially before the levels needed for pulpal anesthesia, which takes several minutes and will wear off first (usually within an hour of a standard lidocaine/epinephrine LA). Disinfection of mucosa prior to LA is not required; however, sterile disposable needles are absolutely mandatory because of risks of cross-infection. For use of LA for children, see p. 78. Faints, p. 505.

Sedation—nitrous oxide-oxygen

Nitrous oxide-oxygen sedation is the most commonly used and safest form of sedation in dentistry. It has two aspects: **1** the delivery of a mixture of nitrous oxide and O_2, and **2** a semi-hypnotic patter from the doctor administering the sedation. In dentistry, two different techniques of nitrous oxide sedation have been described: **1** inhalational sedation with a fixed concentration of nitrous oxide, and **2** titrating nitrous oxide to the patient. In our view the titration technique is the most useful one.

Nitrous oxide

Nitrous oxide has both sedative and analgesic properties; the former is the most useful. The analgesic effect requires high levels of nitrous oxide. It is an inert gas that does not enter any of the body's metabolic pathways and is distributed as a poorly soluble solution. This allows very rapid distribution; peak saturation is reached within 5 min and is similarly eliminated (90% in 10 min).

Indications It is of particular value in anxious patients undergoing relatively atraumatic procedures and in children, for whom the benzodiazepines are less suitable.

Contraindications There are few, but upper airway obstruction, e.g., a cold, is one. First-trimester pregnancy makes the procedure difficult and preexisting vitamin B12 deficiency would C/I its use. Other C/I, e.g., complex medical history, are relative and may limit nitrous oxide use in a dental practice but not in the hospital.

Nitrous oxide pollution This is the major problem associated with nitrous oxide use. It is essential to have a scavenging system in place as nitrous oxide accumulation can lead to B12 deficiency and demyelination syndromes. There is a real potential hazard to pregnant staff working in confined conditions with this gas.

Aim

The goal is to produce a comfortable, relaxed, *awake* patient who is able to open their mouth on request with no loss of consciousness or the laryngeal reflex. During the procedure, patients will experience general relaxation and a tingling sensation often in the fingers or toes, and describe feeling mildly drunk. There is often a sense of detachment and distortion of the sense of time. Rarely, patients may dream despite being awake, and these can be sexual fantasies, which is another reason for always having a second person in the room at all times.

Technique

A nitrous oxide machine will not deliver less than 30% O_2. Start by delivering 100% O_2 via a nasal mask and set flow control to match their tidal volume (flow rates 6–8 1/min for adult, 4 1/min for child). Then give 10% nitrous oxide for 1 min, ↑ (if needed) to 20% for 1 min, ↑ to 30% (if needed) for 1 min, and so on. Most patients achieve adequate levels of sedation at 20–30%; some may require less, a few a bit more. Remember that nitrous sedation relies on the reassuring banter of the operator more than any of the other sedation technique, and many view this as hypnosedation. Give LA and carry out Rx. To discontinue, turn flow to 100% O_2 and oxygenate patient for 5 min. Then remove mask and get the patient to sit in a recovery room for 10 min, by which time 90% of the nitrous oxide will have been blown off and they will be safe to leave the operating room.

Sedation—benzodiazepines

General pointers, problems, and hints

Benzodiazepines are both sedative and hypnotic drugs useful for sedation of patients. Two techniques are generally used: oral and IV.

Elderly patients tend to be very sensitive to benzodiazepines and doses are best halved in the >60 age group initially. Interestingly, children show not only resistance to these drugs but sometimes paradoxical stimulation, and benzodiazepine sedation is not recommended for those <16 years.

Postoperative drowsiness is perhaps the biggest problem, as patients may be influenced by, e.g., diazepam, for up to 24 h after administration (this time is ↓ with midazolam). There is also a re-sedation effect caused by enterohepatic recirculation.

IV sedation This is the most efficient and effective method of extending the use of LA in dental Rx; however, it requires substantial skill and confidence in venepuncture and administration of the drugs; ∴ an inexperienced operator and a patient with needle phobia form relative C/I, as do inability to be accompanied, the need to be in a responsible position within 24 h of sedation (e.g., looking after young children on one's own, driving, etc.), patients with liver or renal impairment, glaucoma, psychoses, pregnancy, or a demonstrated allergy to the benzodiazepines.

Certain drugs interact, including cimetidine, disulfiram, anti-parkinsonian drugs, other sedatives, narcotic analgesics, antiepileptic drugs, antihistamines, and antihypertensives. Patients on these may be best treated (and then cautiously) in a hospital environment. Patients addicted to alcohol or other drugs may require a substantial dose modification, usually a big ↑. Those being sedated need to give written informed consent. Always provide written postoperative instructions because patients will not remember verbal ones. The role of the doctor administering sedation is supported by a second appropriate person, i.e., one trained in CPR, who must be present. At no time should the patient lose consciousness during IV sedation. The addition of any drug, especially opioids, converts a technique with a wide safety margin into one with a very narrow margin and confers no routine advantage.

Multiple drug techniques should be used by trained anesthesiologists. There is no need to starve patients prior to being sedated, although many local policies dictate this and oral medication should be continued. Rectal sedation is popular in some countries, using a prepackaged solution of diazepam given PR dose 2–10 mg.

Flumazenil A specific benzodiazepine reversal agent. *Dose:* 200 µg IV over 15 sec followed by 100 µg at 60-sec intervals until reversal occurs. **Note:** This drug has a shorter half-life than the drugs it will reverse, ∴ multiple doses may be required. Patients **should never** be reversed, then left unsupervised. This is an essential emergency drug for IV sedation.

Benzodiazepines—techniques

Oral sedation

This is of use for managing moderately anxious patients. There are problems, however, with absorption time and the risk of sedation occurring too early or too late. There is again a risk of patients having sexual fantasies under the influence of these drugs. Two drugs are used:

Temazepam 30 mg, 1 h pre-Rx produces a degree of sedation similar to that seen with IV techniques.

Diazepam, either divided regimen, 5 mg night before, 5 mg morning of Rx, and 5 mg 1 h pre-Rx; *or* as 10–15 mg 1 h prior to Rx. Both drug and technique are highly variable in consistency and quality of sedation achieved. Both doses may have to be modified depending on the size and age of the patient.

IV techniques

A far greater control of the duration and depth of sedation can be consistently achieved with this approach. It gives excellent sedation with detachment for ~30 min with amnesia for the duration of Rx. The major disadvantage is a potential for respiratory depression, post-Rx drowsiness, and amnesia (a reversal agent is available but not suitable for routine reversal of conventional sedation, see p. 580). Skill with venepuncture is a prerequisite of the technique. Diazepam has been entirely superseded by diazepam in lipid emulsion (diazemuls) as diazepam is not water-soluble and is very irritant.

Midazolam A water-soluble benzodiazepine of roughly double the strength of diazepam. It has a much shorter half-life, with no significant metabolites, creating a quicker and smoother recovery, and it is more amnesic than diazepam. It is supplied in both 2 ml and 5 ml ampoules, both containing 10 mg midazolam (5 ml ampoule is preferable, as it is easier to control the increments, given at 1 mg/increment). It is the drug of choice.

Diazepam Diazepam is metabolized to desmethyldiazepam, which has a long half-life. It is presented in an ampoule containing 10 mg diazepam, given in slow IV increments (usually 2.5 mg via a butterfly) until signs of sedation are observed. The suggested maximum dose is 20 mg.

IV technique

Relax the patient and have them sitting in the chair. Place a tourniquet around the most convenient arm and ask them to dangle the arm at their side. Any useful veins on the dorsum of the hand will become quickly evident. While this is happening, get your equipment ready: sticky tape, spirit wipe, butterfly, and drug in syringe. Look at the hand; is there a reasonable straight segment of vein? (If not, cut your losses and look elsewhere.) If there is, secure the hand with your nondominant hand, palmar surface to palmar surface, with your thumb in a position to tense the skin overlying the selected vein. Stroke the back of the hand and tap the vein to engorge it. Prepare the skin with alcohol wipe; get your assistant to help remove the needle cover and inform the patient there will be a slight scratch. Introduce the butterfly tip at a shallow angle through skin, then ↓ the angle further and move along the line of the vein until it has entered, as revealed by a flashback into the extension tubing. Then introduce the length of the needle along the vein carefully, so as to avoid cutting through, and secure with tape. Remove air by aspirating blood into the tubing and release tourniquet. Place the patient in the supine position and give a small bolus (2–3 mg diazepam, 1–2 mg midazolam). Wait for 1 min and then give further increments until an adequate level of sedation is achieved. Leave the butterfly in to maintain venous access. Loss of laryngeal reflex constitutes oversedation and means you must stop and ensure that the airway is patent, only proceeding if there is no respiratory depression and the airway can be protected.

Monitoring A second appropriate person must be present. Pulse and BP should be monitored. Pulse oximetry is mandatory. An itchy nose is an early sign of "complete" sedation. Hiccups constitute oversedation.

Post-sedation Allow time for recovery (30–60 min) in calm surroundings. The patient must be accompanied home and forbidden to drive or assume a responsible position for 24 h.

Anesthesia—drugs and definitions

Sedation is a triad of depressed consciousness, muscle relaxation, and analgesia.

IV anesthetic agents

Thiopental (dose 4 mg/kg) Although an ultra-short-acting barbiturate anesthetic, its half-life is 6–12 h. It is a poor analgesic and relatively sparing to the laryngeal reflexes, requiring a greater depth of anesthesia to prevent laryngospasm. It is highly irritant on injection but cheap and very popular as an inpatient induction agent. It will abolish epileptic seizures in induction doses.

Propofol (dose 2.5 mg/kg) A true ultra-short-acting anesthetic as it is completely metabolized within minutes. It is less irritant than the others and is the drug of choice for day-case anesthesia.

Etomidate (dose 0.3 mg/kg) An IV induction agent often used for patients with compromised cardiovascular systems. It can be associated with involuntary movements, cough, and hiccup. Avoid in traumatized patients.

Ketamine (dose 1–2 mg/kg) Can be given IM at higher doses (unique among anesthetic agents for this). It tends to maintain the airway and causes little respiratory depression. Its use is limited by a high incidence of severe nightmare hallucinations in adults, which are eased by midazolam.

Inhalational anesthetics

Nitrous oxide An excellent analgesic but weak anesthetic, mainly used to supplement other inhalational anesthetics or in RA. A problem is created by its rapid excretion if used for perianesthetic analgesia; it wears off rapidly, so it has no postoperative analgesic benefits.

Halothane Largely superseded by newer agents, it is a weak analgesic, causing hypotension and dysrhythmias. The concomitant use of injected epinephrine should be avoided in non-ventilated patients breathing halothane as it ↑ risk of ventricular fibrillation (VF). It is very rarely hepatotoxic after repeated anesthetics in adults, and extremely rarely used de novo.

Enflurane A weaker anesthetic than halothane but less likely to produce dysrhythmias or hepatitis. Avoid in epileptics.

Sevoflurane A newer agent with rapid onset and recovery. It is good for inhalation induction and has become increasingly the inhalational agent of choice.

All inhalational agents cause muscle relaxation.

Muscle relaxants

These are used to create laryngeal relaxation for intubation; this stops patients breathing, and they must then be ventilated until the agent wears off or is reversed.

Succinylcholine Used for emergency cases for rapidly securing airway. It is a short-acting depolarizing muscle relaxant, with quick, good recovery but cannot be reversed. The main problems for the patient are muscle pains, which arise 24–48 h after administration. These can be very severe and are more likely in the ambulant. It can also cause severe bradycardia, especially on a repeat dose in children. It is metabolized by plasma cholinestese, absence of which can lead to succinylcholine sensitivity (p. 488). It causes an ↑ in K^+, ∴ know U&Es in all but very routine cases.

Pancuronium, atracurium, vecuronium, and rocuronium All non-depolarizing muscle relaxants; slower acting and longer lasting, but can be reversed using neostigmine.

Analgesics Opioids are mainstay, and include the following:
- Morphine; long acting, mainly used for postoperative analgesia
- Fentanyl; first of the short-acting opioids
- Alfentanil; purely used as anesthetic opioid due to short duration
- Remifentanil; continuous infusion needed because of ultra-short duration; ideal as anesthesia adjunct but not postoperative pain relief

Anesthesia and the patient on medication

Certain drugs should ring alarm bells when patients require a GA. These include the following:

Monoamine oxidase inhibitors Should be stopped 2 weeks prior to GA.

Antiepileptic drugs Must be continued up to, during, and after GA; however, methohexitone should be avoided.

Antihypertensives Should be continued, but ensure that the anesthesiologist is aware they are being taken.

Bronchodilators Should be continued. Give inhaler with premedication and ensure that nebulizer is available postoperatively.

Cardioactive drugs Should all be continued. Warn the anesthesiologist, as these patients often benefit from a preoperative anesthetic assessment.

Cytotoxics Patients on these rarely need GA, but if they do, they need FBC, U&Es, and LFTs. Suxamethonium should be avoided.

Diabetic drugs For management, see p. 530.

Lithium Measure levels. Omit prior to major surgery.

Oral contraceptives Think about DVT prophylaxis, although experience suggests the risk is remote. The NIH recommends discontinuing 4 weeks prior to major elective surgery; this is generally unnecessary for maxillo-facial/oral surgery. Be guided by local policy. HRT does *not* need to be stopped.

Sedatives and tranquillizers If the patient takes a regular dose these can be maintained, but warn the anesthesiologist.

Corticosteroids Patients on long-term steroids require supplementation; see p. 488, 512, 531.

Oral anticoagulants Stop and heparinize for all major surgery. Monitor clotting. Monitor INR for warfarin.

Anesthesia—hospital setting

With the exception of the outpatient GA service provided by dental hospitals, GA in a hospital setting is similar to that for any other surgical service. The provision for and the care of the patient immediately prior to, during, and after the anesthetic is the domain of the trained anesthesiologist. The input from the hospital junior staff is the same, whether in a dental or surgical specialty, and is mainly covered on p. 518. The fundamental problem for any dental, oral, or maxillofacial anesthetic is that the surgeon and anesthesiologist both need to have access to the same anatomical site: the shared airway. The means by which this is overcome in hospital practice is by endotracheal, particularly nasendotrachea, intubation, muscle relaxation, and ventilation.

Endotracheal intubation secures the airway by placing a tube into the trachea via the nose, mouth, or a tracheostomy. This tube has an inflatable cuff that prevents aspiration of debris and is connected to an anesthetic machine to allow delivery of O_2, nitrous oxide, and an inhalational anesthetic. Most anesthesiologists also use a throat pack to supplement the cuff, **which must be removed at the end of the operation**. Intubation is a specialist skill and must be learned with practice; skilled practitioners can perform blind nasendotracheal intubation, which is of enormous value in cases with trismus; most cases are, however, performed by direct vision of the vocal cords using a laryngoscope with the patient's neck fully extended. The major risk of intubation is intubating the esophagus **and not recognizing it**. Other complications include: traumatizing teeth; vocal cord granulomata; minor trauma to the adenoids; rarely, pressure necrosis of tracheal mucosa; and laryngeal stenosis.

The laryngeal mask airway (LMA) The LMA has become an acceptable method of maintaining the airway. Structurally, it is a curved tube with a large cuff at its end. It is a device inserted orally without direct vision following the normal curve of the pharynx. Its onward progression is stopped by the upper end of the esophagus and at this point the cuff is inflated, forming a seal around the entrance to the larynx. Patients must be starved as it does not protect against aspiration. It occupies a substantial volume in the mouth. The necessity of movement of the LMA to allow surgical access may displace the cuff, possibly causing laryngeal obstruction. The LMA is expensive, but autoclavable up to 40 times. Quite deep anesthesia is required to both pass and maintain the LMA, which may prolong anesthesia inappropriately. The LMA should only be used by those trained in intubation.

Muscle relaxation Essential for successful intubation in elective patients. These drugs are covered on p. 585. For most oral surgery, once the patient is intubated, ventilation is aided by small doses of non-depolarizing muscle relaxant. An alternative is a continuous infusion of a very short-acting opioid (e.g., remifentanil).

Ventilation May be hand or mechanical. The latter is more precise and convenient for the anesthesiologist. It involves a machine providing intermittent +ve pressure ventilation.

Monitoring There are increasingly sophisticated noninvasive techniques available: pulse oximetry to measure the percutaneous saturation of hemoglobin with O_2 (a normal person breathing air will have a saturation >95%); capnograph to measure end-tidal $PetCO_2$ (normal: 5.2 kPa or 40 mmHg); ECG and automatic BP machines. It must be stressed, however, that these machines do not replace, only ↑, the ability of the anesthesiologist to use clinical observation of pulse, color, skin changes, and ventilatory pattern. The minimum standard of monitoring is BP, ECG, SaO_2, and end-tidal CO_2. Patient safety standards, guidelines, and quality assurance measures for the administration of anesthesia in the United States have been developed by the American Society of Anesthesiologists.

Malignant hyperthermia See p. 488.

Anesthesia—practice setting

The ideal team to provide exodontia under GA is a small, skilled group, e.g., anesthesiologist, dentist, and nurse, who have received appropriate postgraduate training and have suitable facilities.

Outpatient anesthesia is given to healthy patients; most anesthetics, from induction to recovery, are a few minutes.

Controversial points

Pollution with anesthetic gases In the hospital environment it is possible to scavenge the majority of gases as patients are either intubated or have an LMA or a relatively leak-proof face mask. This is not the case in dental surgery, as patients are breathing through a nasal mask and, invariably, through their mouths.

Hazards of inhaling anesthetic gases These are not well established. It is true that patients continuously breathing nitrous oxide for 24 h or so begin to have suppression of the bone marrow and that chronic recreational abuse can cause subacute combined degeneration of the spinal cord. The short-term and intermittent long-term effects of exposure to nitrous oxide, halothane, enflurane are, however, simply not known. It remains common sense that no one should work in a polluted atmosphere. OHSA sets standards to ensure that health-care workers are not exposed to any unnecessary risks to their health and safety while in the workplace.

Dental materials

Relevant pages in other chapters: Materials used in endodontics, p. 288.

Principal sources: J. F. McCabe 1998 *Applied Dental Materials*, Blackwell. E. C. Combe 1999 *Dental Biomaterials*, Kluwer. W. J. O'Brien 2002 *Dental Materials and Their Selection*, Quintessence.

Many materials texts list the requirements for an ideal cement, filling material, impression material, etc., and then conclude that it doesn't exist. We will try to resist this temptation.

Properties of dental materials

Definitions

Stress Internal force per unit cross-sectional area acting on the material. Can be classified according to the direction of the force: tensile (stretching), compressive, or shear.

Strain Change in size of a material that occurs in response to a force. It is the change in length divided by the original length.

Yield strength (or elastic limit) The stress beyond which a material is permanently deformed when a force is applied.

Elastic modulus A measure of the rigidity of a material, defined by the ratio of stress to strain (below elastic limit).

Stiffness An indication of how easy it is to bend a piece of material without causing permanent deformation or fracture. It is dependent upon the elastic modulus, size, and shape of the specimen.

Toughness The amount of energy absorbed up to the point of fracture. A function of the resilience of the material and its ability to undergo plastic deformation rather than fracture.

Resilience The energy absorbed by a material undergoing elastic deformation up to its elastic limit.

Hardness Resistance to penetration. A number of hardness scales are in use (e.g., Vickers, Rockwell). Between these scales hardness values are not interchangeable.

Creep The slow plastic deformation that occurs with the application of a static or dynamic force over time.

Wear The abrasion (±chemical) of a substance.

Fatigue When cyclic forces are applied a crack may nucleate and ↑ by small increments each time the force is applied. In time the crack will ↑ to a length at which the force results in # through the remaining material.

Thermal conductivity Ability of a material to transmit heat.

Thermal diffusivity Rate at which temperature changes spread through a material.

Coefficient of thermal expansion The fractional ↑ in length for each degree of temperature ↑.

Wettability Ability of one material to flow across the surface of another, determined by the contact angle between the two materials and influenced by surface roughness and contamination. The contact angle is the angle between solid/liquid and liquid/air interfaces measured through the liquid.

Evaluation of a new material

Before it reaches the dental supply companies a new material should have undergone the following tests:

- *Standard specifications* (i.e., physical properties), e.g., compressive strength, hardness, etc. The actual values obtained are mainly of value in comparing the new material with those already in use and that are performing satisfactorily. Compliance with an international (ISO) standard indicates fitness for dental use.
- *Laboratory evaluation* should be relevant to the clinical situation, but this is easier said than done!
- *Clinical trials* are usually conducted under optimal conditions. Many materials have been less successful under the conditions imposed by clinical practice, particularly those with demanding placement techniques.

Clinically, the important questions to ask pertain to the following:

- Shelf life
- Details of the chemical constituents
- Handling characteristics, e.g., presentation, mixing, working time, setting time, and dimensional changes on setting
- Performance in service
- Cost
- Does the material meet the relevant ISO standard?

Then decide whether this new material has any significant advantages over the material you are familiar with. Being new does not always mean it is better! Always look for research to support the use of a new material.

Amalgam

An *amalgam* is a mixture of Hg and another metal. Dental amalgam is made by mixing together Hg with powdered silver–tin alloy to produce a plastic mass that can be packed into a preparation before setting. Despite toxicity scares and the introduction of universal resin composites, amalgam is still widely used. Since 1984 the American Dental Association (ADA) has recommended the use of pre-encapsulated amalgam alloys.

Types of amalgam

There are two ways of classifying amalgam:

Particle shape Can be lathe cut (irregular), spheroidal, or a mixture of the two. Spheroidal particles give a more fluid mix that is easy to condense, can be carved immediately, and takes 3 h to reach occlusal strength (compared to >6 h for lathe-cut amalgams). Spheroidal amalgams are preferable for large Class V and pinned restorations.

Particle composition The first (conventional) alloys introduced had a low copper content (5%). Research showed that the weakest (tin–Hg or gamma-2) phase of the set amalgam could be eliminated by ↑ the proportion of copper, so a variety of high-copper (6–25%) amalgams have been introduced. These are more expensive but superior in terms of corrosion resistance, creep, strength, and durability of marginal integrity. There are two types of high-copper alloy: (1) a single composition alloy of silver–tin–copper and (2) a blended (dispersion) mix of silver–tin and copper–silver alloys. Of these, (1) is the most resistant to tarnishing.

Handling characteristics

Mixing or trituration This is carried out mechanically and is pre-encapsulated by manufacturer, with an automatic vibrator. The duration of trituration varies from 5 to 20 s.

Condensation Carry out incrementally, either by hand instruments (lathe-cut or spheroidal) or mechanically (lathe-cut only). Both are equally effective but the latter is quicker. Preparations should be overfilled so that the Hg-rich surface layer is removed by carving.

Carving With spherical alloys this can be commenced immediately, but with lathe-cut one a delay of a few minutes is advisable. Burnishing is now back in vogue.

Polishing Polished amalgams look good, but whether polishing is necessary is still the subject of debate. Maximum strength takes 24 h to develop.

Marginal leakage

While amalgam corrosion products will form a marginal seal in time, initial microleakage can be reduced by the use a conventional cavity varnish (e.g., Copalite), however, it is reported to be effective for only a short period of time, as it is prone to dissolve in oral fluids. Recent studies have shown that adhesive resin, dentin bonding systems (DBS) or the DBS–resin liner combinations (e.g., Amalgambond Plus) can be used as cavity liners to provide increased retention of amalgam alloys and to reduce microleakage at the tooth–amalgam interface.[1,2] Bonding agent, such as Panavia-21, is an anaerobic resin adhesive that also bonds to set amalgam.[3] Alternatively, sealing over the completed restoration with a fissure sealant has been suggested, and this is a possible solution to the "ditched" but caries-free amalgam.

Toxicity

According to the ADA, "there is insufficient evidence to justify the claim that Hg from dental amalgam has an adverse effect on the vast majority of patients."[4] In recent studies, no significant differences were found in neuropsychological and neurobehavioral effects between children who received amalgam restorations and those treated with tooth-colored resin restorations.[5,6] The greatest risk appears to be related to the inhalation of Hg vapor, ∴ attention should be paid to the following:

- Avoid spilling Hg.
- Waste amalgam should be stored in a covered plastic container and labeled "amalgam waste" for recycling.
- When removing old amalgams, safety glasses, masks, and high-volume aspiration and a rubber dam are a wise precaution.

Types of amalgam

Average composition (%)	Silver	Tin	Copper	Zinc
Conventional	68	28	4	0–2
High copper	60	27	13	0

Types of amalgam currently available
- Conventional lathe-cut
- Conventional spherical
- High-copper dispersion lathe + spherical
- High-copper single spheroidal
- High-copper single lathe-cut

1 M. Stanin 1988 *JPD* **59** 397.
2 M. E. Korale *Am J Dent* **9** 249.
3 D. C. Watts 1992 *J Dent* **20** 245.
4 ADA Council on Scientific Affairs 2003 *JADA* **134** 1498.
5 D. C. Bellinger 2006 *JAMA* **295** 1775.
6 T.A. DeRouen 2006 *JAMA* **295** 1784.

Resin composites—constituents and properties

The modern resin composite is a mixture of resin and particulate filler, the handling characteristics of which are determined largely by the size of the particles and method of cure.

Constituents

Resin Most resin composites are based on either Bis-GMA or urethane dimethacrylate plus a diluent monomer, triethylene glycol dimethacrylate (TEGDMA).

Filler confers the following benefits on the resin composite:
- ↑ compressive length, abrasion resistance, modulus of elasticity, and # toughness
- ↓ thermal expansion and setting contraction
- ↑ esthetic qualities

Resin composites can be subdivided according to particle size:

Macrofilled (or conventional) Contains particles of radio-opaque barium or strontium glass 2.5–5 µm in size, to give 75–80% by weight of filler. Good mechanical properties, but hard to polish and soon roughens.

Microfilled Contains colloidal silica particles 0.04 µm in size and 30–60% by weight. Retains a good surface polish, but is unsuitable for load-bearing situations, has poor wear resistance, and ↑ contraction shrinkage.

Hybrid Contains a mixture of conventional and microfine particles designed to optimize both mechanical and surface properties. Contains 75–85% by weight of filler.

Most composites are of the hybrid type; however, materials with smaller particles (nanofillers) have recently been introduced.

Initiator/activator

1 Chemically cured: benzoyl peroxide (or sulfinic acid) initiator + tertiary amine activator. **2** Light-cured: amine + ketone activated by blue light (460–70 nm).

Other constituents include pigments, stabilizers, and silane coupler to produce bond between particles and filler.

Important properties of composites

1 Polymerization shrinkage of 1–4%.
2 Thermal expansion is significantly greater than that of enamel or dentin, and without acid-etch bond can result in marginal leakage.
3 Elastic modulus should be high to resist occlusal forces. Modulus of hybrid type is greater than other resin composites, amalgam, or dentin. However, resin composites are still brittle and fracture if used in thin section.
4 Wear resistance is greatest in hybrids.
5 Radio-opacity is particularly useful, especially for posterior resin composites.

Resin composites—practical points

Method of polymerization

Chemical (self-cure) No additional equipment is required, but mixing of two components introduces porosity and the working time is limited.

Light activation provides long working time, command set, and better color stability, but requires a light source, has a limited depth of cure, and the temperature ↑ during setting can be as high as 40°C. Three types of light source are currently available: quartz tungsten halogen (QTH), plasma arc light (PAC), and light-emitting diode (LED). Current evidence suggests that a QTH is the preferred option and that PAC and LED lights confer no advantage at present.

Dual-cure Curing is initiated by a conventional light source, but continues chemically to help ensure polymerization throughout the restoration.

Practical tips

- Replace bulbs every 6–12 months. Some lights correct for the effects of bulb aging.
- Air attenuates light beam, ∴ position as close to tooth as possible.
- Preparations >2 mm depth should be cured incrementally.
- Precautions are necessary to protect eyes from glare, ∴ use safety glasses, have the patient close their eyes and the dental assistant look away. Alternatively, use a hand-held shield or one attached to the light tip.
- Efficiency of light source can be tested by curing a block of composite. Practical depth of cure is half thickness of set material.
- The greater the intensity of the light source the greater the depth of cure.

Finishing Ideally, use a mylar strip to produce the contour of the restoration. Then refine with microfine diamond or multiblade tungsten carbide finishing burs (under water spray), finishing strips, and then polish with aluminum oxide–coated discs (Shofu, Soflex). Shofu points or finishing pastes are useful for inaccessible concave surfaces.

Problems with resin composites

1 They are technique sensitive. Field needs to be dry. Contamination with saliva must be avoided.
2 It is difficult to obtain satisfactory contact points and occlusal stops. Modern placement techniques have largely overcome this.
3 Polymerization shrinkage occurs.
4 Depth of cure of light-cured materials is limited. This is a particular problem in posterior teeth. Indirect composite inlays may circumvent the last two problems (p. 240).

Fissure sealants Composite resins containing little or no filler, which are either self- or light-cured. Clear or opaque types are available, the former having better flow characteristics (whether this is an advantage depends on the position of the tooth). Success depends on being able to achieve good moisture control for the acid-etch bond.

Flowable resin composites are now available. They are predominately resin with a reduced % of filler particles, and consequently shrink considerably on curing. Some advocate using them as liners or in the bottom of proximal preparations, but the high level of shrinkage precludes this. Resin-modified glass ionomer cement (RMGIC) is preferable in proximal preparations, which are below the CEJ (bonded-base approach); however, they have a place in the marginal repair of restorations.

Acid-etch technique

Recent research on this technique would suggest the following:

- Success depends on adequate moisture control, as contact with saliva for as little as 0.5 s will contaminate the etch pattern.
- A prophylaxis prior to etching is not required unless abundant plaque deposits are present.
- 30–50% buffered phosphoric acid provides the best etch pattern.
- An etching time of 15–20 s is adequate for both primary and permanent enamel, and 15 s for dentin is recommended.
- The etch pattern is easily damaged, ∴ using a probe to aid etchant penetration of pits and fissures or applying etchant by rubbing vigorously with a swab of cotton wool is C/I.
- There is no difference in bond strength regardless of whether an etchant solution or gel is used. Gels take twice as long to rinse away but have the advantage of greater viscosity and color contrast.
- Rinse for at least 15 s.
- Remineralization of etched enamel occurs from the saliva, and after 24 h it is indistinguishable from untreated enamel.
- Etched enamel is porous and has a high surface energy. The etch pattern consists of three zones (from surface inwards):

Etched zone (enamel removed)	10 μm
Qualitative porous zone	20 μm
Quantitative porous zone	20 μm

∴ composite resin tags may penetrate up to 50 μm into enamel to give micromechanical retention.

Note: Many of the newer dentin adhesive systems do not have a separate acid-etch stage. These systems use a combination of acidic primers and bonding resins, either as a single stage or applied separately.

Dentin-adhesive systems (dentin bonding agents)

The advantages of bonding to dentin (e.g., preservation of tooth tissue) have fuelled considerable research effort. The problems that have had to be overcome include the high water and organic content of dentin; the presence of a "smear layer" after dentin is cut; and the need for adequate strength immediately following placement, to withstand the polymerization contraction of resin composite. These difficulties have been approached in a number of ways, making the topic of dentin bonding confusing, a situation exacerbated by the pace of new developments and by the claims of the manufacturers.

Indications

- Marginal seal where preparation margin in dentin or cementum, e.g., cervical (Class V), proximal (Class II) box
- Retention and seal of direct resin-composite restorations
- Retention and seal of indirect porcelain and composite inlays
- Dentin adhesives have also been used for repairing # teeth, cementing ceramic crowns and veneers, and as an endodontic sealer.

The smear layer consists of an amorphous layer of organic and inorganic debris, produced by cutting dentin. It ↓ sensitivity by occluding the dentin tubules and prevents loss of dentinal fluid. It purportedly has an ↑ inorganic content compared to dentin. The smear layer is partially or completely removed and/or modified during dentin bonding.

Mechanism of dentin bonding

Most dentin adhesive systems aim to modify and partially remove the smear layer, by the application of an acidic primer. This demineralizes the underlying surface, exposing the collagen and opening up the dentinal tubules. It is important to keep this surface moist to prevent the collagen from becoming flattened (for food readers: the collagen should resemble *al-dente* spaghetti). This layer is then infiltrated using a resin with bi-functional ends: one hydrophilic end, which is able to bond to wet dentin, and one hydrophobic end capable of bonding to the composite resin. In this infiltrated hybrid layer molecular entanglement of the collagen and resin occurs, providing the basis for the bonding system.

Practical points

- Follow manufacturer's instructions.
- For better results use a matched resin-composite and adhesive system.
- When a dentin adhesive is used polymerization shrinkage of resin composite is more likely to result in cuspal deformation and ∴ postoperative pain. An incremental filling and curing technique will help to ↓ this problem.
- Precuring the adhesive bonding agent before placing the composite ↑ bond strength.[1]
- No technique produces zero microleakage.

For a review of adhesive systems and the science of bonding, the articles by Watson and Bartlett and by Kugle and Ferrari are recommended.[2,3]

1 J. F. McCabe 1994 *BDJ* **176** 333.
2 T. F. Watson and D. Bartlett 1994 *BDJ* **176** 227.
3 G. Kugel and M. Ferrari 2000 *JADA* **131** 20S.

Glass ionomers—properties and types

Glass ionomer has been officially renamed *glass polyalkenoate*. However, we have continued with glass inonomer (GI) as abbreviating glass polyalkenoate could lead to confusion with gutta-percha (GP).

Setting reaction

Aluminosilicate glass + polyalkenoic acid → calcium + aluminum polyalkenoates (base + polyacid → polysalt + water).

The set material consists of unreacted spheres of glass surrounded by a silicaceous gel, embedded in metal polyalkenoates. Fluoride is released from the cement to give cariostatic properties.

Presentation

1 Powder + liquid
2 Powder (with anhydrous acid) + water
3 Encapsulated

Itaconic acid is added to ↑ rate of set, and tartaric acid to sharpen set. In some products polymaleic acid replaces polyacrylic and one new material is based on polyvinyl phosphoric acid.

Properties

Adhesion to enamel and dentin occurs by 1 ionic displacement of calcium and phosphate with polyacrylate ions; 2 possible absorption of polyalkenoic acid onto collagen. Some authors recommend preconditioning the dentin, e.g., with 10% polyalkenoic acid (GC Dentin Conditioner) for 30 s. Whether this ↑ adhesion is controversial. GI cement also bonds to the oxide layer on SS and tin.

Cariostatic Due to fluoride release throughout the lifetime of the restoration. GI are also able to take up fluoride when the IO concentration is raised, the "reservoir effect." However, the therapeutic benefit of fluoride release has yet to be shown to be effective.

Thermal expansion Similar to enamel and dentin.

Strength Brittle material. Tensile strength is only 40% of resin composite.

Radiolucent Except for the cermets, which are rarely used.

Abrasion resistance Poor, but ↑ all the time, especially with the high-viscosity versions.

Biocompatibility This is being questioned following reports of pulpal inflammation when used as a luting cement, but this is not a problem clinically.[1]

Applications

GI are unable to match the aesthetics and abrasion resistance of the resin composites, and brittleness limits their use to non-load-bearing situations. However, their adhesive and fluoride-releasing properties have resulted in a range of applications and matching formulations.

1 R. van Noort (ed.) 1994 *J Dent* **22** 8.

Type I Luting cements for crowns, bridges, and orthodontic bands.

Type II Restorative cements. There are two subtypes: (a) esthetic; (b) reinforced. They can also be used as a fissure sealant, for the restoration of deciduous teeth (p. 80) and for repairing defective restorations.

Type III Fast-setting lining materials. Defer placement of amalgam for at least 15 min and composite for 4 min. In load-bearing situations or where lining is exposed to the oral environment (e.g., in sandwich technique), use of a type II reinforced cement or RMGIC is preferable.

Type IV Includes the light-cured and dual-cure GI (use of a light source optimizes the properties of the dual-cure materials, although they will self-polymerize without it). It has been suggested that the light-cured GI have higher bond strengths than that of self-cure GI.[1]

1 C. G. Plant 1988 *BDJ* **165** 54.

Glass ionomers—practical points

Practical tips

- A dry field is essential.
- Encapsulated systems ensure optimal mixing and allow placement via syringe tip, e.g., Ketac-fil.
- Cement should be inserted before its sheen is lost.
- GI sticks to SS, ∴ use powder as a separator.
- Cellulose or soft metal strips provide the best finish.
- Water balance during setting is critical. Absorption of water results in dissolution, and dehydration leads to crazing, ∴ cement must be protected with waterproof varnish (Copalite is not waterproof). Alternatively, use light-cured bonding resin, which acts as a lubricant for finishing and can then be cured.
- Although most manufacturers claim that trimming can be started 10–15 min after placement, it is better to defer for >24 h.

Cermets

These are similar to GI, except that the ion-leachable glass is fused with fine silver powder. Mixing with a polymeric acid gives a cement consisting of unreacted glass particles to which silver is fused, held together by a metal–salt matrix.

Properties
- Adhesion to enamel and dentin
- Radio-opaque
- ↑ wear resistance compared to GI, but have equivalent strength
- Cariostatic

Applications Core buildups; low-stress-bearing restorations; restoration of deciduous teeth.

Cermets, however, are rarely used and have been largely superseded by the RMGICs.

Resin-modified glass ionomers

These allow "command" setting and help overcome the moisture sensitivity and low early mechanical strength associated with conventional GI. The acid–base reaction of GI is supplemented by the addition of 5% resin (HEMA Bis-GMA). The initial set of the material is due to the formation of a polymerization matrix, which is strengthened by the acid–base reaction. They are easier to handle than conventional GI and may be polished immediately after light-curing. The esthetics approach those of resin-based materials, plus they have the advantage of fluoride release.[1] These materials can be used in conjunction with resin composite for placement in deep proximal preparation where the deepest parts of the preparation are below the CEJ. This type of open sandwich restoration fell into disrepute when restorations were placed with traditional GI cement. The development of RMGICs has improved the technique, with good results reported at 7 yr.[2]

Compomer

Another recently introduced hybrid material, it combines the adhesive and fluoride-releasing properties of GI with the abrasion resistance of resin composite and is thus called, with a touch of originality, compomer. It is composed of a single hydrophobic resin filled with acid-leachable glass particles. Compmer is bonded with a bifunctional primer and light-cured. The chemical reaction apparently takes place through uptake of water from saliva leading to fluoride ions leaching out. It is difficult to think of a situation where compomer could be used but a resin composite material could not. It is hard, therefore, to give specific indications for this group of materials except possibly for the restoration of deciduous teeth.

Giomers

This group of materials is more correctly described as resin composites with active filler particles. The filler particles are based on pre-reacted surface or fully reacted GI filler particles, which have been shown to be capable of sustained fluoride release. They may be useful for high-caries-risk individuals.

1 S. K. Sidhu 1995 *Dental Update* **10** 429.
2 J. W. van Dijken 1999 *J Dent Res* **78** 1319.

Cements

These are used for a variety of purposes, including temporary dressings, preparation liners, and as luting agents. With the exception of calcium hydroxide, the materials available are based on combinations of:

Powder Zinc oxide or fluorine-containing aluminosilicate glass (this releases fluoride and is stronger than zinc oxide).

Liquid Phosphoric acid (irritant) or eugenol (↑ solubility, obtundent) or polyalkenoic acid (adhesive).

Setting occurs by an acid–base reaction. The set cement comprises cores of unreacted powder in a matrix of reaction products.

It is now thought that the ability of a cement to prevent microleakage is more important than its setting pH.

Based on zinc oxide-eugenol (ZOE)

ZOE Powder of pure zinc oxide is mixed (in a ratio of 3:1) with eugenol liquid to give zinc eugenolate and unreacted powder. Setting time is 24 h. This is the weakest cement, but the eugenol acts as an obtundent and analgesic, ∴ it is useful as a temporary dressing, but not for RCT, as there is no seal.

Accelerated ZOE Addition of zinc acetate to the powder ↓ setting time to 5 min.

Resin-bonded ZOE Addition of 10% hydrogenated resin to the powder ↑ strength.

EBA (ethoxy benzoic acid) Addition of ortho-ethoxybenzoic acid (62%) to the liquid ↑ strength.

Zinc phosphate The powder consists of zinc and magnesium oxides, and the liquid is 50% aqueous phosphoric acid. The working time is ↑ by adding the powder in small increments. It is popular because of its strength. Although its low-setting pH theoretically C/I its use for vital teeth, in practice this does not seem to be a problem.

Zinc polycarboxylate, e.g., Poly-F, Durelon. The powder is a mixture of zinc and magnesium oxides and the liquid is 40% aqueous polyacrylic acid. Recently, anhydrous acid formulations have been introduced, which are mixed with water. The powder should be added quickly to the liquid. The temptation to remove excess cement should be resisted until it has reached a rubbery stage. It adheres to dentin, enamel, tin, and SS.

Calcium hydroxide Chemically curing types comprise two pastes that are mixed together in equal quantities. One paste contains the calcium hydroxide plus fillers in a non-reacting carrier, and the other has polysalicylate fluid. The set material consists of an amorphous calcium disalicylate complex plus calcium hydroxide and has a pH of 11. In addition to being bacteriostatic, calcium hydroxide can induce mineralization of adjacent pulp. Light-cured formulations that are resin based are available. They have ↓ bactericidal properties, but ↑ strength.

GI (p. 604) This and RMGIC are the preferred luting cements for cast indirect restorations.

Strength Phosphate > EBA or polycarboxylate > resin-bonded ZOE > accelerated ZOE > calcium hydroxide.

Practical points
- Generally, the thicker the mix, the greater the strength.
- Heat ↓ setting time, ∴ a cooled slab is advisable.
- To stop cement sticking to the instruments during placement, dip in cement powder (except calcium hydroxide) or use non-stick instruments.
- When luting, apply cement to crown or inlay before tooth.

Choice of cement

Temporary restorations Choice depends on how long the dressing needs to last and whether any therapeutic qualities are required. Pure ZOE is useful for a tooth with a reversibly inflamed pulp, but resin-bonded ZOE is stronger. GI is preferable for semi-permanent dressings and because it seals the preparation margins.

Luting cement Zinc phosphate, GI, and polycarboxylate are all popular as luting cements. EBA cement is C/I because of ↑ solubility. Composite-based luting systems are available, which are often used in conjunction with dentin adhesive systems. This cement is mandatory for cementing ceramic or porcelain inlays or onlays and ceramic veneers.

Lining cement Choice of lining depends on depth of the preparation and the material being used to restore it.

    Amalgam Minimal: preparation sealer (Gluma Desensitiser); moderate: RMGIC (vitrebond); deep: use a sublining of calcium hydroxide (direct or indirect pulp capping) and any of the cements listed above. Typically, RMGIC is recommended, as it seals as well as lines the preparation.

    Resin composite Dentin adhesive system with direct or indirect pulp capping as indicated.

Pulp capping Hard-setting calcium hydroxide.

Sedative dressing ZOE and/or calcium hydroxide.

Bacteriostatic dressing Calcium hydroxide plus GI (stepwise excavation).

Always follow manufacturer's recommendations for proper handling!

Impression materials

Classification

Non-elastic		Elastic	
Plaster	*Elastomers*	*Hydrocolloid*	
Compound	Silicone	Reversible	
ZOE paste	Polysulfide	Irreversible	
Wax	Polyether		

Elastomers

These are indicated when accuracy is paramount, e.g., crown and bridge work, and implants.

Condensation-cured silicone e.g., Xantopren, Optosil. This material is relatively cheap compared with other elastomers, but is prone to some shrinkage and models should be poured immediately. Addition-cured silicones are preferred.

Addition-cured silicone e.g., Aquasil, President, Dimension. This type of silicone is very stable, which means that impressions can be posted or stored prior to pouring models. A perforated tray is advisable as the adhesives supplied are not very effective. Up to five viscosities are manufactured, allowing a range of impression techniques. *Note:* Powdered latex gloves (now rarely used) can retard setting of putty materials.[1]

Polysulfide e.g., Permalastic. Messy to handle, but useful when a long working time is required. Use with a special tray and, although stable, models should be poured within 24 h. Recommended for dentures only.

Polyether e.g., Impregum. Popular because it uses a single mix and a stock tray. The set material is stiff, and removal can be stressful in cases with deep undercuts or advanced periodontitis. It absorbs water, ∴ do not store with alginate impressions. It can cause allergic reactions. It is routinely used for implant cases and crown and bridgework, especially when there are multiple preparations.

Hydrocolloids

Reversible hydrocolloid is accurate, but liable to tear. It requires the purchase of a water bath. There are potential problems with contamination and breaks in infection control protocols. It is no longer widely used. Impressions must be kept damp and models must be poured as soon as possible.

Irreversible hydrocolloid (alginate) Setting is a double decomposition reaction between sodium alginate and calcium sulfate. It is popular because it is cheap and can be used with a stock tray. It is widely used for impressions for study models, but is not sufficiently accurate for crown and bridge work. Impressions must be kept damp and cast as soon as possible. Alginate can retard the setting of gypsum and affect the surface of the cast.

1 W. W. L. Chee 1992 *J Prosthet Dent* **68** 728.

Impression compound

This is available in either sheet form for recording preliminary impressions, or in stick form for modifying trays. The sheet material is softened in a water bath with warm water (55–60°C/130–140°F) and used in a stock tray to record edentulous ridges. The viscosity of compound results in a well-extended impression, but with limited detail.

Impression waxes

These are produced in four grades. The very soft (orange) type is useful for the correction of small imperfections in ZOE impressions, or for recording -/P free-end saddles.

Zinc oxide pastes

These are dispensed 1:1 and mixed to give an even color. They are used for recording edentulous ridges in a special tray or the patient's existing dentures, but are C/I for undercuts. Setting time is ↓ by warmth and humidity.

Impression techniques

(For crown and bridge work)

▶ Time spent recording a good impression is an investment, as repeating lab work is costly.

Special trays help the adaptation of impression material and ↓ the amount required, i.e., ↑ accuracy and ↓ cost. They can be made in cold-cure acrylic or light-activated tray resin. Special trays are rarely used for crown and bridge work impressions, with stock trays used routinely.

For crown and bridge work an accurate impression of the prepared teeth is required. Usually the palate does not need to be included, so design the special tray accordingly or use a lower stock tray. For the opposing arch, alginate in a stock tray will suffice.

Monophase technique (e.g., polyether) The same mix of medium-viscosity material is used for both a stock tray and syringe.

Double-mix technique (e.g., polysulfide, addition-cured silicone) A single-stage technique necessitating the mixing of heavy- and light-bodied materials at the same time, and use of a special or stock tray.

- Apply adhesive to tray.
- Mix light- and heavy-bodied viscosities simultaneously for 45–60 s.
- Remove retraction cord or preferably leave in place and dry preparation, while dental assistant loads syringe with light-bodied material.
- Syringe light-bodied mix around prep. A gentle stream of air helps to direct material into crevice.
- Position tray containing heavy-bodied material.
- Support tray with light pressure until 2 min after apparent set.

Putty and wash technique (e.g., silicone) The putty and light-bodied viscosities can be used with a stock tray, either

1 *Single-stage,* which is similar to the double-mix technique above, or
2 *Two-stage,* which involves taking an impression of the prep with the putty, using a polythene sheet as a spacer. This is then relined with the light-bodied material, which is also syringed around the prep. The trend is, however, away from putty wash toward monophase or a double-mix technique.

Cost in decreasing order is as follows:

- Addition-cured silicone using putty/reline
- Polyether with special tray
- Addition-cured silicone using double mix and special tray
- Polysulfide with special tray
- Condensation-cured silicone using putty/reline
- Hydrocolloid

Automixing dispensers This double-cartridge presentation is exceptionally popular. The two pastes are extruded and mixed in the nozzle when the trigger is pressed. It appears to be expensive, but ↓ waste and the mixture is void free. Many manufacturers are now producing their materials in this format.

Disinfection of impressions

Impressions should be rinsed to remove debris and then immersed in a solution of sodium hypochlorite (1000 ppm available chlorine) for 10 min.

Casting alloys

An *alloy* is a mixture of two or more metallic elements. The chemistry of alloys is too complicated for this book (and its authors), so for a fuller understanding the reader is referred to one of the source texts.

The properties of an alloy depend on the following:

- Thermal treatments applied to the alloy (including cooling)
- Mechanical manipulation of the alloy
- Composition of the alloy

Note: The properties of an alloy may differ significantly from that of its constituents.

The main examples of alloys in dentistry include amalgam (p. 594), steel burs and instruments, metallic denture bases, inlays, crowns and bridges, and orthodontic wires.

Casting alloys

A warm, moist mouth provides the ideal environment for corrosion. To overcome this problem, dental casting alloys comprise an essentially corrosion-resistant metal (usually gold), with the addition of other constituents to enhance its properties. However, with the exception of titanium, all have the potential to affect hypersensitive individuals.

Additions to gold alloys
    Copper ↓ density, ↓ melting point, ↑ strength and hardness, but ↓ corrosion resistance.
    Silver ↑ hardness and strength, but ↑ tarnishing and ↑ porosity.
    Platinum ↑ melting point, ↑ corrosion, and ↑ tarnish resistance.
    Palladium Similar properties to platinum, but less expensive.
    Zinc or indium Scavenger, preventing oxidation of other metals during melting and casting.

Dental casting gold alloys Noble metal (gold, platinum, palladium, iridium) content must >75%; 65% must be gold. Four types are defined by proof stress and elongation values from type I (low strength for castings subject to low stress) to type IV (extra-high strength).

Dental casting semi-precious alloys have 25–74% noble metal content. Four types are defined by proof stress and elongation properties.
    Silver palladium Palladium (>25%), silver, gold, indium, and zinc. It is cheaper than gold alloys and of equivalent hardness, but less ductile, more difficult to cast, and prone to porosity.
    Nickel chromium 75% nickel, 20% chromium. Used in crowns and bridgework. In the latter ↑ rigidity compared to gold alloys is an advantage. However, castings are less accurate than gold, and nickel sensitivity can C/I its use.
    Cobalt chromium 35–65% cobalt, 20–35% chromium. Modulus of elasticity is twice that of type IV gold alloys. A good polish is difficult to achieve, but durable. Used mainly for P/-.
    Titanium Good biocompatibility; used primarily for implants. Pure titanium casting is still being perfected.

Alloys for porcelain bonding

Requirements:
- Higher melting point than porcelain
- Similar coefficient of thermal expansion to porcelain
- Won't discolor porcelain
- High modulus of elasticity to avoid flexure and fracture of porcelain

Indium is usually added to facilitate bonding to porcelain. Copper is C/I as it discolors porcelain. A matched alloy and porcelain should be used.

High gold ↑ palladium or platinum content (to ↑ melting point) compared to non-porcelain alloys.

Medium gold 50% gold, 30% palladium. This is widely used.

Silver palladium Inexpensive, but care required to avoid casting defects.

Nickel chromium Very high melting point and modulus of elasticity, but casting more difficult. *Note:* Some patients are sensitive to nickel.

Casting

For gold (melting point <950°C/1742 °F)
- Wax pattern and sprue are invested in gypsum-bonded material.
- Wax is burnt out by slowly heating investment mold to 450°C/842°F.
- Alloy is melted either by gas/air torch or electric induction heating and cast with centrifugal force.
- Casting is allowed to cool to below red-heat.
- Quenched. Some alloys are used as cast and others are heat hardened.
- Cleaned with ultrasonics and acid immersion.

For nickel chromium and cobalt chromium alloys (melting points 1200–1500°C/2192-2732°F), you need silica or phosphate bonded investment and either oxyacetylene torch or electric induction heating.

Casting faults A casting may be
- dimensionally inaccurate;
- have a rough surface; or
- be porous, contaminated, or incomplete.

Wrought alloys

Wrought alloys are hammered, rolled, drawn, or bent into the desired shape when they are solid.

Stainless steel (SS) Steel is an alloy of iron and carbon. The addition of chromium (>12%) produces a passive-surface oxide layer that gives SS its name. The SS used in dentistry is also known as austenitic steel (because the crystals are arranged in a face-centered cubic structure) or 18:8 steel (because of the chromium and nickel content) and is available in two forms.

1 Pre-formed sheets for denture bases. The SS is swaged onto the model by explosive or hydraulic pressure. This produces a thin (0.1 mm), light denture base resistant to fracture. It is rarely used today.

2 Wires are produced by drawing the SS through dies of ↓ diameter until the desired size is achieved. This work-hardens the wire, but heat treatments are carried out to give soft, hard, or extra-hard forms. Manipulation of SS wire also work-hardens the wire in the plane of bending, ∴ trying to correct a bend is more likely to result in #. The main applications are orthodontics and partial denture clasps. SS can be welded and soldered.

Soldering SS requires use of a flux to remove the passive oxide layer (this reforms after soldering). The ↓ part of the flame should be used, but do not overheat, as this can anneal and soften the components.

• Melt a small bead of low-fusing silver solder onto the wire.
• Mix up the flux with water to a thick paste and apply to the item to be added.
• Heat up the solder so that wire underneath is a cherry red.
• Bring the fluxed wire into the molten solder and remove the flame at the same time.

This is not easy and requires practice, which explains the popularity of electrical soldering.

Cobalt chromium has a similar composition to the cast form (p. 615).

Cobalt chromium nickel is used in orthodontics as an archwire material. It has the advantage that it can be hardened by heat treatment after being formed. It is also used for post fabrication in post and core crowns.

Titanium Pure titanium is used in implant systems.

Titanium alloys Nickel and titanium alloy (nitinol) is useful in endodontics and orthodontics as it is flexible, has good springback, and is capable of applying small forces over a long period of time. However, it is not easy to bend without #. Titanium molybdenum alloy (TMA) is also used for archwires and has properties midway between those of SS and nitinol.

Gold Expense limits the application of wrought gold alloys to partial denture clasp fabrication.

Alloys for dentures

Cast cobalt chromium is the material of choice for partial denture connectors because of its high proof stress and modulus of elasticity: thin castings are strong, rigid, and lightweight. Although wrought gold alloys are more suitable for clasps, the advantage of being able to cast connector and clasps in one means that cobalt chromium is more commonly used (p. 306). Be aware of nickel allergy.

Ceramics—dental porcelain

Ceramics are simple compounds of both metallic and nonmetallic oxides. Although many of the materials used in dentistry are ceramics, the term is commonly used to refer to porcelain and its derivatives. Dental porcelain actually more closely resembles a glass, and comprises feldspar, quartz (for strength and translucency), and kaolin (for strength and color), plus pigments. Most dental porcelain is reinforced with alumina particles (40–50% by mass) to provide greater strength. Unfortunately, this ↑ the opacity, ∴ the proportion of alumina in enamel porcelains is ↓. During construction of a PJC a platinum matrix is laid down on the die produced from the impression of the prepared tooth to act as a base. The porcelain powder is mixed with water to form a slurry, which is built up in layers onto the foil until the desired shape is achieved. The porcelain is compacted by removing water from the preparation by blotting with absorbent paper or by flicking with a brush. This ↑ firing shrinkage. The crown is then fired to ↓ porosity, which ↑ strength and ↑ translucency. Glazing produces a glossy outer skin that resists cracking and plaque accumulation. It can be added as a separate layer or by firing at a higher temperature after the addition of surface glazes. The platinum foil lining is removed prior to cementation to give space for the cement lute.

Other ceramic crowns have replaced PJC and are built up on a refractory die (dentin-bonded crowns), heat-processed core (Empress), or computer-generated sintered core (Procera).

Properties
- Firing shrinkage 30–40%, ∴ crown must be overbuilt
- Chemically inert provided the surface layer is intact
- Low thermal conductivity
- Good esthetic properties
- Brittle. The main cause of failure is crack propagation that almost invariably emanates from the unglazed inner surface. This can be ↓ by (1) fusion of the inner surface to metal, as in the platinum foil and metal-bonded techniques or (2) by use of an aluminous porcelain core.
- High resistance to wear
- Glazed surface resists plaque accumulation

Ceramics—practical applications

Porcelain jacket crown Now considered somewhat old-fashioned. A core of aluminous porcelain is laid down first, onto which "dentin" and then "enamel" porcelains are built up. For strength a minimum porcelain thickness of 0.8 mm is required and a 90 butt joint at the margin.

Porcelain fused to metal crown The porcelains used for bonding to a metal substructure have additional alkali oxides added to ↑ the coefficient of thermal expansion to almost match the alloys used. Also, a porcelain that fuses below the melting point of the alloy is required. Bonding to the metal occurs by a combination of

- mechanical retention, and
- chemical bonding to the metal oxide layer on the surface of the alloy.

The ↑ strength of porcelain bonded to metal crowns is due to

- the metal substructure supporting the porcelain;
- ↓ crack propagation by bonding the inner surface of the porcelain to metal;
- the outer surface of porcelain being under tension, thus ↓ crack propagation.

Glass ceramic or castable ceramics Semi-crystalline glass, e.g., tetrasilicic fluormica glass (Dicor—no longer in use), was produced by adding a nucleating agent onto which the glass crystals precipitate during cooling. This structure resists crack propagation, having a similar strength to core aluminous porcelain. An additional advantage is that the lost wax process can be used, so compensation for firing shrinkage is not required. A wax pattern is built up by the technician and invested and cast. Following cooling, the casting is reheated to allow crystal growth to occur. The castable ceramics have ↑ translucency compared to porcelain, but dentin color has to be created with surface glazes, which requires time and skill. Glass ceramic crowns are more expensive than PJC but were useful for young translucent teeth. Currently, hot-pressed (IPS-Empress II) and glass-infiltrated (Inceram) ceramics have gained wider acceptance. They do not match the strength of porcelain fused to metal.

All ceramic systems now also include flame-sprayed (Techceram) or CAD-CAM (Procera) alumina cores onto which conventional porcelains are fired.

Porcelain veneers A thin shell of porcelain or castable ceramic (~0.5–0.8 mm thick (p. 258). Their thin section limits their ability to hide underlying tooth discoloration unless they are used with opaque cements.

Porcelain inlays Promising alternative to conventional treatment procedures. Only limited long-term studies are available.

Porcelain repairs can be carried out using composite and a silane coupling agent. A number of proprietary kits are available.

Denture materials—1

Acrylic resin

Acrylic is the most commonly used polymer for denture bases. Not only can it be relined, repaired, and added to comparatively easily, but it is also esthetically pleasing and lightweight. Acrylic is composed of a chain of methacrylate molecules linked together to give polymethylmethacrylate (PMMA).

Presentation usually comprises a liquid and a powder mixed together. The liquid is stored in a dark bottle to ↑ shelf-life.

Powder	Liquid
PMMA beads (<100 mm)	Methylmethacrylate monomer
Initiator, e.g., benzoyl peroxide	Cross-linking agent
Pigments and/or fibers	Inhibitor, e.g., hydroquinone
	Activator (self-cure only)

Manipulation The powder and liquid should be mixed in a ratio of ~2.5:1 by weight. The mix passes through several distinct stages: sandy, string, dough, rubbery, and hard (set).

The dough stage is the best for handling and packing.

In denture fabrication the wax pattern and teeth are invested in plaster. The wax is then boiled out and the plaster coated with sodium alginate as a separator. The resultant space is then filled to excess (to allow for contraction shrinkage of 7%) with acrylic dough under pressure. The acrylic is then polymerized.

Mode of activation

Self-cure acrylics show less setting contraction but more water absorption than heat-cured ones. This may result in the final item being slightly oversized, thus having ↓ retention. Self-cure acrylics are more porous, only 80% as strong, less resistant to abrasion, and contain a greater level of unreacted monomer compared to heat-cured acrylics. The main applications of self-cure acrylics are for denture repairs and relines, and orthodontic appliances, although for the latter the greater strength of heat-cured acrylics is preferable.

Heat-cured Conventionally, polymerization requires heating in a hot-water bath for 7 h at 70°C/158°F, then 3 h at 100°C/212°F. The flask should be cooled slowly to minimize stresses within the acrylic. However, resins with different curing cycles (fast heat-cure) are now available. Microwave energy can be used to cure acrylic resin, but has no advantage over a water bath.

Light-cured resins are supplied as moldable sheets. They are used for denture bases or special trays.

Properties

- The glass transition (or softening) temperature of self-cure acrylic is 90°C/194°F, and for heat-cured, 105°C/221°F.
- Acrylic has poor impact strength and low resistance to fatigue fracture.
- Abrasion resistance is not very good, but usually adequate.
- Good thermal insulator—undesirable as it can lead to the patient swallowing foods that are too hot.
- Low specific gravity (i.e., not too heavy)
- Radiolucent. Attempts to ↑ radio-opacity have not been very successful.
- Acrylic absorbs water, resulting in expansion. Drying out of acrylic should be avoided.
- Residual monomer due to inadequate curing weakens acrylic and can cause sensitivity reaction.
- Good aesthetics

The strength of a denture depends on

1 Design, e.g., adequate thickness, avoidance of notches.
2 Strength of the acrylic, i.e., low monomer content, ↓ porosity, adequate curing. Can be ↑ by using high-impact resin.

Researchers are still evaluating methods of i strength of denture resins. The addition of high-performance fibers (e.g., glass fibers) appears promising.

Denture materials—2

Rebasing

Rebasing a denture base involves replacement of the fitting surface. Rebases can be either

1 Hard: heat or self-cure; or
2 Soft: permanent: heat, self-cure, or light-cured
     temporary (a) tissue conditioner: self-cure
             (b) functional impression material: self-cure

The properties of self-cure materials are generally inferior, ∴ should only be used as a temporary measure.

Hard rebases Heat-cured PMMA is preferred, but requires the patient to do without the denture while it is being added. A self-cure material has obvious advantages, but even the higher acrylics, e.g., butylmethacrylate (peripheral seal), should only be used as a temporary measure as they are weaker than PMMA and discolor.

Soft liners require a material with a glass transition temperature below or at that of the mouth so that it is soft and resilient. Most soft liners are based either on silicone or acrylic (polyethylmethacrylate or PMMA powder plus alkyl methacrylate monomer and a plasticizer), but the recently introduced polyphosphazene fluoroelastomer liners look promising.[1]

Plasticized acrylic	Silicone polymers
Good bond to denture	Bond with denture base is not reliable
Hardens over time	Maintain resilience
More readily distorted	Absorb water: candida colonization
	More elastic

Heat, light, or self-cure types are available. The self-cure materials have inferior properties, but all require replacement during the lifetime of the denture.[2] For cleaning, see p. 328.

Tissue conditioners usually comprise powdered polyethylmethacrylate to which a plasticizing mix of esters and alcohol is added. No chemical reaction takes place, the liquids merely soften the powder to form a gel and leach out over time, resulting in hardening. To ensure maximum tissue recovery, the lining should be a minimum thickness of 2 mm and be replaced every few days—e.g. Coe-soft, Coe-comfort. For cleaning, see p. 328.

Functional impression materials The tissue-conditioning materials are usually used for this purpose, an impression being cast of the fitting surface after a few days of wear.

---

1 F. Kawano 1992 *J Prosthet Dent* **68** 368.
2 E. R. Dootz 1993 *J Prosthet Dent* **69** 114.

Biocompatibility of dental materials

Before a new material can be marketed it must successfully pass both laboratory and clinical trials to evaluate its biocompatibility. Yet, some adverse effects become apparent only after the material has been in clinical use. Unless used with care, many materials may prove a hazard to the patient or the dentist and staff.

Hazards to the patient

Systemic effects

Allergic reactions

- *Amalgam* Although genuine cases of amalgam allergy exist, these are rarer than the tabloid press would suggest. For proven cases resin composite or cast restorations should be used.
- *Nickel* constituent of some alloys can cause contact eczema. Sensitive patients often have a history of allergy to jewelry or watch casings. Alternative alloys are available.
- *Acrylic monomer* can cause an allergic reaction and should be considered in a patient complaining of a "burning mouth." The concentration of monomer is ↑ in poorly cured acrylic and greater in self- than heat-cure. Extended curing, e.g., 24 h, may ↓ concentration of monomer to an acceptable level; if not, a cobalt chrome or SS denture base will be required.
- *Epimine* in polyether impression material.
- If an allergy is suspected, refer to a dermatologist.

Directly toxic

- Beryllium, present in some nickel alloys, is known to be a carcinogen. Provided the alloy is not ground, any risks are confined to the production laboratory. Beryllium-free alloys are becoming ↑ available.
- Fluoride in excess can be toxic (p. 28).

Ingestion or inhalation of air-borne dust must be avoided.

Local effects

Eye damage Curing lamps can cause eye damage from the glare. The simplest solution is to ask the patient to close their eyes and use a shield.

Thermal injury can result, extending **1** to the pulp, e.g., caused by exothermic setting reactions; **2** to the mucosa, e.g., caused by dentures that are thermal insulators, as the patient may swallow drink or food that is too hot, or by the setting reaction of self-cure denture reline materials; **3** to the soft tissues, e.g., by hot instruments.

Chemical injury can be caused by noxious chemicals (e.g., etchant, hydrogen peroxide) being allowed to come into direct contact with the tissues.

Hypersensitivity reactions can occur in response to the materials that cause systemic allergy.

Hazards to staff

In surgery

- Allergic reactions, e.g., topical anesthetics, latex gloves, methyl methacrylate monomer, dentin adhesive systems
- Eye damage from light sources. Use eye protection or shielding.
- Alginate dust
- Mercury vapor
- Nitrous oxide

In the laboratory

- Cyanide solution for electroplating
- Vapors from low-fusing metal dies
- Silica particles in investment materials
- Fluxes containing fluoride
- Hydrofluoric acid used for etching porcelain veneers
- Beryllium in some alloys
- PMMA powders
- Methyl methacrylate monomer
- Casting machines

Jurisprudence

Relevant pages in other chapters: Employment and termination, p. 655; privacy and patient health information, p. 658; infection control, p. 674

Principle resources: B. Pollack 2002 *Law and Risk Management in Dental Practice*, Quintessence. D. Ozar and D. Sokol 2002 *Dental Ethics at Chairside: Professional Principles and Practical Applications*, 2nd ed., Georgetown University Press. N. Schafler 1996 *Dental Malpractice: Legal and Medical Handbook*, 3rd ed., Wiley Law. B. Weinstein 1993 *Dental Ethics*, P. Beemsterboer 2001 *Ethics and Law in Dental Hygiene Practice*. W.B. Saunders.

The law is not always simple to understand. Therefore, some scenarios are presented for clarity.

American system of government

In the American federal system of government, the federal government has limited powers. Most of the power resides with the states. Thus, with very few exceptions, state law regulates the practice of dentistry. Since state laws differ from state to state, this chapter can cover only general principles. Dentists should consult their own state laws for specific information.

Sources of law

The law can be divided into two major categories, criminal and civil law. Civil law is concerned with private rights and remedies. In this chapter we are concerned only with civil law.

Until the modern era, the law was derived from two sources, namely, the legislature, which enacts statutes, and common law. Laws enacted by the legislature are sometimes referred to as *black letter law*. *Common law* is that body of law derived from judges' decisions. This system of laws originated and developed in England and was adopted from the English common law at the time of American independence. Today a third source of law is derived from regulatory or administrative bodies, which are established by acts of the legislature and which create law in the form of rules, regulations, orders, and decisions. A board of dentistry is an example of a regulatory or administrative body or agency.

In order that they may be freely available to the public, laws from all sources, whether passed by the legislature, administrative law bodies or resulting from court decisions, are published. As far as common law is concerned, generally only the decisions of the intermediate and the highest appellate courts are published. Decisions of trial courts (the lower courts) are kept in the court in which the case was heard. Decisions made by appellate courts apply only in the jurisdiction in which the court sits and nowhere else. Decisions of an appellate court are legally binding on the lower courts in the jurisdiction in which the appellate court sits. Intermediate appellate courts are bound by the decision of a state's highest court. Thus, lower courts are bound by the decisions of higher courts, in a practice referred to as *stare decisis* ("to abide by, or adhere to, decided cases"). Researching the law is not easy and special expertise is needed to conduct a search.

Regulation of dental practice

All states regulate the practice of dentistry. The primary purpose behind the regulation of any profession, including dentistry, is the protection of the public's health, safety, and welfare. Dentistry, being a profession, has like all professions been granted the privilege by the legislature of regulating itself. Dentists are granted this privilege by statute, which specifies the composition of the board, the terms of appointment, how often the board is required to meet and certain other details (see M.G.L Ch. 13, § 19, for an example). Boards promulgate rules and regulations concerning the conduct of dentists, the qualifications necessary to obtain a license, how complaints against dentists must be made, continuing education requirements, and the discipline for various violations. The boards have wide latitude to promulgate rules and regulations, but they may not conflict with federal laws or the federal or state constitutions, which take precedence over them. Dentists may be disciplined for a variety of transgressions and these need not be criminal in nature. The grounds for discipline are diverse and typically include a catchall phrase akin to "conduct that undermines the confidence of the public in the profession." Since the loss of a license is a civil proceeding, a dental board need only prove its case by a preponderance of the evidence and does not need to do so beyond a reasonable doubt. Constitutionally, a dentist must be afforded a reasonable opportunity to defend him- or herself. This includes the right to counsel. In cases where the board deems the conduct of a dentist to be an immediate threat to the public's health, safety, and welfare, the board may summarily suspend the license of the dentist. The board must, however, constitutionally grant the dentist a hearing within a fairly short time, typically somewhere in the vicinity of 7 days, although the exact time varies from state to state.

Dentist–patient relationship

The dentist–patient relationship is a contractual and voluntary one. Like most contracts, it need not be in writing. Concerning prospective new patients, the general rule is that a dentist has no obligation to treat anyone. In American jurisprudence, this applies even in emergency situations. Some states, however, have so-called duty-to-rescue statutes requiring a person who knows that another is exposed to grave physical harm to give reasonable assistance to the exposed person to the extent that the aid can be rendered without danger or peril to the rescuer, unless that assistance or care is being provided by others. These statutes typically apply to the general public and not to health-care providers in particular.[1] It is important to note that the freedom to choose to treat a new patient may be circumscribed by the dentist's employer. For example, if an oral surgeon works in a hospital, he or she is obligated to treat anyone seeking emergency oral surgery care when on duty or on call. This obligation derives not from any contractual obligation that the surgeon has with a patient, but rather from the contractual obligation with the hospital, whose contract will specify that one of the surgeon's duties is to treat all emergency oral surgery patients.

The right to refuse treatment to a new patient is circumscribed by laws against discrimination. So, for example, a dentist may not discriminate against someone on the basis of religion, ethnicity, cultural background, etc. Under the American with Disabilities Act (ADA) (42 USC § 12101 et seq), a dentist may also not discriminate against anyone protected under that act. Interestingly, the act protects not only people with actual disabilities but also those who are perceived to have disabilities protected under the act, even though they may not in fact have a protected disability. A dentist may not avoid treating disabled patients by deliberate ignorance. For example, a dentist cannot say that they are unable to treat HIV-positive patients because they do not know how. Treating such patients is part of the everyday practice of dentistry.

Although the dentist–patient relationship is a contractual one, most lawsuits by patients are not brought under contract law but rather on the basis that the dentist was negligent in their treatment. The branch of law that is implicated in these lawsuits is the law of medical malpractice.

---

1 Vt. Stat. Ann., Title 12, § 519; J. Bagby 2000 Note, Justifications for State Bystander Intervention Statutes: Why Crime Witnesses Should Be Required to Call for Help. *Ind L Rev* **33** 571, 574–75.

Malpractice law

Just as dentistry has various specialties, so too does the law have its disciplines. Malpractice falls under that branch of the law known as tort law. A *tort* is a civil or private wrong or injury, other than a breach of contract, for which the court provides a remedy in the form of an action for damages. There is no one body of law that constitutes malpractice law. Malpractice is governed by common law and, to a lesser extent, by statute. In the United States, juries decide the vast majority of trials, including civil ones. The overwhelming majority of malpractice cases are heard in a state court. If certain conditions are met, a case may be heard in federal court. Even then, however, with rare exception the law of a particular state will govern.

Settling a dispute informally

A patient who believes that they have been harmed as a result of a dentist's malpractice or negligence may informally begin a process with the dentist and/or the dentist's insurance company to arrive at a mutually agreeable resolution, which usually involves the payment of money. The process does not have to involve the court system at all. Some complaints are settled in this manner, with or without the assistance of a lawyer representing the patient. A dentist should not wait until a formal legal proceeding has begun before informing their malpractice insurance carrier of a potential problem. Indeed, the dentist should involve the insurer if he or she suspects that a patient complaint may be forthcoming. The insurer can best advise the dentist how to respond and may also make counsel available. According to the dentist's contract with the malpractice carrier, a dentist has an obligation to cooperate with the company. In many states, laws mandate an insurance company to act in good faith toward the patient. This means, among other things, that the insurance company must make a reasonable settlement offer if it determines that the dentist committed negligence. A patient may also seek to have a dental board mediate a dispute, and many dental boards in fact offer such a service, especially concerning disputed fees. A dentist should treat any complaint made against them at the board seriously, and should inform their malpractice carrier. A malpractice insurer may not provide coverage in cases involving the dental board, but can at least help put the dentist in touch with an attorney who is familiar with board practice.

Formally invoking the legal system

The legal system becomes formally invoked when a patient files a complaint in the appropriate court. This complaint is then served, according to the rules of the jurisdiction, on the dentist. Once such a complaint has been filed, both the patient, now known as the *plaintiff*, and the dentist, now known as the *defendant*, must abide by certain formal rules established by the court and/or the legislature. To eliminate or reduce frivolous claims, many states have introduced an additional burden before a medical malpractice lawsuit may proceed. While taking different forms in various states, the hurdle is essentially a screening tribunal. In Massachusetts, members of the tribunal include a judge, who acts as chair, an attorney, and a health-care provider similar to the one being sued. Thus, in the case of a dentist a tribunal will consist of a judge, an attorney, and a dentist; in the case of a nurse it will consist of a judge, an attorney, and a nurse. Based on the plaintiff's presentation, the tribunal must decide whether "the evidence presented if properly substantiated is sufficient to raise a legitimate question of liability appropriate for judicial inquiry or whether the plaintiff's case is merely an unfortunate medical result" (M.G. L. Ch. 231, § 60B).

The statute of limitations

One of the most basic rules of malpractice is the statute of limitations. The statute of limitations establishes the time frame within which a patient must initiate a suit against a dentist or lose their right to a remedy. The purpose of the statute of limitations is to prevent the threat of a lawsuit from lasting forever, to prevent memories from fading before a matter is heard, and to allow the parties to get on with their lives. The burden of proving that the statute of limitations has run rests on the dentist. A state may follow one of two basic rules concerning the statute of limitations. According to one rule, the patient must bring suit within a certain time period following the act of negligence. This rule, the occurrence rule, is not concerned with whether the patient knew or should have known of the alleged malpractice. According to the second rule, the so-called discovery rule, a patient must bring suit within a certain period of time from the time they knew or should have known of the occurrence of the alleged malpractice.[1] Under the discovery rule, it is possible for the threat of a lawsuit to hang over a dentist for the rest of his or her life. Most states follow the discovery rule. If a dentist fraudulently conceals facts, it may extend the statute of limitations. To avoid the threat of a lawsuit continuing forever under the discovery rule, many states also have a statute of repose. This statute establishes an outer maximum time limit or "ceiling" during which a plaintiff must initiate a suit against the dentist, regardless of when the patient knew or should have known of the alleged malpractice. Once the statute if repose has run, the plaintiff is barred from suing.

The plaintiff's burden

In order to prevail in a malpractice action, the plaintiff must prove certain elements by a preponderance of the evidence. The meaning of preponderance of the evidence is somewhat subjective, but in a general sense it means that the jury must be persuaded that the facts are more probably one way (the plaintiff's way) than another (the defendant's)—i.e., on a scale of 1 to 100, 51% or better in favor of the plaintiff. The elements of a malpractice claim that the plaintiff must prove are depicted in the figure below.

---

1 M.G.L. c.260, § 4; Riley v. Presnell, 409 Mass. 239 (1991).

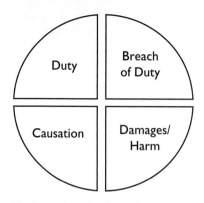

The elements that a plaintiff in a malpractice suit must prove.

The dentist–patient relationship Courts are generally quite liberal in finding that a dentist–patient relationship existed, so this element usually does not involve much argument. On occasion, however, it can be problematic to determine whether or not such a relationship existed. A typical example of this is a telephone call from a prospective new patient. Depending on the precise facts of what transpired during the call, a dentist–patient relationship may or may not be deemed to have existed. The dentist does not need to receive payment in order for a dentist–patient relationship to be established. A relationship may even be established outside the dental office, for example, at a social occasion. A visit by an individual to a dentist where the dentist speaks to the patient but does not examine them and does not accept them as a new patient probably does not result in a relationship. Once the dentist examines the patient, however, a dentist–patient relationship exists, at least as far as that examination is concerned, even if the dentist declines to undertake any future work, for example, because he or she feels that the work is beyond his ability.

The standard of care The second element, namely, that the dentist breached the duty or standard of care, is typically heavily litigated, with each side bringing in its expert witness to bolster its side of the argument. States follow one of two rules in determining the appropriate standard of care.

- *Locality rule* The older rule is known as the locality rule and is followed today in only a minority of jurisdictions. According to this rule, a physician is bound to exercise that skill only which physicians of ordinary ability and skill, practicing in similar localities, with opportunities for no larger experience, ordinarily possess.[1] According to this rule, a dentist is not bound to exercise the caring skill possessed by dentists practicing in larger cities or academic centers. The so-called locality rule was followed by all states for many years. With changes in

1 Small v. Howard, 128 Mass 131 (1880).

communication, the availability of textbooks, continuing-education courses, and the ability to travel to conferences, many courts later decided that this rule was antiquated. They saw no need to restrict the standard of care of dentists to the locality in which they practice.

- *Reasonably prudent practitioner standard* Most states have now switched to a different rule in which a dentist is required to exercise the degree of care and skill of the average qualified practitioner, taking into account the advances in the profession.[2] This rule not only eliminates the locality rule, but the words "taking into account the advances in the profession" are in essence a requirement for continuing education. The modern rule is sometimes referred to as the reasonably prudent practitioner standard. There is increasingly a move toward states accepting a national standard of care. This is especially true with regard to specialists, as specialty examinations are conducted by specialty boards on a national basis. For example, Massachusetts requires that the care and treatment rendered by a specialist must be in accordance with the standard of care and skill of the average member of the medical profession practicing that particular specialty.[3]

- *Respectable minority* Some states follow the so-called respectable minority rule. According to this rule, a physician does not incur liability merely because he or she chooses to pursue one of several recognized courses of treatment. Courts are not always clear in defining what " respectable" means, but the general consensus seems to be that " respectable" refers both to the number of dentists following the minority rule, as well as to their standing in the professional community. The respectable minority rule reflects the reality that some practitioners have a different approach to the same problem. The rule still requires that the care rendered by these practitioners must comply with the standard of care of the minority.[4]

- *Standard of care established by the profession* With rare exception, the standard of care is established by the profession itself and not by the court. For an example of the latter, see Nelson's discussion of a case in Washington state.[5] A good example of the fact that the profession establishes that standard of care is the current use of CT scans in planning implant surgery. Some dentists always use a CT scan for the placement of even a single implant. Others rarely or never use it, even when placing multiple implants. If a patient who was injured as a result of implant surgery were to bring a malpractice claim against the dentist for failing to use advanced radiographic imaging in planning the implant surgery, the court will not dictate that the dentist should have used it. Instead, the court will leave it up to the jury to decide what the current standard of care is. In practice, the jury will decide this based on expert witness testimony from both the dentist's and plaintiff's expert witnesses. While professional organizations may publish their

2 Brune v. Belinkoff, 354 Mass 102 (1968).

3 Stepakoff v. Kantar, 393 Mass. 836 (1983).

4 Henderson v. Heyer-Schulte Corp. of Santa Barbara, 600 S.W.2d 844 (Tex Civ. App. 1980); Jones v. Chidester 610 A.2d 964 (Pa. 1992).

5 L. J. Nelson III 2002 *Seattle University Law Review* **25** 775, discussion of Helling v. Carey, 83 Wash. 2d 514, 519 P.2d 981 (1974).

own standards of care, these standards are not controlling in a court of law, but experts may use them as one factor on which they base their opinion. With a few exceptions, a patient must have an expert witness to establish that a dentist committed malpractice. One example where an expert is not required is when an instrument is left inside the patient, for example, when a surgeon leaves a clamp inside the patient and then sutures up the patient.

Damages and causation The third element of a malpractice, that the patient suffered damage as a result of the dentist's breach of duty, is one that is also rarely heavily litigated. Far more heavily argued over is the fourth element, namely, whether the damage occurred as a result of the breach of the dentist's duty, an issue known as causation. The following scenario is an example. Assume that during an examination a dentist misses a palatal ulcer that ought to have raised a reasonably prudent dentist's suspicions. Assume further that another dentist notices the ulcer 8 months later and performs a biopsy, with the pathologist's report coming back as squamous cell carcinoma. In order to treat the cancer, the patient undergoes a hemimaxillectomy. The dentist will argue that the 8-month delay caused the patient no greater damages than if the cancer were diagnosed 8 months earlier, as the treatment—hemimaxillectomy—would have been the same at the earlier date. The patient, on the other hand, will argue that if the true nature of the lesion had been known 8 months earlier, the treatment would have involved only partial loss of the palate and not half of the maxilla. The critical question is thus whether the fact that the first dentist missed the diagnosis "caused" the additional harm or damage to the patient in the form of greater loss of the patient's maxilla.

The issue of causation is extremely complicated and is the subject of numerous legal treatises. We have probably all heard the old adage that lawyers say: "Never admit to anything." The reason that lawyers admonish their clients never to admit to anything is that any admission on the part of an individual is admissible in a legal proceeding. Thus, a statement by the dentist, "I messed up," or "I used the wrong instrument," would be admissible against them and the jury will hear it as evidence. However, the dentist may not realize that even though things did not go as planned, he or she did not in fact do anything wrong, or that any wrongdoing on their part probably made no difference to the outcome. Consider, for example, a dentist who, while performing endodontic therapy, separates a file in the tooth. The dentist may say, "I should have known that file was too old to use again," or "I tried to turn it too hard and I broke it." Such a statement would be an admission by the dentist that they did something they should not have done. Assume now that the dentist's attorney gets the case and sends it for an expert opinion. The expert, after looking at all the facts and examining the radiographs, writes an opinion stating that the root was so badly dilacerated that there was no chance of a successful outcome, even had an experienced endodontist performed the procedure. Thus, the tooth was doomed from the outset and the fact that the dentist separated the file made no difference to the ultimate outcome of extraction. At time of trial, however, the jury will hear the dentist's admission and may decide that the dentist's expert is just a hired gun trying to cover up for the dentist.

Comparative negligence Under the doctrine of comparative negligence a patient may be negligent and thus partially or fully to blame for any damage that occurred. The patient's negligence is known as contributory negligence. While states' laws differ on the effect of contributing negligence, two commonly followed rules are that any financial recovery by the patient will be reduced in proportion to the patient's negligence or, if the patient's negligence exceeds a certain amount—usually more than 50%–the patient will recover nothing (M.G.L. Ch 231, § 85). Examples of patient actions that may constitute negligence include poor home care and multiple missed appointments.

Patients have an obligation to follow the reasonable recommendations of their dentist. Noncompliant patients can be difficult to deal with. However, it is important to make sure that the patient understands the reasons for the necessity of following the dentist's directions. For example, should a dentist note an ulcer in a patient's mouth, it may not be sufficient to simply tell the patient to return for a follow-up visit in 10 to 14 days. The patient probably does not understand the implications of a non-healing ulcer. While the dentist does not want to frighten a patient unnecessarily, he must give the patient sufficient information to get across the need to follow the dentist's directions. In the case of the ulcer, the dentist may, for example, tell the patient that it is necessary to biopsy the ulcer if it has not healed in approximately 14 days to rule out anything serious. A dentist should make reasonable efforts to contact a patient to remind the patient that it is necessary to come in for a visit, the extent of the effort depending on the nature of the reason for the visit. If, for example, the reason is to rule out a malignancy, the dentist should make a greater effort than if the reason for a needed visit is a routine scaling. For serious matters such as ruling out the treatment of a malignancy, it is best to send a letter by certified mail, with return receipt requested to the patient's address of record. Under the doctrine of mitigation of damages, in some states a patient who suffers damages at the hands of a dentist has an obligation to mitigate the damage. In Massachusetts "if the condition of the person claiming damages would be improved by having an ordinary operation which a reasonably prudent man in the circumstances would submit to, a refusal would be evidence of an unreasonable failure to lessen the amount of the damages."[1]

Informed consent

Although part of the law of malpractice is subject to the standard of care, the doctrine of informed consent is sufficiently unique to justify treating it as a separate entity. While informed consent is required as a matter of (malpractice) law and serves as a liability prevention measure, some believe that its most useful purpose is that patients who understand what is happening to them and endorse the method chosen to treat them do better clinically. These people feel that this placebo effect is the strongest reason for a well-done informed consent.

1 Baglio v. N.Y. Central R.R., 180 N.E.2d 798 (Mass. 1962); see also Weinstock v. Ott, 444 N.E.2d 1227 (Ind. App. 1983).

Contrary to popular belief, informed consent does not usually have to be in writing. Some jurisdictions may require written informed consent for certain, usually surgical, procedures, but this is by far the exception. States follow one of two standards concerning informed consent.

Professional community standard The older professional community standard is physician centered and requires a dentist to disclose to the patient only such information as is customarily disclosed by dentists in similar circumstances.[1] In these jurisdictions, a dentist can ascertain what information he or she needs to provide a patient simply by asking fellow dentists what they tell patients concerning the same or similar procedures.

Patient-centered standard In most states, professional community standard of informed consent has been replaced by the patient-centered standard. According to this more modern standard, dentists must disclose in a reasonable manner all significant medical information that they possesses or reasonably should possess, that is material to an intelligent decision by the patient whether to undergo a proposed procedure.[2] Under this standard, a court is not concerned with what other dentists customarily tell their patients, although this may be some evidence of what is reasonable. As part of the informed-consent process, a dentist should disclose not only the risks and benefits of the proposed treatment but also the risks and benefits of refusing treatment. No court following the patient-centered standard has attempted to define every detail that a dentist has to tell a patient to obtain informed consent, but they do recognize that there are limits to what a patient can reasonably expect of a dentist in this regard.

Recognizing that it is easy for patients to complain after the fact that they would not have undergone a procedure that went awry if they had known of a particular risk, courts following the modern standard have built in a significant safeguard for the practitioner, holding that there is no tort liability unless the unrevealed risk that should have been made known materializes. An example illustrates just what this means. Assume that a patient undergoes third-molar extraction. The dentist warns the patient of the risk of hemorrhage, but does not warn the patient of the risk of infection. Following the extraction, the patient dies of hemorrhage. The patient's estate cannot sue the dentist on the theory that had the patient been told of the risk of infection, he would not have consented to procedure. The reason that the estate cannot use this theory is that infection, the unrevealed risk, was not at issue. Many jurisdictions have built in an additional safeguard, namely, the patient must show that had the proper information been provided neither the patient nor a reasonable person in similar circumstances would have undergone the procedure.

1 R. Shrugue and K. Linstromberg 1992 The Practitioner's Guide to Informed Consent. Defense Law Journal **41** 73–125.
2 Harnish v. Children's Hosp. Med. Center, 387 Mass. 152 (1982).

Termination of the dentist–patient relationship

At some time every dentist is confronted with the situation of having a patient that he or she would prefer not to see. As long as the reason for wishing to dismiss the patient is not discriminatory (e.g., because of race, religion, etc.), a patient may be dismissed for any reason, including not paying their bills, refusing to cooperate, or being rude or threatening to staff.

The dentist–patient relationship may be terminated in one or four ways:

- The patient dismisses the dentist.
- By mutual consent of the patient and dentist
- The dentist brings the case to its conclusion.
- The dentist withdraws from the case.

While dismissal of the dentist by a patient might be hardest on the ego, it is the easiest way to terminate the relationship as the patient has unilaterally done so. From a malpractice perspective, the most problematic way to terminate the relationship is when the dentist withdraws from a case. This is especially true when the patient would like the relationship to continue. Withdrawal from a case is more likely than any other way of terminating the relationship to result in abandonment of a patient. Patient abandonment is the unilateral withdrawal by a dentist from a patient's care without first formally transferring that care to another qualified dentist who is acceptable to the patient.[1]

Terminating the case by bringing it to its conclusion may also, depending on the circumstances, be problematic. If a patient is referred by a general dentist to a prosthodontist for a crown on tooth #9 and no other treatment, and the prosthodontist completes the treatment, the case can be said to have been brought to its conclusion. The prosthodontist probably has no obligation to see the patient again, with the possible exception that if tooth #9 should require additional prosthodontic care he would be obliged to see the patient. When the situation involves more general work, such as that performed by a general dentist or a full-mouth rehabilitation done by a prosthodontist, the situation is different. Typically, a dentist and dental specialists who see patients on a long-term basis have a recall system. This being the case, it is difficult for them to argue that the case has been brought to its conclusion, as care is really ongoing in the form of regular follow-up.

No matter how the dentist–patient relationship ends, it is always good practice for the dentist to send a letter to the patient. The letter should be written in friendly terms, and should state that the dentist will no longer be treating the patient. The dentist should give the patient the contact information for the local dental society that can help him or her find a new treating dentist and/or to offer to assist the patient to identify prospective new dentists. It is also advisable to offer to continue to see the patient for a reasonable period of time to give the patient sufficient

1 E. D. Pellegrino 1995 *Ann Intern Med* **122** 377.

time to find a new dentist. What constitutes a reasonable period of time varies, depending on circumstances. In a large city with many dentists, a couple of weeks might be sufficient. In a remote area with few dentists, months may be reasonable, and if a dentist is the only practitioner in a wide radius, the dentist may have no choice but to keep seeing the patient, at least until the current treatment plan has been completed.

Liability

An individual may be responsible for the negligence of another under the theory of vicarious liability. One form of vicarious liability is that of respondeat superior, which means "let the master answer." Respondeat superior may apply, for example, in the case of a hygienist who commits negligence. Courts will look to various factors to determine if vicarious liability should be applied in a particular case. A dentist may be responsible for acts of negligence committed by his or her partner. A dentist may also be responsible for negligent referral if the dentist refers a patient to a practitioner whom the dentist knows or has reason to know is incompetent. Although negligent referral can only arise as a result of another dentist's negligence, strictly speaking, negligent referral is not a case of liability for the actions of another, but is a tort in and of itself, even though the referring dentist may be held monetarily liable for the negligent act of the other dentist.

Patient records

Good record keeping is essential to successful treatment of a patient. This is especially true if a patient transfers from one dentist to another or is referred between practitioners, for example, for specialty care.

- Records should be complete, and legible.
- The record should not include financial information, which should be kept separately.
- No disparaging remarks should be made in the record.
- The dentist should sign each entry immediately following the last word of that entry. No blank spaces where words can later be added between the last word of an entry and the signature should be left.
- Words should not be whited or crossed out, nor should words be interlineated.
- Any changes to an entry should be made by an additional entry in the form of an addendum to a previous entry.
- All entries should be dated. Poor records may cause the dentist's malpractice carrier to decide that a case is indefensible and may compel them to settle a claim that the dentist may regard as non-meritorious.
- Records must be kept for a certain period of time as specified by state law.
- The physical record belongs to the dentist, but the information contained in them belongs to the patient.

Thus, while a patient is not entitled to the original record, he or she is entitled to a copy of both the written record as well as any X-rays, test results, photographs, casts, etc. The patient's entitlement is valid even if there is an outstanding financial obligation, the law taking the position that the patient's health comes first and the dentist can always pursue legal action to recover money owed.

- The dentist may charge a reasonable fee for reproducing or copying the record.
- The dentist may have a reasonable amount of time to duplicate a patient's record.
- All requests for copies of the record should be in written form. With the advent of privacy laws such as the Health Insurance Portability and Accountability Act (HIPAA) it is advisable to have written record requests.
- The dentist should keep the patient's written request as part of the patient's record.

When buying or selling a practice, it is imperative to spell out clearly in the contract how records are to be handled. Typically, contracts specify or assume that the records will transfer to the buyer. For the seller, however, this could prove problematic down the road. State law requires a dentist to keep patient records for a specified period of time, and transferring them prior to this time may violate the law. It is possible too that some patients would not want their records transferred to the buyer, placing the seller in breach of his or her duty of confidentiality. Ideally, the seller should write all patients a letter explaining his or her plan to sell the practice and asking their written permission to transfer their records to the buyer. The letter should also give patients the option of asking that the records be sent to them or a dentist of their choice. Finally, in the event the seller gets sued, the seller may not have access to the records in order to defend himself if he has transferred them to the buyer. Thus, if the records have been transferred, the contract should spell out that the buyer will keep the records for a certain number of years and will grant the seller access to them in the event the latter issued.

Emergencies

As far as existing patients are concerned, a dentist has both a legal and ethical obligation to ensure that emergency care is available for their patients at all times and during any absences.

- The dentist is not obligated to be personally available at all times, but must make reasonable arrangements for patients to be seen in emergencies or during the dentist's absence.
- The dentist should have a publicly listed telephone number and an answering service or answering machine that directs the patient to a number to call for immediate care in the event of an emergency.
- It is not acceptable to simply direct patients to the nearest hospital emergency room unless the dentist has made formal arrangements with the hospital. Most hospitals are not equipped to provide appropriate dental care. Unfortunately, too many dentists do not take the obligation to provide emergency care seriously enough.[1]

1 B. Friedland and Katzman 2005 *J Mass Dent Soc* **54(3)** 22.

Consent for children

Individuals under the age of 18 cannot give legal consent for treatment. Either a parent or someone with legal responsibility must give consent on behalf of the child. With older children, it may be reasonable to obtain the child's assent to treatment in addition to a parent's or guardian's consent.

- Consent to treatment does not need to be obtained in an emergency (M.G.L. c. 112, § 12F). In the case of an avulsed tooth, for example, where time is of the essence, the dentist will legally be permitted to go ahead and provide such treatment as is customarily provided under the circumstances.
- State law grants certain minors the status of an emancipated minor, which gives them the right to make their own decisions. Examples are minors who are married, who are pregnant or have children of their own, and who are in the military (M.G.L. c. 112, § 12F). Dentists should check their own state law to determine which minors may give consent.
- It is also important to realize that minors may not be bound by any contracts they might make. Thus, dentists who undertake work on a minor with only the latter's consent may find themselves unable to collect their fee. Under the doctrine of contracts for necessaries, there is usually an exception for work performed as part of emergency treatment. Emancipated minors are be bound by contracts they enter into.
- As far as consent to treatment is concerned, incompetent adults are treated similarly to children. However, the law may treat previously competent adults differently from those who were never competent. A dentist who treats incompetent adults should check the state law for guidance on how to proceed and may even need to request an opinion from an attorney specializing in this aspect of the law.

Insurance

No dentist should practice without malpractice insurance. In some states it may be a condition of licensure that a dentist has insurance coverage. While Massachusetts does not require malpractice coverage as a condition of licensure for dentists, it does do so for physicians (MGL Ch. 112 §2). There are two primary forms of insurance coverage, an occurrence and a claims-made policy. It is important understand the difference between the two.

- An *occurrence policy* covers losses that happen during a given period of time, the policy term. The loss can be reported years later, but the key is when it happened. If it happened while the policy was in effect, the dentist is covered. Thus, if a dentist is sued after retiring, he or she will be covered by the occurrence policy that was in effect at the time of the alleged malpractice or occurrence.

- A *claims-made policy* covers claims made during a given period of time. The loss may have happened many years ago, but if it is reported during the current policy term, there is coverage based on the policy now in effect.

- Occurrence forms are considered more valuable as they respond to claims even years later.

- A claims-made policy has no guarantee of continued insurability, so if an insurance company cancels a dentist's policy, the dentist may not have coverage in the future for activities in the past.

- A dentist who is considering getting a claims-made policy should, at a minimum, inquire into the following: retrospective date, extended reporting periods, and tail coverage.

An important caveat concerning insurance is to keep in mind that malpractice insurance covers only malpractice and not liability due to other causes, such as a patient slipping and falling. A dentist should be sure to have appropriate general liability insurance as well.

National practitioner data bank

As part of the Health Care Quality Improvement Act of 1986, the federal government instituted the National Practitioner Data Bank (42 USC § 11101). The NPDB was enacted because the U.S. Congress believed that the increasing occurrence of medical malpractice litigation and the need to improve the quality of medical care had become nationwide problems that warranted greater efforts than any individual state could undertake. The intent is to improve the quality of health care by encouraging state licensing boards, hospitals and other health care entities, and professional societies to identify and discipline those who engage in unprofessional behavior; and to restrict the ability of incompetent physicians, dentists, and other health-care practitioners to move from state to state without disclosure or discovery of previous medical malpractice payment and adverse action history.

- Adverse actions can involve licensure, clinical privileges, professional society membership, and exclusions from Medicare and Medicaid. The NPDB specifies the kind of information that must be reported.
  These include medical malpractice payments, adverse actions taken by hospitals and other health-care entities, the voluntary surrender of clinical privileges, and actions taken by dental boards of registration and professional societies.
- Health care–related civil judgments and criminal convictions that must be reported to the NPDB include criminal convictions, civil judgments, injunctions, and nolo contendere/no contest pleas related to health care.
- A denial of privileges because a practitioner fails to meet initial credentialing criteria is not reportable.
- Although the NPDB states that malpractice payments are reportable, a court has ruled that payment from personal funds is not reportable.[1] Personal funds mean that the payment is made from the dentist's personal bank account, and not from the funds of the practice, corporation, or partnership. Refunds are not reportable if a patient makes a request for a refund orally and the practitioner makes payment personally.
- The NPDB protects dentists who make a payment by stating that payments made in settlement of malpractice actions or claims shall not be construed as creating a presumption that malpractice has occurred.
- The NPDB further states that waiver of an outstanding debt is not considered a payment by the practitioner.

Access to information in the NPDB is available to entities that meet certain eligibility requirements. In order to access information, entities must first register with the NPDB. Dentists may access their own information. This is done online (http://www.npdb-hipdb.hrsa.gov/welcomesq.html).

---

1 American Dental Association v. Shalala, 3 F.3d 445 (DC Cir. 1993).

Forensic dentistry

Forensic dentistry is a branch of forensic medicine that deals with teeth and marks left by teeth.

Identification Because the dental tissues survive the effects of fire, water, and time well, dental identification is helpful where other means of distinguishing a person have been lost, e.g., following incineration or burial. Not only can the teeth be used to indicate the approximate age of a victim, but also the condition of the dentition, including any filled or missing teeth, can be compared with dental records to aid identification. Occasionally dentists are called upon to assist in the identification of a victim. Remember that dental treatment may have been carried out subsequently and that additional restorations or missing teeth may not match dental records precisely. This does not necessarily exclude identification. Information can also be obtained from studying the skull and jaw bones, e.g., age, gender, racial origin, and the time elapsed since death. Comparative radiographs may be as individual as fingerprints. From a forensic point of view the value of accurate up-to-date records, and identification marks in dentures, are self-evident.

Occasionally, a practitioner is asked by the police to reveal the dental records of a missing person. The advice of a lawyer should be sought, as legally a patient's confidential records should not be revealed without a court order.

Bite marks in inanimate objects left at the site of a crime have on occasion contributed to the conviction of the perpetrator. If the "evidence" is a perishable foodstuff, then a permanent record can be made by casting in either stone or rubber base material, following photography.

Bite marks in human skin can occur in assault or non-accidental injury cases. Considerable aggression is required to penetrate the skin. It is important to first establish any identifying features of the teeth that caused the bite and then compare them with the dentition of any suspects. Good photographs, including a linear scale, are essential, and if the victim is alive, they need to be repeated in 24 h since the clarity of the bite may improve with time. In addition, any saliva associated with the mark can be analyzed to assist in the identification of an assailant.

Practice management

Principal sources: K. J. Lewis 1989 *Practice Management for Dentists*, Wright. R. Rattan 1996 *Making Sense of Dental Practice Management*, Radcliffe Medical Press. J. O. Forrest 1984 *A Guide to Successful Dental Practice*, Wright. http://www.ada.org

Management skills

There are numerous dental management courses offered to dentists and office staff through weekend seminars and online courses. Although it may be easy to dismiss them as a way of making a quick profit (for the person giving the course), in fact we can benefit tremendously by applying some of the fundamental principles that are commonly taught in these courses.

What are the benefits of good management? ↑ communication, ↑ efficiency, ↓ stress, and ↑ job satisfaction for the entire dental team. A happy practice environment is not only a pleasant to work in, but the ambience will also be conveyed to the patients.

Keys to successful management

Good communication and organization skills While the benefit of good communication with patients is acknowledged, the importance of communication with other members of the dental team often receives less emphasis. For teamwork to be successful, all staff should help to create a vision for the practice as well as have an opportunity to participate in the development of office policies and procedures. This type of task usually requires establishing some time within the work week for staff meetings. It is helpful if these meetings have structure. This does not mean that the dentist dominates the proceedings; rather, all staff should be encouraged to submit ideas for an agenda. On occasion, guidance might be necessary to assure that these meetings are positive.

Delegate those tasks that do not require your training and expertise. In addition to ↓ stress and freeing you for the more demanding tasks, this also ↑ job satisfaction for the staff, provided they are given the training and time to manage their new responsibilities—e.g., having the hygienist do the background research necessary to decide which new ultrasonic scaler to purchase. Try to develop a detailed job description for each member of the staff. This empowers your staff to maximize the notion that what they do is not only essential for the office but may also result in a renewed sense of dedication and commitment.

Teamwork The importance of building a mutually supportive team can readily be appreciated by the doctor, the staff, and the patients. Successful leadership involves encouraging staff to develop their potential as both individuals and valued members of the team, as well as encouraging a discussion on what the goals are and how to achieve them. Motivation to work as a team can be fostered by monetary incentives linked to the performance of the practice, but it is wise to explore what motivates individual members of the team, as money is not always the most important motivator.

Staff training This should involve not just the newly appointed members of the team. Training and motivating current staff to extend their skills will allow the delegation of new tasks to each staff member. Effective patient management and communication skills for both administrative and clinical staff should also be developed. A manual of procedures and routines applicable to the practice is a must, and staff should be encouraged to contribute and help update this manual periodically. In-house training days with speakers either from within the practice or invited are recommended, as is participation in local, regional, and national meetings.

Salary Motivation and commitment can often be achieved through financial incentives. Therefore, by structuring payment to comprise **1** a fixed hourly rate; **2** an individual bonus, related to attendance, sickness record, and productivity paid as a percentage of the hourly rate; and **3** a group bonus that is a fixed proportion of the profits of the practice, all staff have incentive to reduce overhead and improve efficiency, while reducing the stress of everyday practice.

Complaints Because patients are paying for their treatments, they will have ↑ expectations for the service provided. In a large proportion of cases, a potential problem can be prevented through good communication.

Employment and termination

Hiring

1 Define what tasks the practice would like the new staff to perform. Decide on the criteria for an ideal candidate, as this will aid the selection process later.

2 Draw up a job description. Consider including details of the practice philosophy, the role of the new staff in the team, required skills, in-job training to be provided, hours of work, pay, and other benefits.

3 Advertise the job in the local press and on an Internet job search site. Remember to include a realistic closing date for applications.

4 Establish a short-list of potential candidates.

5 Interview candidates, preferably with two or three people on the panel. This should be structured so that candidates are asked the same questions, to aid comparison. Notes should be taken, because after several interviews the distinction between candidates may become obscured. When a suitable person is found, the job offer should be made in writing, subject to references and recommendations. If no suitable person is found, go back to step **1** and reassess the requirements and consider rewriting job descriptions as necessary.

6 Write a provisional contract, including how assessment is to be carried out at the end of the trial period (usually 6–8 weeks is long enough). Both employee and employer should retain a signed copy.

7 Orient and train the newly hired staff, giving time for feedback in both directions.

8 Before the end of trial period, reassess. If both parties are satisfied, formal contract should be signed.

9 When recruiting staff, do not discriminate on grounds of disability, sex, gender reassignment, race, religion, marital situation, or whether or not they have children.

Note: Train employees thoroughly to ensure that they understand your practice vision, philosophy, and policies. Always put all matters regarding employment in writing.

Termination

Frustration and possible lawsuits can be initiated by improperly conducted employee terminations. Employee termination generates stress for the person being dismissed, the dentist who orders the dismissal, and the remaining staff who might be threatened by such a proceeding. The American Dental Association (ADA) has produced catalog resources that will give guidance on employee employment and termination.[1] Both from a practical and emotional point of view, dismissal of staff is not easy and if taken to court will be expensive.

---

1 http//www.ada.org

When problems arise with an employee, to prevent a claim of unfair dismissal, use the following guidelines:

1 Be honest and completely clear about the reasons for dismissal. Avoid personal accusations that might degrade or humiliate the individual. Tell employee formally (with either warning or disciplinary action) that their conduct is unsatisfactory, giving a timetable for improvement, advice, and assistance. Make sure they are familiar with office policies and expectations, as well as with the consequences for noncompliance.

2 Give written warning that if there is no improvement, dismissal will follow.

3 Keep complete and accurate records to protect the interests of both parties involved.

4 After firing an employee, document the termination in writing immediately, detailing the conversation, reactions, and even emotional tone of both parties. This is essential for response to any future challenge to the termination.

Note: Federal law requires a 60-day advance notification of employees affected by layoffs and plant or office closings.

Right to job security

This right protects the employee from "termination at will" or the previously customary employer practice of discharging an individual for virtually any reason. Legislation, including Title VII of the Civil Rights Act of 1964 and more recent anti-discriminations laws, should be reviewed and respected.

Privacy and patient health information

The Health Insurance Portability and Accountability Act of 1996 (HIPAA)[1]

The HIPAA is a federal law that protects the privacy and security of individually identifiable health information through a privacy rule and a security rule. This applies to all patient information, called *PHI* (protected health information), in any forms such as electronic, paper, or oral. This law was enacted to restore public trust in the health-care industry as patient records could be unknowingly transmitted to other parties without a patient's consent.

PHI is any information that could be used to identify a patient. For example:

- Patient demographic information (e.g., name, date of birth, Social Security number, address, or insurance)
- Medical records (e.g., medical record number, medical history, diagnosis, or treatment)
- Payment information (e.g., bills or receipts)
- Ancillary services (e.g., radiographs or labs)

Note: All PHI must be treated as confidential. This protection includes information relating to the past, present, and future physical or mental health of a person. This protection also includes information generated in the context of clinical research.

Who must follow this law?

- Most doctors, nurses, pharmacies, hospitals, clinics, nursing homes, and other health-care providers
- Health insurance companies, health maintenance organizations (HMOs), and most employer group-health plans
- Certain government programs that pay for health care, such as Medicare and Medicaid

What information is protected?

- Information that doctors, nurses, and other health-care providers put in a patient's medical record
- Conversations a doctor has about a patient's care or treatment with nurses, dental assistants, and others
- Information about a patient in a patient's health insurer's computer system.
- Patient's billing information

Providers and health insurers who are required to follow this law must comply with a patient's right to

- See and get a copy of their records
- Have corrections added to their health information
- Receive a notice that tells patients how their health information may be used and shared
- Get a report on when and why their health information was shared for certain purposes

1 http://www.hhs.gov/ocr/hipaa/

What are the HIPAA penalties?
1 Civil penalties for rule noncompliance
   - Fines of up to $25,000/person/year for violation of a single standard
   - Privacy enforced by Department of Health and Human Services (DHHS) Office for Civil Rights
   - Security enforced by DHHS Office of HIPAA Standards
2 Criminal penalties for wrongful disclosure of PHI
   - Fines of up to $250,000 and 1–10 years imprisonment
   - Enforced by the Department of Justice

Documentation
- Privacy and security rules require written policies and procedures available in the workforce as needed.
- Policies and procedures and other rule-related documents must be kept at least 6 years from last use.
- Know the rules before destroying the documents.

What does this mean for you?
- Be careful with all patient information, in any form. Ask yourself the following:
   - Am I allowed to have this information? Is it required for me to do my job?
   - Is the person with whom I am about to share this information allowed to receive it? Do they need the information to do their job? Is there a new procedure I need to follow?
   - If I were the patient, and this was my information, how would I feel about it being shared?

Patient privacy is
- Ensuring computer security
- Sending and receiving faxes and e-mail
- Disposing of information
- Using and disclosing patient information
- Conducting everyday work practices

In your everyday work practices
- Think about how and when you disclose patient information.
- Look for opportunities to reduce unnecessary uses and/or disclosure.
- Watch where you talk about your patients.
- Only discuss patients with others responsible for a patient's treatment or services or with someone a patient has given you permission to speak to.
- Talking about an identified patient in any other circumstances is prohibited.

Financial management

Find a good accountant and a supportive financial institution, preferably on the recommendation of another practitioner. It is advisable to develop a structured system for dealing with fees and payments, tailored to the individual practice, that is well understood and adhered to by all staff.

Delegating many aspects of calculating and collecting fees from patients to motivated staff should make the practice more cost-effective. However, failure to monitor the situation adequately can, at best, result in a false sense of security.

Overhead By making subtle changes in how your practice operates financially, you can show improvement in profitability by reducing unnecessary costs. According to the ADA Survey of Dental Practices, published in 2004, average overhead represented 60.5% of general practice revenues.[1] Thus, you should aim to keep the overhead percentage at 60% or less.

Bookkeeping is time consuming, but necessary. Many bookkeeping tasks can be performed using dental practice management software that is integrated with a practice management system. This software should provide easy access to a few key reports that are frequently assessed:
- Accounts receivable (total amount of money owed by patients, insurance companies, or other third parties)
- Bank deposits
- Patient lists
- Income and expenditures. This should include all monies received and all bills paid (e.g., lab fees, wages) and be compiled monthly by the principal, to develop a feel for the financial situation. It is wise to seek the advice of your accountant on the methodology, since accurate accounts will make their job easier and reduce the cost of their services.
- Even petty cash transactions should be recorded, together with relevant receipts. The large bills are best stored in a separate, locked box.
- Wages

Banking It is advisable to bank all monies at the end of each day, as the bank statement then indicates daily receipts. Accept payments by cash, check, or credit card to encourage settlement of accounts. Although credit cards incur a commission, patients may elect to use this form of payment. It is good policy to negotiate overdraft facilities in advance to cover those occasions when cash-flow problems arise.

Budgeting An annual forecast and budget should be prepared jointly with the accountant because a well-prepared budget allows a practice to reduce unnecessary overhead while improving the efficiency and performance of the practice.

Bad debts These can often be prevented by having a definite office policy regarding late payments that is announced to patients and adhered to—e.g., payment in part at the beginning of treatment and the balance on

1 http://www.ada.org

completion or payment in full up front. In addition, have the patient acknowledge and agree to be responsible for the total fee in the absence of insurance coverage. At the treatment plan presentation appointment, the patient should receive a written estimate and be reminded when payment is due. If a patient forgets to pay, at the last visit they should be asked to sign a form confirming that the treatment has been satisfactorily completed and that they agree to pay within 7 days. If payment is still not forthcoming, reminders should be sent out at 7, 14, and 28 days. If there is still no response, notify the debt collectors.

Taxes This is really where a good accountant is important. By providing an accountant with information on income and expenditures on a monthly basis, he or she will be able to provide advice on what to do before the end of the financial year to minimize your tax liability.

Insurance This is essential for property, contents, equipment, indemnity, staff, loss of income, and personal coverage.

Running behind schedule

Running behind schedule occasionally happens to everyone. A common reaction is to cut corners, a strategy that should never be used. Another response to being overstressed is to try too hard to hurry, not pausing to plan time effectively. There are no immediate simple solutions, but if another member of the staff is available, e.g., a hygienist or dental assistant, you may be able to delegate some simple tasks.

If running behind becomes a habit, it is imperative to stop and reassess your working practices before your patients or staff become annoyed. The first step is to re-evaluate the time allocated for each common procedure—are you being realistic? If the answer is yes, then the problem lies with the receptionist's perceptions of your superhuman abilities, and some gentle re-education or reminder is necessary. After erring on the generous side for the length of time required for each treatment, go through the appointment book and block out some buffer zones in each session for emergencies, doing paperwork, or, if for no other reason, a breather. The frequency and length of these will depend on the severity of the original problem.

Some additional hints to ↓ everyday stress:
- Have an appointment book, divided into 10-min units to provide flexibility; 15-min units often cause either under- or overscheduling of patients.
- A working day comprising a longer morning (high-revenue procedures) and a shorter afternoon (routine procedures) can be more productive.
- If you are so busy that longer procedures have to be booked well in advance, designate some specific sessions for them each month (thus ↓ the temptation to squeeze them in).
- For busy sessions, try to use two or more dental chairs.
- For last-minute cancellations, have a list of patients who are willing to come in at short notice (call list).
- Define the working day and try not to extend beyond this.
- Coffee breaks and lunchtime should not always be used to catch up on other work. Be kind to yourself and your staff, and take a break.

Emergency appointment This should be booked for a patient who needs to be seen as soon as possible; a patient who attempts to negotiate to make an earlier appointment to meet his or her time demand is not considered an emergency. If buffer zones are built into your timetable, scheduling the true emergencies should not be a problem. For emergencies that might occur during nonworking hours, there should be a telephone number for patients to contact you or a designee for advice and treatment.

Marketing

Advertising Announcement of your practice can be accomplished in many different formats. It is a means of letting the public know about the philosophy of your practice and the services available to the community. Apart from the traditional yellow pages listing, promotion of your service can be publicized by the following means:

• Brochures and informational packets can be distributed to existing patients and be used as possible sources of new recruits.
• Hosting an open house. This will allow apprehensive patients to find out about your office atmosphere without the need to have an examination or treatment. Also invite business, educational, and community leaders to visit your office and prepare a brief presentation about something special in your office.
• Community or school presentation. Contact community and school organizations in your area, and offer oral health education.
• Practice Web site. With ↑ popularity of the Internet, this can be an efficient and dynamic medium for practice promotion.
• Advertising in local publications or via direct mail, but follow the ADA and state guidelines on advertisement.
• The best advertisement is a satisfied patient who will recommend you by word of mouth.

First appearances count This starts before the patient arrives for their first appointment, as most patients will make their initial contact by phone. The phone should always be answered promptly, in person (not by an answering machine), with a friendly and welcoming greeting. When the prospective patient arrives, the external and internal décor, together with the warm welcome they receive, will play a role in determining a patient's impression of the professionalism of the practice. The reception and waiting areas should appear cozy and inviting. Choose light, warm colors and comfortable seating to give a relaxing ambience. Plants, provided someone remembers to water them, also help. A small area for children to play with toys and some books are good practice builders. A range of interesting magazines and practice brochures on different aspects of dental care and health should be available.

Staff The receptionist must be friendly and helpful at all times. It is worth spending some time with the receptionist to decide on common responses to some of the more common problems that arise (e.g., dealing with the angry patient) and ↑ their knowledge of dental technologies available so that patients' queries can be answered correctly. It is also helpful if the receptionist can ask new patients how they heard about the practice, to better target future marketing strategies. The presentation and attitude of all the staff are of vital importance. An attractive and functional uniform in the practice color bearing the practice logo might be useful as well.

Emergencies Although it is tempting to exclude non-registered patients from receiving emergency treatment, it is a good practice-builder to see new patients in discomfort, as some of them need immediate attention and may become patients of your practice.

Market research It is vital to know your patient base. Is there a significant group that may need special attention (e.g., elderly or young families)? What extra services would your patients like to see (e.g., implants or veneers)? What do they feel about your office hours—is there another group of patients who might attend if the office hours were extended or changed?

Note: Remember, the most important marketing aid is, without doubt, the personal touch.

Practice brochures

What information to include?

Pertinent information:
- Practice name, address, and telephone number
- Name and credentials of all the dentists
- Hours of operation
- Dental services provided (e.g., sedation, implant surgeries, etc.)
- Any foreign languages spoken by the dentist and staff

Further *optional* information can be included in the brochures:
- Practice philosophy
- Map showing location of practice
- E-mail and Web site addresses
- Emergency arrangements and contact phone number
- Further information on the special interests of the dentists, both dental and nondental
- Illustrations of the practice, and photos of staff and facilities
- Details of charges for broken appointments, if applicable
- Methods of payment accepted

How to set about producing a brochure Broadly speaking, there are two approaches: either get professional help (e.g., consultant, designer, photographer, or printer), or do it yourself, using a commercially available printing package. However, the two are not mutually exclusive and all practices should at least consider getting advice from a designer.

Prior to seeking help, it is important to have some idea of what you want. For example:
- Only one brochure, or the first of a series?
- What is your potential market (young families with small children, older professionals and their families)?
- Black and white, or two or more colors?
- Glossy booklet or a trifold?
- How much money do you want to spend?
- How many copies do you need (to avoid being led astray by the bulk discounts)?
- How is the brochure to be distributed?

It is wise to shop around and examine the work of several professionals before choosing your brochure(s).

Design and layout The brochure creates the impression of a caring practice and informs patients about the services available to them. The key to success is simplicity. One helpful tip is to have a practice logo and/or house style (or colors), replicated in other items of practice stationery. This idea of a corporate image is not new and has worked well in the business world. A designer will be able to suggest styles and layouts best suited to your projected market, and help with the content of the text.

Sponsorship This is worth considering, to give full flight to your creative aspirations. Try approaching toothbrush manufacturers, dental supply companies, or local firms that you deal with on a regular basis.

Points to watch

- Don't advertise services or goods in which you are not proficient.
- Don't include names of practice staff other than dentists, as there might be employee turnover.
- Be legal, decent, honest, and truthful.

Computers and dental practice

Computers and dental practice

Commonly used dental software programs are becoming user friendly (getting easier to learn and use) and are becoming essential tools to carry out daily operations. As with any other new tasks, it will take specific training to become familiar with the new program, but excellent training and technologic support is usually available from vendors. Today there are many opportunities to incorporate digital technology into your office. For example, digital radiographs and clinical photographs can be electronically stored in the patient's clinical record, printed, and given to the patient for review, or e-mailed to specialists for consultations or insurance companies for claim review. An integrated program allows several functions to operate simultaneously without having to change from one package to another. Integrated dental software can run any kind of dental-related functions, providing full clinical and administrative capabilities in one system. For example, digital records are safer and more efficient than traditional paper records because backup copies could be stored away from the office and you can save the office space by eliminating patient chart files.

The cost of the necessary computers, monitors, printers, and scanners, etc. to update your office informational technology has fallen to very reasonable price points. There are many payment and lease plans available that will allow for flexible monthly payment schedules.

Where to go for advice?

- Dental computer specialist—generally worth the extra expense
- Business computer specialist
- Local retailers
- Colleagues
- Teach yourself, but be careful, because computers can be addictive.

Choosing a system It is important to decide what you want the computer to do and how much you are prepared to spend. If an (expensive) multi-function practice management system is being considered, then the choice of hardware is less important and is often dictated by the software package. However, if a more cautious approach is planned (starting with intraoral cameras only), then the choice of computer and operating system is more important. In this case, a computer with the largest memory you can afford and a good-quality inkjet or laser printer is advisable. An agreement providing on-site maintenance in case of breakdown is a necessity, and training and data backup are essential.

Digital radiographic imaging

Digital radiographic imaging has the potential to improve the way clinical data are collected, evaluated, and presented. In addition, digital radiographic imaging is safer for the staff and patient because radiation exposure is greatly reduced. Traditional film-based imaging requires chemical processing and is a limited visual aid for the patient. Also, the diagnostic quality of digital radiographic imaging is equal to that of the traditional film method. There are different digital systems available for dentistry, and it is advisable to consult with different company representatives and colleagues prior to purchasing a system.

Starting your dental career[1]

Deciding on how you will begin practicing dentistry can be the most important decision to make prior to graduating from dental school. There are many different practice options to choose from, including academic, hospital-based, and private practices. In addition to the many different career options to choose from, many new graduates decide to go into practice as an employee, independent contractor, or owner.

Associateship Almost 2/3 of recent graduates have decided to seek associateship after graduation. They have found that associateships give them an attractive alternative to starting their own practice, especially while coping with their high dental-education debt. As an associate, you will be able to earn income and gain hands-on technical experience without the financial impact of starting your own practice. Plus, you may have the option of buying into the practice a few years down the road.

Independent contracting Some graduates who do not want all the responsibility of practice ownership, but want to build their own practice seek out the opportunity to serve as an independent contractor in another practice. The key difference between being an associate and being an independent contractor is the degree of autonomy—independent contracts are responsible for building their own patient base and have control over the dental care they provide. Thus, independent contractors generally take their patient records with them when they leave a practice.

Practice ownership Being your own boss and managing your own staff is a big responsibility. Not only do you have to have the clinical expertise to practice dentistry, but you also need to know how to operate business. You can buy into an existing practice, buy out the owner (or partner) of a practice, start your own practice from scratch, or share space in another office. There are many things to consider as you pursue practice ownership:
- Selecting the proper location (e.g., city or suburb)
- Deciding if you are going to purchase an existing practice or open a new practice
- Securing capital
- Selecting staff
- Developing management systems (e.g., record, inventory, OSHA/infection control, financial, and payment)
- Determining your marketing approach

Dental education and research The benefits offered to faculty members can definitely make it worth the effort. Not only do you get to work with outstanding researchers and students, but most faculty members receive benefits including continuing education, paid vacation, paid sick time, health insurance, retirement plans, life insurance, malpractice insurance, and disability insurance.

---

1 http://www.ada.org/prof/ed/careers/infopaks/

Researching the market

To develop the potential of a practice it is essential to fully evaluate its present position. By simply going through the manual or computer records and looking at the geographical spread and socioeconomic groups you can gain an appreciation of the existing patient base. If most patients are part of a family group, then future developments need to provide advantages for parents and children—e.g., if changing to independent practice, then to a family-based capitation scheme, might be more applicable. Also, the potential for attracting new patients to the practice and the competition from other practices in the area for these and existing patients should be assessed.

Business planning

Two practical business-planning tools are

1 The planning cycle:

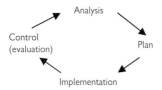

2 A SWOT analysis is a consideration of the Strengths, Weaknesses, Opportunities, and Threats to and of a business.

Fee setting

This difficult exercise should be carried out in conjunction with the advice of the practice accountant. The following will need to be calculated:
• Practice overhead
• Profit desired (realistic expectation)
• Inflation
• Number of sessions worked per week

From this the target hourly rate can be calculated. However, local market conditions need to be considered, which may necessitate a little rounding of the profits desired. Once a realistic hourly rate has been calculated, fees can then be determined for each procedure by the average amount of time taken, to develop a fee schedule. Don't forget the laboratory fees for the procedures that require them.

Evidence-based medicine and dentistry[1]

Evidence-based medicine and dentistry (EBM/D) involves making clinical decisions based on the best available evidence, which should include sound research, epidemiology, basic science, and clinical experience.

Clinical effectiveness This involves using clinical interventions that have been shown to be effective by both research and audit. The gold standard for research is a well-planned randomized, controlled, clinical trial (RCCT), but in many areas of clinical practice evidence from such trials is not available. In the meantime, clinicians should continue to carefully evaluate the techniques they use and the results of studies reported in the literature, although the sheer volume of scientific literature makes keeping up to date a difficult task. Review articles are helpful, but in the past have tended to be rather subjective.

Systematic review is a method of collating and assessing the results of research on a particular topic. This implies that a thorough search for suitable articles and indeed unpublished work has been made and explicit criteria used to decide whether an article should be included or rejected.

Meta-analysis A systemic review that uses special statistical methods to combine the results of several studies. Only RCCTs should be included. By considering a number of studies, the effects (and side effects) of a Rx are magnified as the sum total of subjects is effectively ↑. Whether the findings are consistent for different population groups or for Rx variations can also be evaluated. For example, if this technique had been used to evaluate the results of research into the use of streptokinase in treatment of myocardial infarction, a positive benefit would have been demonstrated almost 20 yr before it became apparent from individual studies.

The Cochrane collaboration This aims to collate the results of systematic reviews in all areas of health care and ensure that the findings are kept up to date. The results can be accessed electronically in the Cochrane library, which is available via the Internet. An Oral Health Group is currently investigating several topics of interest to the dental specialties.

Clinical guidelines are defined as "systematically developed statements which assist clinicians and patients in making decisions about appropriate treatment for specific conditions."[2] They may be developed nationally or locally, but should always be seen as guidance and are therefore aids to, but not a substitute for, clinical judgment. To be effective, clinical guidelines should be brief, practical, and based on the results of sound research. They should be reviewed regularly in light of new research and their effectiveness audited. Clinical guidelines can be drawn up by any group of clinicians.

---

1 D. L. Sackett 1997 *Evidence-Based Medicine*, Churchill Livingstone.
2 T. Mann 1996 *Clinical Guidelines*, NHS Executive.

Infection control

In 1991, the Occupational Safety and Health Administration (OSHA) issued the Bloodborne Pathogens Standard to help protect workers from transmission of bloodborne pathogen diseases.[1] For example, the OSHA Bloodborne Pathogens Standard defines personal protective equipment (PPE) as "specialized clothing or equipment worn by an employee for protection against a hazard. General work clothes (e.g., uniforms, pants, shirts or blouses) not intended to function as protection against a hazard are not considered to be PPE."[2]

The Centers for Disease Control and Prevention (CDC) in its 2003 Infection Control Guidelines for Dentistry also addressed the issue of PPE.[3] Primary PPE used in oral health-care settings includes gloves, surgical masks, protective eyewear, and protective clothing such as gowns and jackets. It is imperative that heath-care workers (HCWs) review individual state laws and consult with their board of registration in dentistry to determine their legal obligation in regard to these guidelines.[4]

Of note is the distinction between OSHA and the CDC: (1) while CDC guidelines are designed to protect both the patient and the HCW, OSHA regulations apply only to HCWs; (2) while guidelines by the CDC or other advisory agencies do not carry the weight of law, a regulatory agency such as OSHA has the authority to require and enforce compliance.[4]

Currently there are no OSHA standards or directives specific to dentistry. However, exposure to numerous biologic, chemical, environmental, physical, and psychological workplace hazards can apply to dentistry.[5] When a specific standard does not exist for a situation, the OSHA General Duty Clause applies. The clause states that each employer "shall furnish…employment and a place of employment which are free from recognized hazards that are causing or are likely to cause death or serious physical harm to its employees." In addition to the General Duty Clause, a number of other standards are frequently cited for dentistry. These include the following:[5]

• Bloodborne pathogens
• Hazard communication
• Occupational exposure to hazardous chemicals in laboratories
• Medical services and first aid
• Respiratory protection
• Personal protective equipment
• Formaldehyde
• Portable fire extinguishers
• Nitrous oxide

1 Occupational Safety and Health Administration 1991 *Fed Regist* **56** 645175.
2 Occupational Safety and Health Administration 2001 *Fed Regist* **66** 5318.
3 Centers for Disease Control and Prevention 2003 *MMWR Morb Mortal Wkly Rep* **52** 1.
4 H. Bednarsh 2004 *Compendium* **25** 6.
5 C. J Palenik 2005 *Compendium* **26** 6.

2003 CDC infection control recommendations for dental health-care settings[1]

I. Personnel health elements of infection-control program
   A. General recommendations
   B. Education and training
   C. Immunization programs
   D. Exposure prevention and postexposure management
   E. Medical conditions, work-related illness, and work restrictions
   F. Records maintenance, data management, and confidentiality

II. Preventing transmission of bloodborne pathogens
   A. Hepatitis B vaccination
   B. Preventing exposures to blood and other potentially infectious materials

III. Hand hygiene
   A. General considerations
   B. Special considerations for hand hygiene and glove use

IV. PPE
   A. Masks, protective eyewear, and face shields
   B. Protective clothing
   C. Gloves
   D. Sterile surgeon's gloves and double gloving during oral surgical procedures

V. Contact dermatitis and latex hypersensitivity
   A. General recommendations

VI. Sterilization and disinfection of patient-care items
   A. General recommendations
   B. Instrument processing area
   C. Receiving, cleaning, and decontamination work area
   D. Preparation and packaging
   E. Sterilization and unwrapped instruments
   F. Sterilization monitoring
   G. Storage area for sterilized items and clean dental suppliers

VII. Environmental infection control
   A. General recommendations
   B. Clinical contact surfaces
   C. Housekeeping surfaces
   D. Spills of blood and body substances
   E. Carpet and cloth furnishings
   F. Regular medical waste

VIII. Dental-unit water lines, biofilm, and water quality
   A. General recommendations
   B. Boil-water advisories

[1] http://www.cdc.gov/OralHealth/Infectioncontrol/guidelines/

IX. Special considerations
   A. Dental handpieces and other devices attached to air and water lines
   B. Dental radiology
   C. Aseptic technique for parenteral medications
   D. Single-use (disposable) devices
   E. Preprocedural mouth rinses
   F. Oral surgical procedures
   G. Handling of biopsy specimens
   H. Handling of extracted teeth
   I. Dental laboratory
   J. Laser and electrosurgery plumes, surgical smoke
   K. *Mycobacterium* tuberculosis
   L. Creutzfeldt-Jakob disease and other neurodegenerative diseases
   M. Program evaluation

Highlights from the 2003 CDC infection control recommendations

Hand hygiene[1] For routine or nonsurgical dental procedures, workers should wash visibly soiled hands with soap (either antimicrobial or nonantimicrobial) and water. If hands are not visibly soiled, antimicrobial soap and water, plain soap and water, or an alcohol-based hand rub may be used.

Gloves Hand washing does not replace the need to wear gloves in situations where there is a risk of contact with blood, saliva, mucous membranes, or exudates.[1] Gloves should be removed after a procedure and changed between patients and should not be washed for use on multiple patients. It is also strongly recommended that lotions be used to prevent skin dryness. Those with an allergy to latex can try vinyl or nitrile gloves.

Immunization Even though effective infection control might limit the potential for microbial disease transmission in clinical settings, all susceptible staff who have potential occupational exposure to blood and other possibly infectious materials, including saliva, must be offered the hepatitis B vaccination series.[2] Generally, vaccination includes three injections. The first two are given 4 weeks apart. The final injection is administered 4 to 6 months after the first. The duration of vaccine immunity remains unknown. Current data indicate that protection lasts for at least 14 years if the initial immune response was appropriate.[3] You must keep documentary evidence of immunization and response for all staff. Staff should also be immunized against illnesses such mumps, measles, rubella, and varicella. Employees can decline to take the hepatitis B vaccination; however, they must sign a declination form, which must be kept on file by the employer.

1 C. Eva 2004 *Compendium* **25** 11.
2 Centers for Disease Control and Prevention 2003 *MMWR Recomm Rep* **52** 1.
3 C. J. Palenik 2004 *Compendium* **25** 17.

Sterilization[1] The instrument-processing area must be organized so that contaminated items are not confused with sterilized items. Instruments need to be cleaned completely of visible debris using an ultrasonic cleaner or instrument washer. Processing the packaged instruments through a heat sterilizer (steam, dry heat, or unsaturated chemical vapor) kills any microbes that remain on the instruments. The use and functioning of the sterilizer are monitored by mechanical, chemical, and biological means (spore testing), and records are kept to document these evaluations.

Needlestick injuries[2] Planning and advance preparation are essential for post-exposure management, and each practice should have a written, comprehensive program that explains what to do and where to go in the event of an exposure. In general, puncture wounds and other injuries to the skin should be washed with soap and water. A qualified medical health-care professional should evaluate any occupational exposure involving blood or other potentially infectious material, including saliva in dental settings, regardless of whether blood is visible.

1 J. A. Harte 2004 *Compendium* **25** 24.
2 L. G. DePaola 2004 *Compendium* **25** 38.

Syndromes of the head and neck

Principal sources: R. J. Gorlin 2001 *Syndromes of the Head and Neck*, 4th ed., OUP

Syndromes of the head and neck

The aim of this section is neither to bemuse the reader nor to demonstrate esoteric knowledge, although both may appear to occur. The real importance behind the learning of names associated with conditions that may be of relevance to, or be picked up by, clinical examination of the head and neck is that, once learned, some difficult diagnostic problems can be quickly solved and appropriate Rx instituted. We have retained eponyms where relevant (although this is not in keeping with current fashion) as they are, we feel, easier to learn and certainly more fun. Examiners have a tendency to remember their favorite eponymous syndrome, and it helps to at least agree on the name. We have, however, avoided the use of the possessive when using eponyms because invariably others were involved in describing or elucidating the condition and the syndrome does not belong to the individual(s) associated with it. The following list is in no way comprehensive but takes you through conditions met by the authors either in their clinical practice or in examinations and could ∴ be considered worth knowing about.

Definitions

Malformation A primary structural defect resulting from a localized error of morphogenesis.

Anomaly A malformation *and* its subsequently derived structural changes.

Syndrome A recognized pattern of malformation, presumed to have the same etiology but not interpreted as the result of a single localized error in morphogenesis.

Association A recognized pattern of malformation not considered to be a syndrome or an anomaly, *at the present time.*

Syndromes

Albright syndrome (McCune–Albright syndrome) Consists of polyostotic fibrous dysplasia (multiple bones affected), patchy skin pigmentation (referred to as *café-au-lait* spots), and an endocrine abnormality (usually precocious puberty in girls). Facial asymmetry affects up to 25% of cases.

Apert syndrome is a rare developmental deformity consisting of a craniosynostosis (premature fusion of cranial sutures) and syndactyly (fusion of fingers or toes). Severe mid-face retrusion leads to exophthalmos of varying severity. Early surgical intervention may be indicated for raised intracranial pressure or to prevent blindness from subluxation of the globe of the eye.

Behçet syndrome (pronounced behh-chet, after Turkish doctor Hulusi Behçet) is, classically, oral ulceration, genital ulceration, and uveitis. Clinical Δ can be made on finding any two of these. It is, in fact, a multisystem disease of immunological origin, although no hard diagnostic tests are yet available. It tends to affect young adults, especially males, and there is an association with HLA-B5. It undergoes spontaneous remission, although a variety of drugs, including thalidomide, are in use to treat it. See also p. 434.

Binder syndrome Maxillonasal dysplasia, severe mid-facial retrusion, and absent or hypoplastic frontal sinuses are the main features. There is no associated intellectual defect.

Chediak–Higashi syndrome is a combination of defective neutrophil function, abnormal skin pigmentation, and ↑ susceptibility to infection (leading to severe gingivitis, periodontitis, and aphthae in young children). It is a genetic disease.

Cleidocranial dysostosis (cleidocranial dysplasia) is an autosomal dominant inherited condition consisting of hypoplasia or aplasia of the clavicles, delayed ossification of the cranial fontanels, and a large, short skull. Associated features are shortness of stature, frontal and parietal bossing, failure to pneumatize the air sinuses, a high, arched palate and/or clefting, mid-face hypoplasia, and failure of tooth eruption with multiple supernumerary teeth. Many of the teeth present have inherent abnormalities such as dilaceration of roots or crown gemination. Hypoplasia of $2°$ cementum may occur. The condition mainly, though NOT exclusively, affects membranous bone.

Cri du chat syndrome is a chromosomal abnormality caused by deletion of part of the short arm of chromosome No. 5, resulting in microcephaly, hypertelorism, and a round face with a broad nasal bridge and malformed ears. Associated laryngeal hypoplasia causes a characteristic shrill cry. There is associated severe mental retardation.

Crouzon syndrome is the most common of the craniosynostoses. It is an autosomal dominant condition consisting of premature fusion of cranial sutures, mid-face hypoplasia, and, due to this, shallow orbits with proptosis of the globe of the eye. Radiographically the appearance of a "beaten copper skull" is characteristic. The enlarging brain is entrapped by the prematurely fused sutures, and ↑ intracranial pressure can lead to cerebral damage and resulting intellectual deficiency. This and the risk of blindness justify early craniofacial surgery to correct the deformity.

Down syndrome (trisomy 21) is the most common of all malformation syndromes, affecting up to 1:800 births. Risk ↑ with maternal age. Down's children account for 1/3 of severely mentally handicapped children. Facial appearance is characteristic with brachycephaly, mid-face retrusion, small nose with flattened nasal bridge, and upward sloping palpebral fissures (mongoloid slant). There is relative macroglossia and delayed eruption of teeth. Major relevant associations are heart defects, joint hyperflexibility, esophageal atresia, anemia, and an ↑ risk of acute lymphocytic leukemia. Most Down's children and adults are extremely friendly and cooperative.

Eagle syndrome is dysphagia and pain on chewing and turning the head associated with an elongated styloid process.

Ehlers–Danlos syndrome A group of disorders characterized by hyperflexibility of joints, ↑ bleeding and bruising, and hyperextensible skin. There appears to be an underlying molecular abnormality of collagen in this inherited disorder. Bleeding is more common in type IV, early-onset periodontal disease in type VIII. Pulp stones may be seen in all types.

Frey syndrome (Lucie Frey, a Polish physician) is a condition in which gustatory sweating and flushing of skin occur. It follows trauma to skin overlying a salivary gland and is thought to be due to post-traumatic crossover of sympathetic and parasympathetic innervation to the gland and skin, respectively. Its frequency following superficial parotidectomy ranges from 0% to 100%, depending on which surgeon you are talking to, but is almost certainly present in all cases to some degree if looked for carefully enough (use starch–iodine test).

Gardener syndrome This comprises multiple osteomas (particularly of the jaws and facial bones), multiple polyps of the large intestine, epidermoid cysts, and fibromas of the skin. It shows autosomal dominant inheritance. The discovery on clinical or X-ray examination of facial osteomas mandates examination of the lower gastrointestinal tract, as these polyps have a tendency toward rapid malignant change.

Goldenhar syndrome is a variant of hemifacial microsomia and consists of microtia (small ears), macrostomia, agenesis of the mandibular ramus and condyle, vertebral abnormalities (e.g., hemivertebra), and epibulbar dermoids. Also, cardiac, renal, or skeletal abnormalities can occur. Most patients have normal mental capabilities, but 10% are mentally handicapped.

Gorlin–Goltz syndrome (multiple basal cell nevi syndrome) See p. 496. Consists of multiple BCCs (epitheliomas), multiple jaw cysts (odontogenic kerato-cysts), vertebral and rib anomalies (usually bifid ribs), and calcification of the falx cerebri. Frontal bossing, mandibular prognathism, hypertelorism, hydrocephalus, eye, and endocrine abnormalities have also been noted.

Graves' disease Autoantibodies to thyroid stimulating hormone (TSH) cause hyperthyroidism with ophthalmopathy; women age 30–50 years are commonly affected; exophthalmos can be helped by a craniofacial approach to orbital decompression.

Heerfordt syndrome (uveoparotid fever) is sarcoidosis with associated lacrimal and salivary (especially parotid) swelling, uveitis, and fever. Sometimes there are associated neuropathies, e.g., facial palsy.

Hemifacial microsomia Prevalence: 1 in 5000 births. It is bilateral in 20% of cases. Congenital defect is characterized by a lack of hard and soft tissue on affected side(s), usually in the region of the ramus and external ear (i.e., first and second branchial arches). A wide spectrum of ear and cranial deformities is found.

Histiocytosis-X This is really three broad groups of diseases with the histological feature of tissue infiltration by tumor-like aggregates of macrophages (histiocytes) and eosinophils.
- *Solitary eosinophilic granuloma* Mainly affects males <20. The mandible is a common site. It responds to local Rx.
- *Hand–Schüller–Christian disease* Multifocal eosinophilic granuloma causing skull lesions, exophthalmos, and diabetes insipidus. It affects a younger group, and may respond to cytotoxic chemotherapy.

- *Letterer–Siwe disease* Rapidly progressive, disseminated histiocytosis. Associated pancytopenia and multisystem disease can occur, and it can be fatal.

Horner syndrome consists of a constricted pupil (miosis), drooping eyelid (ptosis), unilateral loss of sweating (anhydrosis) on the face, and occasionally sunken eye (enophthalmos). It is caused by interruption of sympathetic nerve fibers at the cervical ganglion 2° to, e.g., bronchogenic carcinoma, invading the ganglion or neck trauma. This syndrome scores high on the "worthwhile" rating.

Hurler syndrome is a mucopolysaccharidosis causing growth failure and mental retardation. A large head, frontal bossing, hypertelorism, and coarse features give it its classical appearance. Multiple skeletal abnormalities (dysostosis multiplex), corneal clouding, and serum and urinary acid mucopolysaccharide abnormalities also occur.

Hypohydrotic ectodermal dysplasia Hypodontia is found in association with lack of hair, sweating, and saddle nose.

Klippel–Feil anomaly is the association of cervical vertebral fusion, short neck, and low-lying posterior hairline. A number of neurological anomalies have been noted, and unilateral renal agenesis is frequent. Cardiac anomalies sometimes occur.

Larsen syndrome is a mainly autosomal dominant condition, with a predilection for females, consisting of cleft palate, flattened facies, multiple congenital dislocations, and deformities of the feet. Sufferers are usually of short stature. The larynx may be affected.

Lesch–Nyhan syndrome is a defect of purine metabolism causing mental retardation, spastic cerebral palsy, choreoathetosis, and aggressive self-mutilating behavior (particularly involving the lips).

MAGIC syndrome stands for Mouth And Genital ulcers and Interstitial Chondritis and is a variant of the Behçet syndrome group.

Marfan syndrome is an autosomal dominant condition characterized by tall, thin stature and arachnodactyly (long, thin, spider-like hands), dislocation of the lens, dissecting aneurysms of the thoracic aorta, aortic regurgitation, floppy mitral valve, and high, arched palate. Joint laxity is also common. This condition is highly prevalent among top-class basketball and volleyball players, for obvious reasons.

Melkerson–Rosenthal syndrome consists of facial paralysis, facial edema, and fissured tongue. It is probably a variant of the group of conditions now known as orofacial granulomatosis.

Multiple endocrine neoplasia (MEN) A group of conditions affecting the endocrine glands. MEN IIb is of particular relevance, as it consists of multiple mucosal neuromas that have a characteristic histopathology, pheochromocytoma, medullary thyroid carcinoma, and a thin, wasted appearance. Calcitonin levels are elevated if medullary thyroid carcinoma is present. Index of suspicion should be high in tall, thin, wasted-looking children and young adults presenting with lumps in the mouth. Biopsy is mandatory and if histopathology is suggestive the thyroid must be adequately investigated. This is another "worthwhile" syndrome.

Orofacial–digital syndrome is one of the many CLP syndromes, all of which are associated with hypodontia (laterals especially) and supernumeraries. This one has finger abnormalities as well.

Papillon–Lefevre syndrome is palmoplantar hyperkeratosis and juvenile periodontitis, which affects both 1° and 2° dentition. Normal dental development occurs until the appearance of the hyperkeratosis of the palms and soles, then simultaneously an aggressive gingivitis and periodontitis begin. The mechanism is not well understood.

Patterson–Brown–Kelly syndrome (Plummer–Vinson syndrome) is the occurrence of dysphagia, microcytic hypochromic anemia, koilonychia (spoon-shaped nails), and angular cheilitis. The dysphagia is due to a post-cricoid web, usually a membrane on the anterior esophageal wall, which is premalignant. The koilonychia and angular cheilitis are 2° to the anemia but may be presenting symptoms. The main affected group is middle-aged women, and correction of the anemia may both relieve symptoms and prevent malignant progression of the web.

Peutz–Jeghers syndrome is an autosomal dominant condition of melanotic pigmentation of skin (especially perioral skin) and mucosa, and intestinal polyposis. These polyps, unlike those of the Gardener syndrome, have no particular propensity to malignant change, being hamartomatous, and are found in the small intestine. They may, however, cause intussusception or other forms of gut obstruction. Ovarian tumors are sometimes associated with the condition (10% of women with Peutz–Jeghers).

Progeria is probably a collagen abnormality. It causes dwarfism and premature aging. Characteristic facial appearance occurs from a disproportionately small face with mandibular retrognathia and a beak-like nose, creating an unforgettable appearance; death occurs in the mid-teens.

Ramsay Hunt syndrome is a lower motor neuron facial palsy, with vesicles on the same side in the pharynx, in the external auditory canal, and on the face. It is thought to be due to herpes zoster of the geniculate ganglion.

Reiter syndrome consists of arthritis, urethritis, and conjunctivitis. There are frequently oral lesions, which resemble benign migratory glossitis in appearance but affect other parts of the mouth. The condition is probably an unwanted effect of an immune response to a low-grade pathogen; however, some still believe it to be a sexually transmitted disease, although there is no hard evidence for this.

Robin sequence Named after Pierre Robin (and mistakenly called Pierre Robin syndrome at times). This is micrognathia, cleft palate, and glossoptosis. There is a huge number of associated anomalies. Catch-up growth occurs.

Romberg syndrome (hemifacial atrophy) consists of progressive atrophy of the soft tissues of half the face, associated with contralateral Jacksonian epilepsy and trigeminal neuralgia. Rarely, half the body may be affected. It starts in the first decade and lasts ~3 yr before it becomes quiescent.

Sicca syndrome (primary Sjögren syndrome) is xerostomia and keratoconjunctivitis sicca, i.e., dry mouth and dry eyes. There is an ↑ risk of developing parotid lymphoma with this condition. Interestingly, although Sicca syndrome has certain serological abnormalities in common with systemic connective tissue disorders such as rheumatoid arthritis, it does not have any of the symptomatology (unlike Sjögren syndrome).

Sjögren syndrome (secondary Sjögren syndrome) In addition to dry eyes and dry mouth this has both the serology and symptomatology of an autoimmune condition, usually rheumatoid arthritis, but sometimes SLE, systemic sclerosis, or primary biliary cirrhosis. Actual swelling of the salivary glands is relatively uncommon and late-onset swelling of the parotids may herald the presence of a lymphoma.

Stevens–Johnson syndrome A severe version of erythema multiforme, a mucocutaneous condition that is probably autoimmune in nature and precipitated particularly by drugs. Classical signs are the target lesions, concentric red rings that affect especially the hands and feet. Stevens–Johnson syndrome is said to be present when the condition is particularly severe, and is associated with fever and multiple mucosal involvement. Viral infections, e.g., herpes simplex, are the second most common cause.

Stickler syndrome Perhaps the most common syndrome associated with cleft palate (20%). Consists of flat mid-face, cleft palate, myopia, retinal detachment, hearing loss (80%), and arthropathy. Thirty percent of Robin sequence patients have Stickler syndrome, ∴ examine eyes.

Sturge–Weber anomaly is due to a hamartomatous angioma affecting the upper part of the face, which may extend intracranially. There may be associated convulsions, hemiplegia (on the contralateral side of the body), or intellectual impairment. The risks of surgery are obvious.

Treacher–Collins syndrome (mandibulofacial dysostosis) basically involves defects in structures derived from the first branchial arch. It is inherited as an autosomal dominant trait with variable expressivity, and consists of downward-sloping (antimongoloid slant) palpebral fissures, hypoplastic malar complexes, mandibular retrognathia with a high gonial angle, deformed pinnas, hypoplastic air sinuses, colobomas in the outer third of the eye, and middle and inner ear hypoplasia (and hence deafness). Thirty percent of patients have cleft palates and 25% have an unusual tongue-like projection of hair pointing toward the cheek. Most have *completely normal intellectual* function, which may be missed because they are deaf and "funny-looking kids" (how would you like to be called a funny-looking dentist or doctor?). These people may well miss out on fulfilling their potential because of society's (and some professionals') attitude toward deformity. This syndrome is a prime indication for corrective craniofacial surgery.

Trotter syndrome is unilateral deafness, pain in the mandibular division of the trigeminal nerve, ipsilateral immobility of the palate, and trismus, due to invasion of the lateral wall of the nasopharynx by malignant tumor. Pterygopalatine fossa syndrome is a similar condition in which the first and second divisions of the trigeminal are affected.

von Recklinghausen neurofibromatosis/syndrome Multiple neurofibromas with skin pigmentation, skeletal abnormalities, CNS involvement, and a predisposition to malignancy are the basics of this syndrome. It undergoes autosomal dominant transmission and has a large and varied number of manifestations. Lesions of the face can be particularly disfiguring.

Useful information and addresses

Tooth notation

American

Permanent teeth

R $\dfrac{1\ \ 2\ \ 3\ \ 4\ \ 5\ \ 6\ \ 7\ \ 8\ \ \vert\ \ 9\ \ 10\ \ 11\ \ 12\ \ 13\ \ 14\ \ 15\ \ 16}{32\ \ 31\ \ 30\ \ 29\ \ 28\ \ 27\ \ 26\ \ 25\ \ \vert\ \ 24\ \ 23\ \ 22\ \ 21\ \ 20\ \ 19\ \ 18\ \ 17}$ L

Deciduous teeth

R $\dfrac{A\ B\ C\ D\ E\ \vert\ F\ G\ H\ I\ J}{T\ S\ R\ Q\ P\ \vert\ O\ N\ M\ L\ K}$ L

FDI

Permanent teeth

R $\dfrac{18\ \ 17\ \ 16\ \ 15\ \ 14\ \ 13\ \ 12\ \ 11\ \ \vert\ \ 21\ \ 22\ \ 23\ \ 24\ \ 25\ \ 26\ \ 27\ \ 28}{48\ \ 47\ \ 46\ \ 45\ \ 44\ \ 43\ \ 42\ \ 41\ \ \vert\ \ 31\ \ 32\ \ 33\ \ 34\ \ 35\ \ 36\ \ 37\ \ 38}$ L

Deciduous teeth

R $\dfrac{55\ \ 54\ \ 53\ \ 52\ \ 51\ \ \vert\ \ 61\ \ 62\ \ 63\ \ 64\ \ 65}{85\ \ 84\ \ 83\ \ 82\ \ 81\ \ \vert\ \ 71\ \ 72\ \ 73\ \ 74\ \ 75}$ L

Zsigmondy–Palmer, Chevron, or Set Square system

Permanent teeth

R $\dfrac{8\ \ 7\ \ 6\ \ 5\ \ 4\ \ 3\ \ 2\ \ 1\ \ \vert\ \ 1\ \ 2\ \ 3\ \ 4\ \ 5\ \ 6\ \ 7\ \ 8}{8\ \ 7\ \ 6\ \ 5\ \ 4\ \ 3\ \ 2\ \ 1\ \ \vert\ \ 1\ \ 2\ \ 3\ \ 4\ \ 5\ \ 6\ \ 7\ \ 8}$ L

Deciduous teeth

R $\dfrac{e\ \ d\ \ c\ \ b\ \ a\ \ \vert\ \ a\ \ b\ \ c\ \ d\ \ e}{e\ \ d\ \ c\ \ b\ \ a\ \ \vert\ \ a\ \ b\ \ c\ \ d\ \ e}$ L

Because of the difficulties of including the grid notation in written documents, it is common practice to indicate the quadrant by abbreviating the arch and side. Thus the upper right second premolar is UR5 and likewise the lower left second deciduous molar is LLE.

European

Permanent teeth

R $\dfrac{8+\ 7+\ 6+\ 5+\ 4+\ 3+\ 2+\ 1+\ \vert\ 1+2+3+4+5+6+\ 7+8}{8-\ 7-\ 6-\ 5-\ 4-\ 3-\ 2-\ 1-\ \vert\ 1-2-3-4-\ 5-\ 6-\ 7-8}$ L

Deciduous teeth

R $\dfrac{05+04+03+02+01+\ \vert\ +01+02+03\ +04\ +05}{05-\ 04-\ 03-\ 02-\ 01-\ \vert\ -01\ -02\ -03\ -04\ -05}$ L

Some qualifications in medicine and dentistry

BA	Bachelor of Arts
BC/BCh/BS	Bachelor of Surgery
BChD/BDS	Bachelor of Dental Surgery
BS	Bachelor of Science
DBA	Doctor of Business Administration
DDes	Doctor of Design
DDS/DDSc	Doctor of Dental Surgery/Science
DMD	Doctor of Dental Medicine (Dentariae Medicinae Doctorae; Latin)
DMSc	Doctor of Medical Sciences
DPhil	Doctor of Philosophy
DPH	Doctor of Public Health
DSc	Doctor of Science
EdD	Doctor of Education
EdM	Master of Education
JD	Juris Doctor
LLM	Master of Laws
MBA	Master of Business Administration
MBBCh/MBChB	Bachelor of Medicine and Bachelor of Surgery
MD	Doctor of Medicine
MDS	Master of Dental Surgery
MDentSci/MDSc	Master of Dental Science
MDesS	Master of Design Studies
MMSc	Master of Medical Sciences
MPA	Master in Public Administration
MPH	Master of Public Health
MPhil	Master of Philosophy
MPP	Master in Public Policy
PhD	Doctor of Philosophy (Philosophiæ Doctor; Latin)
SD	Doctor of Science
SJD	Doctor of Judicial Science
SM	Master of Science

Bur numbering systems

Maximum diameter of bur head	ISO	USA/UK		
		Round	Inverted cone	Flat fissure
0.6	006	½	½	
0.8	008	1	1	½
0.9	009			1
1.0	010	2	2	2
1.2	012	3	3	3
1.4	014	4	4	4
1.6	016	5	5	5
1.8	018	6	6	6
2.1	021	7	7	7
2.3	023	8	8	8
2.5	025	9	9	9
2.7	027	10	10	10
2.9	029	11		11
3.1	031	12		12

File sizes (for endodontic therapy)

Size	Tip diameter	ISO color
08	0.08	gray
10	0.10	purple
15	0.15	white
20	0.20	yellow
25	0.25	red
30	0.30	blue
35	0.35	green
40	0.40	black
50	0.45	white
55	0.50	yellow
60	0.55	red
70	0.60	blue
80	0.70	green
90	0.80	black
100	0.90	white
110	1.00	yellow
120	1.10	red
130	1.20	blue
140	1.30	green
	1.40	black

Local anesthetic color codes

Product		PMS® color
Lidocaine 2% with epinephrine		Red 185
Lidocaine 2% with epinephrine 1:50,000		Green 347
Lidocaine plain		Light Blue 279
Mepivicaine 2% with levonordefrin 1:20,000		Brown 471
Mepivicaine 3% plain		Tan 466
Prilocaine 4% with epinephrine 1:200,000		Yellow 108
Prilocaine 4% plain		Black
Bupivacaine 1.5% epinephrine 1:200,000		Blue 300
Articaine 4% with epinephrine 1:100,000		Gold 871

Manufacturers of American Dental Association–accepted local anesthetics must use a uniform cartridge color-coding system for identifying specific local anesthetics and local anesthetic/ vasoconstrictor combinations. The system formally went into effect in June 2003. The color code consists of a 3 mm band 15 mm from the stopper end of the cartridge.

* Pantone Matching System (PMS) Pantone, Inc.

File sizes (for endodontic therapy)

Size	Tip diameter	ISO color
08	0.08	gray
10	0.10	purple
15	0.15	white
20	0.20	yellow
25	0.25	red
30	0.30	blue
35	0.35	green
40	0.40	black
45	0.45	white
50	0.50	yellow
55	0.55	red
60	0.60	blue
70	0.70	green
80	0.80	black
90	0.90	white
100	1.00	yellow
110	1.10	red
120	1.20	blue
130	1.30	green
140	1.40	black

Local anesthetic color codes

Product	PMS* color
Lidocaine 2% with epinephrine	Red 185
Lidocaine 2% with epinephrine 1:50,000	Green 347
Lidocaine plain	Light Blue 279
Mepivicaine 2% with levonordefrin 1:20,000	Brown 471
Mepivicaine 3% plain	Tan 466
Prilocaine 4% with epinephrine 1:200,000	Yellow 108
Prilocaine 4% plain	Black
Bupivacaine 1.5% epinephrine 1:200,000	Blue 300
Articaine 4% with epinephrine 1:100,000	Gold 871

Manufacturers of American Dental Association–accepted local anesthetics must use a uniform cartridge color-coding system for identifying specific local anesthetics and local anesthetic/vasoconstrictor combinations. The system formally went into effect in June 2003. The color code consists of a 3 mm band 15 mm from the stopper end of the cartridge.

* Pantone Matching System (PMS) Pantone, Inc.

Wire gauges

Size on wire gauge	Diameter	
	Inches	Millimeters
14	0.080	2.0
19	0.040	1.0
20	0.036	0.9
21	0.032	0.8
22	0.028	0.7
23	0.024	0.6
24	0.022	0.55
25	0.020	0.5
26	0.018	0.45
27	0.0164	0.4
28	0.0148	0.37
29	0.0136	0.35
30	0.0124	0.3

Passing exams

Preparation First, there is unfortunately no substitute for the sheer hard work of studying, and to have a chance of doing adequately well this should start well before the exam. Beware of those who try to impress by saying they have passed every exam, first time, having only started studying the night before. These people are not superintelligent (in fact, their behavior suggests the reverse), they have probably only been lucky—to date!

Equally well, the human brain is not a computer, and studying for hours, day in day out, could result in "burnout." Each person needs to find their own method, but a break of 5–10 min every hour along with a complete hour off after 3 hours' work has succeeded for others.

It is important to be sure that you are studying the correct material in sufficient depth. One way of ensuring this is to go over past questions. If some are tackled under exam conditions, this also gives practice in exam technique.

Immediate pre-exam period If your nerve is strong enough, it is probably wise to stop working 2–3 days before the exams start and have a rest, doing something that you enjoy. Most people baulk at this suggestion but see the logic as that of a marathon runner resting before an important race. Studying the night before is akin to an élite runner going out the night before the Olympic marathon and running 26.2 miles just to make sure he or she can cover the distance.

Written exams It is important to know beforehand how many questions you have to answer and ∴ how long can be spent on each. Do not be tempted to overrun your time for each question. Spend a few minutes deciding which questions to answer and in what order. It is better to tackle your best question second, thus allowing the butterflies to settle. Read each question carefully, and periodically stop to check that you are answering the actual question, not the one you'd like to answer. A rough plan helps to produce a more logical essay and provides an *aide-mémoire* in case of panic halfway through. Write neatly.

Multiple-choice exams are often used by instructors, but feared by students. If they involve negative marking, a careful approach is required for success.
- Do the necessary revision; it is impossible to waffle hopefully round the subject in a multiple-choice exam.
- Go through the paper, only answering those questions of which you are completely sure.
- Count up the number you have answered and see if it is over the pass mark. If yes, stop there.
- If you have not answered enough, go back through the paper, only answering those questions that you are nearly sure of. DO NOT look at the questions you have previously answered, as usually your first instinct is right.
- Stop there, as the next step is to guess—which is usually counterproductive.

Clinical exams Turn up neatly dressed, with a clean gown. Although some patients are regularly wheeled out for exams, many may be almost as nervous about what is going to happen as you are. Many patients can give helpful hints toward their diagnosis and management if asked the right questions. Some students spend most of their time with the patient, scribbling furiously, and do not leave themselves any time to think. Present the patient to the examiners in a logical fashion, i.e., starting with their name and age, chief complaint, history of their present illness, and not the radiographs. Be sure to review the patient's medical history.

Objective structured clinical examinations (OSCEs) have been developed to evaluate the clinical competence of medical and dental students in both undergraduate and postgraduate curricula. This type of exam is so-called because they should have the following qualities:

Objective—independent and competent examiners should have agreed on what skills are being examined, with agreed grading scales.

Structured—have agreed criteria (in advance) for the correct answer for each element of the exam.

Clinical—to test clinical and practical competence, including communication and problem-solving skills.

Examination—this may include evaluation of written responses and/or observation by an examiner.

They usually comprise a series of stations, each testing a different clinical skill. A set time is allocated to each station. The clinical proficiencies tested may include taking a history from a "patient." Actors are often hired to pose as patients rather than using actual patients. This allows the actor to use a uniform script, which permits students to develop a diagnosis. An examiner may be present who observes, evaluates, and grades the student's responses and actions at a particular station.

GOOD LUCK!

Web-based learning

Definitions

Web-based learning is one type of distance education that ↓ the barriers of time and space to learning—"anytime, anywhere learning." It is a component of the broader term *e-learning*, defined as the use of electronic technology and media to deliver, support, and enhance teaching and learning. This encompasses the Internet, Intranet, and the World Wide Web.

In education, the Web is increasingly used both to support lectures and as a means of delivering online learning programs. These may be interactive, with online activities, such as self-assessments, animations, video, and simulations, that can be more enjoyable and meaningful to learners. Discussion forums via e-mail, video conferencing, and live lectures are all possible through the Web. Another advantage is that Web pages and a virtual learning environment may contain hyperlinks to other parts of the Web, thus enabling access to a vast amount of Web-based information.

Glossary

e-conferencing Use of online presentations and discussion forums in real time or stored as downloadable files on a Web site so that participants need not travel.

Hyperlinks Links in Web pages that enable the user to access another Web page either on the same or a different site with just one mouse click.

Internet Global network of computers divided into subsets (e.g., the Web or e-mail systems). Computers are linked to the Internet via host computers, which link to other computers via dial-up (e.g., via a modem), broadband, and network connections.

Internet service provider (ISP) links the home user to the Internet. The ISP maintains a network of personal computers that are permanently connected to the Internet.

Intranet A network of computers that share information, usually within an organization. Access normally requires a password and is limited to a defined range of users, e.g., the university or company-based network.

Managed learning environment provides an integrated function, with administrative tools such as student records, and links with other management information systems.

Search engines (such as Google, Ask, Yahoo) can be used to find information.

Videostreaming The process by which video images are able to be stored on and downloaded from the Web. This might be done in real time (such as a conference) or the images may be used asynchronously.

Virtual learning environment A set of electronic teaching and learning tools. Principal components can map a curriculum, track student activity, and provide online student support and electronic communication.

World Wide Web (WWW) Use of the Internet to present various types of information. Web sites or home pages may be accessed with the aid of a browser program (such as Internet Explorer, Firefox, Netscape, or Safari). All such programs use HTML (hypertext mark-up language).

Advantages

- Information in different formats, i.e. audio, visual
- Provides a central and comprehensive way of delivering course materials
- Resources can be made available from any location and at any time.
- Can widen access, e.g., to part-time, mature, or work-based students
- Can encourage more independent and active learning
- Can provide a useful source of supplementary materials to conventional programs

Disadvantages

- Access to computers can be difficult for some.
- Some sites are bandwidth intensive and require broadband connections.
- Learners find it frustrating if they cannot access graphics, images, and videoclips because of non-user-friendly software and limitations in the hardware.
- It is difficult to write good material that maintains interest and motivation.
- Personal passwords are needed to access selected sites.
- Information varies in quality and accuracy. It requires guidance or use that is limited to accredited sites, e.g., official organizations or education establishments.
- Potentially, Web-based learning can be extremely nonproductive and time-wasting, depending on one's learning style.

Summary

At the undergraduate level, e-learning is becoming engrained in the curriculum. At the postgraduate level it has great potential for continuing education (CE) and for providing resources, online logbooks, and competency assessments. At present, however, it is limited by current software and variable access to hardware. Also, newer technologies are not necessarily better (or worse) for teaching or learning than older technologies, they are just different. Therefore, it is necessary to pick and choose to find what is right for you.

Dentistry and the World Wide Web

As anyone who has surfed the Web will know, it is a big world out there, and new Web sites are constantly appearing; the following is at best a sampler of interesting sites. If you have time on your hands then type the subject that interests you into a search engine...and stand back. For a more academic approach seek the advice of a librarian, as they are often delighted to help you find reputable sites and sources of information. Happy surfing!

Academy of Dental Materials: www.academydentalmaterials.org
Academy of General Dentistry: www.agd.org
Academy of Osseointegration: www.osseo.org
American Academy of Endodonitists: www.aae.org
American Academy of Esthetic Dentistry: www.estheticacademy.org
American Academy of Implant Dentistry: www.aaid.com
American Academy of Oral and Maxillofacial Radiology: www.aaomr.org
American Academy of Pediatric Dentistry: www.aapd.org
American Academy of Periodontology: www.perio.org
American Association for Dental Research: www.iadr.com
American Association of Oral and Maxillofacial Surgeons: www.aaoms.org
American Association of Orthodontics: www.aaomembers.org
American Association of Poison Control Centers: www.aapcc.org
American Association of Public Heath Dentistry: www.aaphd.org
American College of Prosthodontis: www.prosthodontics.org
American Dental Assistants Association: www.dentalassistant.org
American Dental Association: www.ada.org
American Dental Education Association: www.adea.org
American Dental Hygienists' Association: www.adha.org
American Dental Society of Anesthesiology: www.adsahome.org
Association for Medical Education and Research in Substance Abuse: amersa.org
Bad Breath Research: www.tau.ac.il/~melros/
British Medical Association: www.bma.org.uk
International Association for Dental Research: www.iadr.com
Clinical evidence: a compendium of research findings on clinical questions: www.clinicalevidence.org
Cochrane Collaboration: www.cochrane.co.uk

Dental Schools in the United States and Canada
United States
Arizona School of Dentistry and Oral Health: www.atsu.edu/asdoh
Baylor College of Dentistry, a member of the Texas A&M University System Health Science Center: www.tambcd.edu
Boston University, Goldman School of Dental Medicine: dentalschool.bu.edu
Case School of Dental Medicine: dental.case.edu
Columbia University College of Dental Medicine: dental.columbia.edu
Creighton University School of Dentistry: cudental.creighton.edu

Harvard School of Dental Medicine: www.hsdm.harvard.edu
Howard University College of Dentistry: www.dentistry.howard.edu
Indiana University School of Dentistry: www.iusd.iupui.edu
Loma Linda University School of Dentistry: www.llu.edu/llu/dentistry
Louisiana State University School of Dentistry: www.lsusd.lsuhsc.edu
Marquette University School of Dentistry: www.marquette.edu/dentistry
Medical College of Georgia School of Dentistry: www.mcg.edu/SOD
Medical University of South Carolina College of Dental Medicine:
etl2.library.musc.edu/dentistry
Meharry Medical College School of Dentistry: dentistry.mmc.edu
New York University College of Dentistry: www.nyu.edu/dental
Nova Southeastern University College of Dental Medicine:
dental.nova.edu
Ohio State University College of Dentistry: dent.osu.edu
Oregon Health & Science University School of Dentistry:
www.ohsu.edu/sod
Southern Illinois University School of Dental Medicine:
www.siue.edu/sdm
Stony Brook University: www.hsc.stonybrook.edu/dental
Temple University School of Dentistry: www.temple.edu/dentistry
Tufts University School of Dental Medicine: www.tufts.edu/dental
University at Buffalo: www.sdm.buffalo.edu
University of Alabama at Birmingham School of Dentistry:
www.dental.uab.edu
University of California, Los Angeles School of Dentistry:
www.dent.ucla.edu
University of California, San Francisco School of Dentistry:
dentistry.ucsf.edu
University of Colorado School of Dentistry: www.uchsc.edu/sod
University of Connecticut School of Dental Medicine: sdm.uchc.edu
University of Detroit Mercy School of Dentistry: dental.udmercy.edu
University of Florida College of Dentistry: www.dental.ufl.edu
University of Illinois at Chicago College of Dentistry:
dentistry.uic.edu
University of Iowa College of Dentistry: www.dentistry.uiowa.edu
University of Kentucky College of Dentistry: www.mc.uky.edu/Dentistry
University of Louisville School of Dentistry: www.dental.louisville.edu
University of Maryland, Baltimore College of Dental Surgery:
www.dental.umaryland.edu
University of Medicine and Dentistry of New Jersey, New Jersey Dental
School: dentalschool.umdnj.edu
University of Michigan School of Dentistry: www.dent.umich.edu
University of Minnesota School of Dentistry: www.dentistry.umn.edu
University of Mississippi School of Dentistry:
dentistry.umc.edu/sda/servlet/Home
University of Missouri-Kansas City School of Dentistry:
dentistry.umkc.edu
University of Nebraska Medical Center, College of Dentistry:
www.unmc.edu/dentistry

University of Nevada, Las Vegas School of Dental Medicine:
www.unlv.edu
University of North Carolina at Chapel Hill School of Dentistry:
www.dent.unc.edu
University of Oklahoma College of Dentistry: dentistry.ouhsc.edu
University of the Pacific Arthur A. Dugoni School of Dentistry:
dental.pacific.edu
University of Pennsylvania School of Dental Medicine:
www.dental.upenn.edu
University of Pittsburgh School of Dental Medicine: www.dental.pitt.edu
University of Puerto Rico, School of Dentistry: dental.rcm.upr.edu
University of Southern California School of Dentistry:
www.usc.edu/hsc/dental
University of Tennessee College of Dentistry: www.utmem.edu/dentistry
University of Texas Health Science Center at Houston Dental Branch:
www.db.uth.tmc.edu
University of Texas Health Science Center at San Antonio Dental:
dental.uthscsa.edu School
University of Washington School of Dentistry: www.dental.washington.edu
University of West Virginia: www.hsc.wvu.edu/sod
Virginia Commonwealth University School of Dentistry:
www.dentistry.vcu.edu

Canada

Dalhousie University Faculty of Dentistry: www.dentistry.dal.ca
McGill University Faculty of Dentistry: www.mcgill.ca/dentistry
University of Alberta Faculty of Dentistry: www.dent.ualberta.ca
University of British Columbia Faculty of Dentistry: www.dentistry.ubc.ca
University Laval Faculty of Dentistry: www.fmd.ulaval.ca/
University of Manitoba Faculty of Dentistry: www.umanitoba.ca/dentistry
University of Montreal Faculty of Dentistry: www.medent.umontreal.ca
University of Saskatchewan College of Dentistry: www.usask.ca/dentistry
University of Toronto Faculty of Dentistry: www.utoronto.ca/dentistry
University of Western Ontario Faculty of Dentistry:
www.schulich.uwo.ca/dentistry
Epocrates®: www.epocrates.com

Evidence-based courses, links, and guides

www.shef.ac.uk/scharr/ir/scebm.html
FDI World Dental Federation: www.fdiworldental.org
Journal of the American Dental Association: www.jada.ada.org
Journal of Dental Research: jdr.iadrjournals.org
National Institutes of Health: www.nih.gov
Postdoctoral Application Support Service (PASS): www.adea.org/PASS/
Postdoctoral Dental Matching Program: www.natmatch.com/dentres
Physicians' Desk Reference: www.pdr.net
The Associated American Dental Schools Application Service (AADSAS):
aadsas.adea.org
U.S. Census Bureau: www.census.gov
U.S. Department of Health and Human Services: www.hhs.gov
U.S. Food and Drug Administration: www.fda.gov

For when it all gets a bit stressful, try the following:

www.weather.gov
www.ahajokes.com
www.bored.com
www.extremeironing.com
www.lastminute.com
www.lovelaughs.com
www.multimap.com
www.oofun.com

Note: All of these URL addresses were correct at press time.

Index